Pharmaceutical Calculations

MITCHELL J. STOKLOSA, Ph.C., B.S., A.M., Sc.D.

Dean of Students and Professor of Pharmacy,
Massachusetts College of Pharmacy,
Boston, Massachusetts

Lea & Febiger
Philadelphia

Library of Congress Cataloging in Publication Data

Stoklosa, Mitchell J.
    Pharmaceutical calculations.

    First ed. by W. T. Bradley and C. B. Gustafson; 2d-5th ed. by W. T. Bradley, C. B. Gustafson, and M. J. Stoklosa.
    1. Pharmaceutical arithmetic.   I. Bradley, Willis T.   Pharmaceutical calculations. I. Title. [DNLM: 1. Mathematics. 2. Pharmacy. QV16 S874p 1974]
RS57.S86 1974   615'.4'01513   73–12909
ISBN 0–8121–0468–4

Fifth Edition, 1968

Reprinted March, 1970

Reprinted June, 1972

Sixth Edition, 1974

Reprinted March, 1975

Reprinted March, 1976

The use of portions of the text of the United States Pharmacopeia, Eighteenth Revision, official September 1, 1970, is by permission received from the Board of Trustees of the United States Pharmacopeial Convention. The said Board is not responsible for any inaccuracies of the text thus used.

Permission to use portions of the text of the National Formulary, Thirteenth Edition, official September 1, 1970, has been granted by the American Pharmaceutical Association. The American Pharmaceutical Association is not responsible for any inaccuracy of quotation or for false implications that may arise by reason of the separation of excerpts from the original context.

Preface

The Sixth Edition of this text marks the twenty-ninth year of its publication. Since the format of the book has been highly satisfactory for teaching purposes and for use as a source of reference, the general plan of previous editions has not been altered, and the basic substance and method have been retained without any drastic innovations.

The entire content has been critically reviewed. A substantial portion of the material has been rearranged and some topics that were previously included in the appendices are now presented in separate chapters. A new chapter dealing with buffers and buffer solutions has been added. The chapter on electrolyte solutions has been extended and the appendix concerned with dispensing problems has been revised and expanded to include problems dealing with units of potency and parenteral additives. Many problems have been deleted, others have been rewritten and updated, and new ones have been introduced. The problems at the end of the book that are available for review and test purposes have been thoroughly revised with the elimination of a number of the older ones.

As in prior editions, theoretical discussion has been kept at a minimum and included only when it was felt to be necessary for the sake of clarity and understanding of the problems and their solutions. Once again, the aim has been to teach by practice rather than precept: a sample problem of each type sets the pattern with a recommended solution and alternate methods when available. Practice problems at the end of each chapter and section, half of them with answers for the purpose of checking, give the student an opportunity to prove his mastery of the method of his choice.

The introductory material dealing with certain fundamentals of measurement and calculation is intended to be a review of basic arithmetic principles with which the student should be thoroughly familiar at the outset. The main body of the text thereafter shows a logical development of topics, and the self-explanatory character of every section and the solution of examples of typical problems in full permit any arrangement of study that suits the requirements of a separate or integrated course in pharmaceutical calculations. In keeping with the original purpose of the book, the new edition continues to emphasize the practical aspects of the arithmetic of pharmacy.

The author acknowledges with gratitude the helpful comments and suggestions offered by his colleagues and fellow teachers in the preparation of this revision, and he expresses his deepest appreciation to all who contributed in any way to make the book more useful both to students and practitioners.

Boston, Massachusetts   M. J. S.

Contents

Chapter 1

Some Fundamentals of Measurement and Calculation

NUMBERS AND NUMERALS

A *number* is a total quantity, or amount, of units. A *numeral* is a word or sign, or a group of words or signs, expressing a number.

For example, *3*, *6*, and *48* are arabic numerals expressing numbers that are respectively *three times, six times,* and *forty-eight times* the unit *1*.

KINDS OF NUMBERS

In *arithmetic*, which is the science of calculating with positive, real numbers, a number will usually be (a) a natural or *whole* number, or *integer*, such as *549*; (b) a *fraction*, or subdivision of a whole number, such as $\frac{4}{7}$; or (c) a *mixed* number, consisting of a whole number plus a fraction such as $3\frac{7}{8}$.

A number such as *4*, *8*, or *12*, taken by itself, without application to anything concrete, is called an *abstract* or *pure* number. It merely designates how many times the unit *1* is contained in it, without implying that anything else is being counted or measured. An abstract number may be added to, subtracted from, multiplied by, or divided by any other abstract number. The result of any of these operations is always an abstract number designating a new total of units.

But a number that designates a quantity of objects or units of measure, such as *4 grams, 8 ounces, 12 grains*, is called a *concrete* or *denominate* number. It designates the total quantity of whatever has been measured. A denominate number may be added to or subtracted from any other number of the same denomination; but a denominate number may be multiplied or divided only by a pure number. The result of any of these operations is always a number *of the same denomination*.

Examples:

> 10 grams + 5 grams = 15 grams
> 10 grams − 5 grams = 5 grams
> 300 grains × 2 = 600 grains
> 12 ounces ÷ 3 = 4 ounces

If any one rule of arithmetic may take first place in importance, this is it: *Numbers of different denominations have no direct numerical connection with each other and cannot be used together in any arithmetical operation.* We shall see again and again that if quantities are to be added, or if one quantity is to be subtracted from another, they must be expressed in the same denomination. And when we apparently multiply or divide a denominate number by a number of different denomination, we are in fact using the multiplier or divisor as an abstract number. If, for example, *1 ounce* costs *5 cents* and we want to find the cost of *12 ounces*, we do not multiply *5 cents* by *12 ounces*, but by the abstract number *12*.

ENUMERATION AND NOTATION

The really primitive arithmetical operation is *enumeration*, the simple act of *counting*. The really primitive method of *notation*—the *recording* of a number—is the *tally*, originally a notch on a stick and later any mark used to keep score.

We learn by experience in childhood that "counting by ones" is slow and tedious when the total count is large. "Counting by twos" reduces the task by 50%. "Counting by tens" saves us 90% of our trouble. When you want to collect one hundred from a supply of tablets, therefore, your spatula will likely pick off at least two or three at a time.

Now, if "counting by ones" is inefficient, "*recording* by ones" is virtually useless. A notch on his long rifle for each bear may have pleased Daniel Boone, but no pharmacist would be pleased to find a hundred notches cut along the edge of a prescription to designate the desired number of tablets. Small wonder that primitive people, when not driven by necessity, have been known to shrug off the problem with "one—another—another—*many!*" And small wonder, too, is the great antiquity of this familiar method of tallying votes "by fives":

AYES ╫╫ ╫╫ ╫╫ ///   . . . etc.

NOES ╫╫ ╫╫ || . . . etc.

People early discovered the advantage of using a different *sign* for each successive number in their count (as they might have cut differently shaped notches on a stick to record different totals). This removed the need for a *recount* each time they consulted the record. The ancient Hebrews and Greeks, for example, matched their count with the letters of their alphabets. We still often use this device for counting subdivisions (as in some of the practice problems in this book), and the device works very well—until we run out of letters.

We can use our so-called "Arabic numerals" for the same limited purpose, but if this were the only use we made of them we might as well have stayed with the alphabet. We certainly should have needed a great many more figures than *0, 1, 2, 3, 4, 5, 6, 7, 8*, and *9*.

The fact is that our numerical system of notation, while on the surface a seemingly static report of quantities, actually records an intricate, dynamic pattern of mental calculation involving both multiplication and addition. Oddly enough, most of us, for our ordinary purposes, do the required "mental arithmetic" quite unconsciously. We can glance at "*2 × 12*" and instantly equate it with "*24*"; our instant equation has allowed no time for thought about what we have done. We think *with* our figures but seldom think *about* them.

In handling elementary problems like "*2 × 12*" we can easily follow the correct pattern of procedure without seeing it. But when we tackle more advanced problems, without the pattern we are lost.

For *your* own sake, therefore, it will pay you to give careful attention to the following discussion, as well as to the examples and exercises. Adopt as your own everything that you do not already know.

Begin by pondering three features that make our system of notation so remarkably useful:

1. Our notation is *positional* in that the value of a numeral depends upon its *location* in a row. For example, "*5*" appearing by itself means *five*, but when you see "*55*" you do not interpret it to mean *five and five* or *five times five* but *fifty and five*—for the "*5*" on the left means *five tens* or *fifty*. Any unoccupied space in the row is marked by the sign *0*.

2. Our *zero* can indicate more than merely an empty space in the row. It may significantly report a real value found by actual count or measurement (see p. 15).

3. We use the number *ten*, not the number *one*, to serve as a handy "base of operations." In other words, we "record by tens" in what mathematicians call a *Denary System of Notation*.[1] In this system we may quickly soar into a realm of high numbers that "counting by ones" or "recording by ones" could never reach.

---

[1] "Denary" is from a Latin word meaning "by *tens*" and applies properly to the whole numbers to the left of our "decimal point." "Decimal" is from a Latin word meaning "by *tenths*" and applies properly to the decimal *fractions* to the right of the point (see p. 11).

When told that there is nothing logical or necessary in our use of *ten* as a base, people who have never before given any thought to the matter sometimes react as if a rug had been pulled from under their feet. *Ten,* they insist, is *the* natural base. But *two, five, twelve, twenty, sixty—any* quantity greater than *one* may be chosen arbitrarily to serve in a similar way. We happen to use *ten* because our ancestors did, and it may be that they chose it because men have always liked to count with their ten fingers. Some mathematicians used to champion a base of *twelve* on the ground that it is evenly divisible by *twelve, six, four, three, two,* and *one,* and (they argued) the greater the number of even divisions of the base, the more often calculations will "come out even."[1] For obscure and probably mystical reason the ancient Babylonians sometimes used a base of *sixty,* bequeathing to us our sixty-minute hour and our sixty-second minute.

Perhaps nothing can strengthen and sharpen one's grasp of the Denary System more effectively than a brief plunge into some other system. If you have never taken the plunge, you will find the next section alien to your habitual thinking. A first reading may make you feel insecure, but you should be able to read it a second time through with confidence.

BUILDING ON A BASE

Whatever our base, we may express an unlimited number of quantities by using a limited number of symbols. All that we require is a set of individual figures representing the whole numbers (*1, 2, 3,* etc.) between *zero* and our base, *and not including the base itself.* With base *ten* we need *nine* digits; with base *twelve* we should need *eleven;* if we were Babylonians using base *sixty* we should need an unwieldy set of *fifty-nine.*

When the individual figures stand alone, they represent only their individual values. But move a figure one space to the left (marking its original location with a *zero*), and now it represents *its own value times the base.* So the base itself is expressed always as *10.*

You almost certainly have misread the previous sentence. The odds are that you pronounced (or felt) it to mean "... is expressed always as *ten.*" That is exactly what it means when our base is *ten.* But to make the expression "*10*" hold true for *any* base you must interpret it to mean "... is expressed always as *one times the base plus nothing.*" More briefly, in any system *10* means "*the base.*"

Examples:

> *With base two:*   *10 = 1 × base + 0 = two*
> *With base twelve:* *10 = 1 × base + 0 = twelve*
> *With base twenty:* *10 = 1 × base + 0 = twenty*

[1] The concept of "significant figures" (see p. 14) has weakened this argument, since every measurement is only an approximation, however close.

In each system, remember, we use only enough digits to reach the base, starting from *0*. So, for practice, let us begin to build (and *think*) with base *five:*

$$0 = zero$$
$$1 = one$$
$$2 = two$$
$$3 = three$$
$$4 = four$$
$$10 = five$$

We have reached our base. From this point on we shall get nowhere unless we completely shed and leave behind the language of base *ten*. Just as *10* here means *1 × base + 0*, or simply *five*, so *11* must be interpreted to mean *1 × base + 1*, or *six*. And so on, up to *ten*, which will be written *20*, interpreted as *2 × base + 0* and therefore pronounced *ten:*

$$11 = six$$
$$12 = seven$$
$$13 = eight$$
$$14 = nine$$
$$20 = ten$$

Caution: If you read the figures as *"eleven, twelve, thirteen, fourteen, twenty"* you have left the game. In base *five* the left-hand column says nothing but *"six, seven, eight, nine, ten."*

As we continue, we shall find that the same four digits and *zero* will permit us to express in two spaces all successive quantities up to but *not including the base times itself*. This is expressed as *100*, not meaning a hundred, but *base × base + 0*, or, more analytically, *one times the base squared plus nothing times the base plus nothing*. Pronounce it *"twenty-five":*

$$21 = eleven$$
$$30 = fifteen$$
$$40 = twenty$$
$$44 = twenty-four$$
$$100 = twenty-five$$

It works out beautifully that we *never* need more than the four digits and *zero* to continue an upward count toward infinity. Each time we reach a higher power of *five* we express it by entering *1* a new space to the left and entering to its right the required number of zeros:

$101 = 1 \times base\ squared + 1 = twenty\text{-}six$
$200 = 2 \times base\ squared + 0 = fifty$
$300 = 3 \times base\ squared + 0 = seventy\text{-}five$
$444 = 4 \times base\ squared + 4 \times base + 4 = one\ hundred\ twenty\text{-}four$
$1000 = 1 \times base\ cubed + 0 \quad = one\ hundred\ twenty\text{-}five$

It may be interesting to note that when you express *any* power of your base, the *number* of zeros to the right of *1* tells at a glance which power it is *One zero* indicates the *first* power, etc.:

$10 = 1 \times base\ to\ the\ first\ power \quad = five$
$100 = 1 \times base\ to\ the\ second\ power = twenty\text{-}five$
$1000 = 1 \times base\ to\ the\ third\ power \quad = one\ hundred\ twenty\text{-}five$
$10000 = 1 \times base\ to\ the\ fourth\ power = six\ hundred\ twenty\text{-}five$
Etc.

Practice Problems

1. Interpret the following notations in terms of the systems indicated, and then give their values in words:

Ternary System (base *three*)	*Quinary System* (base *five*)	*Duodenary System* (base *twelve*)
(a) 10	(e) 10	(i) 10
(b) 20	(f) 20	(j) 20
(c) 100	(g) 100	(k) 100
(d) 110	(h) 110	(l) 110

2. Express these quantities in the following systems:

Ternary System	*Quinary System*	*Duodenary System*
(a) Four	(e) Seven	(i) Fifteen
(b) Seven	(f) Twelve	(j) Thirty
(c) Ten	(g) Twenty-eight	(k) Two hundred
(d) Fifteen	(h) Fifty	(l) Seventeen hundred twenty-eight

THE BINARY-DIMIDIAL SYSTEM

If you kept your confidence in the preceding section, you should be ready for quick comprehension of the simplest yet clumsiest system of all: the *Binary System*, the language of the electronic computer, using base *two*. When confronted by the machine, you have no choice. It is the man who must yield and agree to communicate in the only system the machine can use. Here the usable figures are limited to *1* and *0*, which in the "yes-no language" of the computer mean "current on" and "current off."

Were it not for the machine, this system would have little but curiosity value. By "perceiving" and calculating with something approaching the speed of light, the machine can gulp in the expression *11110110000* as a very acceptable recording of the year nineteen hundred and sixty-eight. To you, this may seem a pretty unlikely way of recording it. But do not underestimate the power of two. With the rapid expansion of our reliance on computers you will hear more and more frequent reference to the Binary System. In the course of your career you may one day find yourself actively involved in it.

So, let us at least count to *sixteen*, then make a nodding acquaintance with the available fractions, and finally try our hand at a few elementary calculations.

The Count:

Recite this series like a member of a chorus.

$$0 = zero$$
$$1 = one$$

$$10 = 1 \times base + 0 = two$$
$$11 = 1 \times base + 1 = three$$

$$100 = 1 \times base\ squared + 0 = four$$
$$101 = 1 \times base\ squared + 1 = five$$
$$110 = 1 \times base\ squared + 1 \times base + 0 = six$$
$$111 = 1 \times base\ squared + 1 \times base + 1 = seven$$

$$1000 = 1 \times base^3 + 0 = eight$$
$$1001 = 1 \times base^3 + 1 = nine$$
$$1010 = 1 \times base^3 + 1 \times base + 0 = ten$$
$$1011 = 1 \times base^3 + 1 \times base + 1 = eleven$$
$$1100 = 1 \times base^3 + 1 \times base^2 + 0 = twelve$$
$$1101 = 1 \times base^3 + 1 \times base^2 + 1 = thirteen$$
$$1110 = 1 \times base^3 + 1 \times base^2 + 1 \times base + 0 = fourteen$$
$$1111 = 1 \times base^3 + 1 \times base^2 + 1 \times base + 1 = fifteen$$

$$10000 = 1 \times base^4 + 0 = sixteen$$

The Fractions:

Our Denary System includes a *decimal point* to the right of which the *tenths* begin. In the Binary System, such a point, marking where the *halves* begin, should be called a *dimidial point* (from the Latin word meaning "by halves").

It may never have occurred to you that if you record a single *decimal* remainder, you *imply* that your record is sufficiently precise to the nearest *tenth* (remind yourself that there are exactly *nine* fractional tenths). If you record your remainder in *two* spaces, you imply that your precision requires a record to the nearest *hundredth* (there are *ninety-nine* in all), and similarly three spaces imply a precision to the nearest *thousandth* (there are *nine hundred and ninety-nine*), etc.

The Binary System offers a parallel scheme. But here the fractions are expressed in roots of *two*. Here the first space to the right of the point records to the nearest *half* (there is only *one* of these!), two spaces record more precisely to the nearest *fourth* (there are *three,* including a more precise restatement of our *half*), three spaces to the nearest *eighth* (there are seven), etc.

And this is how the system of dimidial fractions may be charted:

1.0	= *two* halves (*one* to the nearest half)
0.1	= *one* half
1.00	= *four* quarters (*one* to the nearest quarter)
0.11	= *three* quarters
0.10	= *two* quarters (a more precise half)
0.01	= *one* quarter
1.000	= *eight* eighths (*one* to the nearest eighth)
0.111	= *seven* eighths
0.110	= *six* eighths
0.101	= *five* eighths
0.100	= *four* eighths (still more precise half)
0.011	= *three* eighths
0.010	= *two* eighths
0.001	= *one* eighth
1.0000	= *sixteen* sixteenths (*one* to the nearest sixteenth)
0.1111	= *fifteen* sixteenths
Etc.	

To add binary quantities:

Addition with base *two* is as simple as *1 + 1, if* you remember that the answer is *10.*

Example:

What is the total of 101.1, 1010, and 11.11?

```
    101.1    (five and a half)
   1010.     (ten)
     11.11   (three and three quarters)
  ─────────
  10011.01   (nineteen and a quarter), answer.
```

The first column on the right totals *1*, which you enter below. The second from the right totals *10* (*two*); so you enter the *0* and carry the *1* over to the third column, which totals *11* (*three*). Enter *1* and carry over *1* to the fourth column, which likewise totals *11*, entered as *1* with a carry-over of *1*. The fifth totals *10* (*two*), and the sixth therefore totals *10*, which you enter below.

To subtract binary quantities :

Subtraction involves a complication. What have you actually *done* when you record that *10 — 1 = 1?* Since *1* cannot be substracted from *0*, you must "borrow from the left" as you do in the Denary System. But here you are borrowing not Denary's *10* (*ten*) but Binary's *10* (*two*). When the space to the left provides the *1* you have to borrow, you must mentally replace it with *0*.

When the space to the left has only *0* to offer, you must first fill this space by borrowing from further to the left; but since you have mentally filled this space with *10* (*two*), of which you have then borrowed only *1*, you must mentally replace its original *0* with the *1* you do not use. (This replacement corresponds to the mental *9* replacing a *0* in the Denary System.)

Examples:

$$\begin{array}{cccc}
10\ (two) & 100\ (four) & 1000\ (eight) & 1100\ (twelve) \\
-\ \ 1\ (one) & -\ \ 1\ (one) & -\ \ 11\ (three) & -\ 101\ (five) \\
\hline
1\ (one) & 11\ (three) & 101\ (five) & 111\ (seven)
\end{array}$$

If uncertain of yourself, you may want to divide the minuend[1] into components containing such *1's* as your subtrahend[2] requires. Adapting the last example, you may rewrite the minuend *1100* (*twelve*) in the form of a column of addends:[3]

$$\begin{array}{l}
\ \ 111\ (seven) \\
+\ \ \ \ 1\ (one) \\
+100\ (four) \\
-101\ (five) \\
\hline
\ \ 111\ (seven),\ answer.
\end{array}$$

To multiply binary quantities :

Multiplication offers no difficulty.

[1] From Latin, "that which is to be diminished."
[2] Latin, "that which is to be taken away."
[3] Latin *addenda*, "things to be added."

Example:

Multiply 1100 by 101.

$$
\begin{array}{r}
1100 \ (twelve) \\
\times \ \ 101 \ (five) \\
\hline
1100 \\
0000 \\
1100 \\
\hline
111100 \ (sixty), \ answer.
\end{array}
$$

To divide binary quantities:

"Long division" can follow the pattern we use in the Denary System.

Example:

Divide 10010 by 11.

$$
\begin{array}{r}
110, \ answer. \\
11)\overline{10010} \\
\underline{11} \ \ \ \ \ \ \\
11 \ \ \ \\
\underline{11} \ \ \ \\
00
\end{array}
$$

You can trace this process as follows: "*11* (*three*) goes into *100* (*four*) once." Enter the *1* above. Enter *11* (*three*) below *100* (*four*) and subtract, getting a difference of *1*. Bring down *1* to make *11* (*three*). "*11* (*three*) goes into *11* (*three*) once." Enter *1* above and *11* below and subtract, getting *0*. Enter the final *0* above.

Practice Problems

1. Without reference to the text, express the quantities from *one* to *sixteen* in the Binary System.

2. Do the same with the dimidial fractions descending from *seven-eighths* to *one-eighth*.

3. Add in the Binary System:

    (a) 110 + 10   (d) 1001 + 111 + 1
    (b) 100 + 11   (e) 111 + 11 + 11
    (c) 101 + 101   (f) 1011 + 100 + 111

4. Subtract in the Binary System:

    (a) 1000 − 100   (d) 1011 − 110
    (b) 11 − 1   (e) 1100 − 1011
    (c) 1010 − 110   (f) 10000 − 1001

5. Multiply in the Binary System:

    (a) 11 × 10   (d) 11 × 110
    (b) 100 × 11   (e) 11 × 11
    (c) 101 × 101   (f) 111 × 11

6. Divide in the Binary System:

    (a) 1001 ÷ 11   (d) 1100 ÷ 100
    (b) 1010 ÷ 10   (e) 1100 ÷ 110
    (c) 1100 ÷ 11   (f) 10000 ÷ 100

The Denary-Decimal System

We have considered the development of a system of numerical notation in terms of the powers and roots of *any* base other than *one*. It may interest you to note that no such system could develop from base *one* itself. Since *1 × 1 = 1*, and *1 ÷ 1 = 1*, the powers and roots of *one* all remain the same, and hence, with *one* as a base, the signs *10, 100, 1000* and *0.1, 0.01*, etc., would all mean *one*.

We have given passing attention to the Binary System since it has responded to the call of the computer and serves indispensably in an increasingly important area of applied mathematics. But you may be reassured that in the world of science, as in all ordinary human affairs, nothing threatens to displace your familiar Denary-Decimal System—or the Metric System of Weights and Measures erected on the same base.

Ten as a notational base is small enough to permit calculation with a manageable set of nine digits plus *zero*, yet large enough to express easily read quantities into the millions (or millionths) and beyond.[1]

The practical range of this system is represented by the following scheme (which can be extended, of course, to the left or right into even higher or lower reaches):

[1] For the expression of extraordinarily large or small quantities see Exponential Notation (Chapter 14, p. 241).

Scheme of the decimal system:

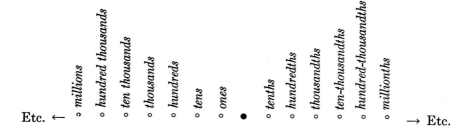

Over-familiarity can breed inattention. Inattention can lead to misunderstanding and error. It will pay you, therefore, to remind yourself occasionally of the structure of this excellent system. When you read, say, that a 1970 survey showed *51,102* community pharmacies in the United States, even though you unhesitatingly think "fifty one thousand one hundred two" you may profit by consciously recognizing that the figures express the sum of these quantities:

$$5 \times 10^4 \text{ or } 50000 \text{ or five } ten\ thousands$$
$$+\ 1 \times 10^3 \text{ or } 1000 \text{ or one } thousands$$
$$+\ 1 \times 10^2 \text{ or } 100 \text{ or one } hundreds$$
$$+\ 0 \times 10^1 \text{ or } 00 \text{ or zero } tens$$
$$+\ 2 \times 10^0 \text{ or } 2 \text{ or two } ones$$

ROMAN NUMERALS

The Romans could express a fairly large range of numbers by use of a few letters of the alphabet in a simple "positional" notation indicating adding to or subtracting from a succession of primitive bases extending from *one* through *five, ten, fifty, one hundred, and five hundred* to *one thousand*.

Roman numerals can merely record quantities: they are of no use in computation. They customarily designate quantities on prescriptions when ingredients are measured by the common or apothecaries' systems.

To express quantities in the roman system, these eight letters of fixed values are used:[1]

ss = ½	V or v = 5	L or l = 50	D or d = 500
I or i = 1	X or x = 10	C or c = 100	M or m = 1000

[1] Physicians tend to use capitals except for the letter *i*, which they dot for the sake of clarity; and many use *j* for a final *i*. Following the Latin custom, they put the symbol for the denomination first and the roman numeral second. Dates are customarily expressed in capitals.

Other quantities are expressed by combining these letters by the general rule that when the second of two letters has a value equal to or smaller than that of the first, their values are to be added; but when the second has a value greater than that of the first, the smaller is to be subtracted from the larger. This rule may be illustrated as follows:

(1) Two or more letters express a quantity that is the *sum* of their values *if they are successively equal or smaller in value:*

ii = 2	xx = 20	ci = 101	dc = 600
iii = 3	xxii = 22	cv = 105	mi = 1001
vi = 6	xxxiii = 33	cx = 110	mv = 1005
vii = 7	li = 51	cl = 150	mx = 1010
viii = 8	lv = 55	cc = 200	ml = 1050
xi = 11	lx = 60	di = 501	mc = 1100
xii = 12	lxvi = 66	dv = 505	md = 1500
xiii = 13	lxxvii = 77	dx = 510	mdclxvi = 1666
xv = 15	lxxxviii = 88	dl = 550	mm = 2000

(2) Two or more letters express a quantity that is the *sum* of the values remaining *after the value of each smaller letter has been subtracted from that of a following greater:*

iv = 4	xxxix = 39	xcix = 99	cdxc = 490
ix = 9	xl = 40	cd = 400	cm = 900
xiv = 14	xli = 41	cdi = 401	cmxcix = 999
xix = 19	xliv = 44	cdxl = 440	MCDXCII = 1492
xxiv = 24	xc = 90	cdxliv = 444	MCMLXXIII = 1973

Practice Problems:

1. Write the following in roman numerals:

    (*a*) 18.   (*d*) 126.   (*g*) 84.
    (*b*) 64.   (*e*) 99.   (*h*) 48.
    (*c*) 72.   (*f*) 37.   (*i*) 1984.

2. Write the following in arabic numerals:

    (*a*) Part IV.   (*c*) MCMLIX.
    (*b*) Chapter XIX.   (*d*) MDCCCXIV.

3. Interpret the *quantity* in each of these phrases taken from prescriptions:

    (*a*) Caps. no. xlv.
    (*b*) Gtts. M.
    (*c*) Tabs. no. xlviii.
    (*d*) Pil. no. lxiv.
    (*e*) Pulv. no. xvi.
    (*f*) Caps. no. lxxxiv.

4. Interpret the *quantities* in each of these prescriptions:

    (a) ℞   Zinc Oxide   part. v
               Wool Fat   part xv
               Petrolatum   part. lxxx
               Disp. ℥iv
               Sig. Apply.

    (b) ℞   Dilaudid   gr. iss
               Ammonium Chloride   gr. xl
               Syrup ad   ℥vi
               Sig. ʒss pro tuss.

SIGNIFICANT FIGURES

When we *count* objects accurately, *every* figure in the numeral expressing the total number of objects must be taken at its face value. Such figures may be said to be *absolute*.

But when we record a *measurement*, the last figure to the right must be taken to be an *approximation*, an admission that the limit of possible precision or of necessary accuracy has been reached, and that any further figures to the right would be non-significant—that is, either meaningless or, for a given purpose, needless.

Recognition of this truth is of fairly recent origin. You will find no discussion of significant figures in the old arithmetic texts—and in few recent ones. We are familiar, of course, with phrases like "roughly a yard" and "about a pint" and "a little over a pound"; but most of us find it difficult to grasp the fact that *every* measurement, no matter how precisely made, is only an approximation. Failure to grasp this fact has two unfortunate consequences: it encourages us (1) to retain too many figures in our calculations and thus waste time and run greater risk of careless error and (2) to record results that are invalid.

We should learn to interpret a denominate number like *325 grams* as follows: The *3* means *300 grams*, neither more nor less, and the *2* means *exactly 20 grams more;* but the final *5* means *approximately 5 grams more—* that is, *5 grams plus or minus some fraction of a gram.* Whether this fraction is, for a given purpose, negligible depends upon how precisely the quantity was (or is to be) weighed.

Significant figures, then, are consecutive figures that express the value of a denominate number accurately enough for a given purpose. The accuracy varies with the number of significant figures, which are all absolute in value except the last—and this is properly called *uncertain.*

Two-figure accuracy is liable to a deviation as high as 5% from the theoretic absolute measurement. For example, if a substance is reported to weigh *10 grams* to the nearest *gram,* its actual weight may be anything between *9.5 grams* and *10.5 grams.*

Three-figure accuracy is liable to a deviation as high as 0.5%; four-figure accuracy may deviate 0.05%; and five-figure accuracy, 0.005%.

In scientific work, three-figure or four-figure accuracy is a commonplace; but laymen are often surprised to hear that five-figure, six-figure, and higher degrees of accuracy are rare and are valid only if we have exercised the greatest skill in measuring with the finest instruments.

Any of the digits in a valid denominate number must be regarded as significant. Whether *zero* is significant, however, depends upon its position or upon known facts about a given number. The interpretation of *zero* may be summed up as follows:

Rule 1.   Any zero *between digits is significant.*

Rule 2.   Initial zeros *to the left of the first digit are never significant: they are included merely to show the location of the decimal point and thus give place value to the digits that follow.*

Rule 3.   One or more final zeros *to the right of the decimal point may be taken to be significant.*

Rule 4.   One or more final zeros *in a whole number—that is, immediately to the left of the decimal point—sometimes merely serve to give place value to digits to the left, but the data may show them to be significant.*

Examples:

Assuming that the following numbers are all denominate—

(1)   In *12.5* there are *three* significant figures; in *1.256, four* significant figures; and in *102.56, five* significant figures.

(2)   In *0.5* there is *one* significant figure. The digit *5* tells us how many *tenths* we have. The non-significant *0* simply calls attention to the decimal point.

(3)   In *0.05* there is still only *one* significant figure, and again in *0.005.*

(4)   In *0.65* there are *two* significant figures, and likewise *two* in *0.065* and *0.0065*.

(5)   In *0.0605* there are *three* significant figures. The first *0* calls attention to the decimal point; the second *0* shows the number of places to the right of the decimal point occupied by the remaining figures; and the third *0* significantly contributes to the value of the number. In *0.06050* there are *four* significant figures, since the final *0* also contributes to the value of the number.

(6)   In *20000* there are *five* significant figures; but *20000* ± *50* (or, to express the same quantity another way, *20000 to the nearest 100*) contains only *three* significant figures.

It should go without saying that the ability to make proper and accurate measurements constitutes an essential qualification of a competent pharmacist; but his zeal for accuracy should not blind him to the truth that there is always bound to be a maximum degree beyond which he cannot go—and need not if he could. As already pointed out, one of the factors determining the degree of approximation to perfect measurement is the precision of the instrument used. It would be absurd for a pharmacist to pretend that he had measured *7.76 milliliters* in a graduate calibrated in units of *1 milliliter;* or that he had weighed *25.562 grains* on a balance sensitive to $\frac{1}{10}$ *grain.*

Other Examples:

(1)   If a substance weighs *0.06 gram* according to a balance sensitive to *0.001 gram*, we may record the weight as *0.060 gram*. But if the balance is sensitive only to *0.01 gram*, the value should be recorded as *0.06 gram*, and a record of *0.060 gram* would be invalid.

(2)   Again, when recording a length of *10 millimeters* found by use of an instrument accurate to *0.1 millimeter*, the value may be recorded as *10.0 millimeters.*

(3)   And again, if a volume of *5 milliliters* is measured with an instrument calibrated in *10ths of a milliliter,* the volume may be recorded as *5.0 milliliters.*

We must clearly distinguish *significant figures* from *decimal places*. When recording a measurement, the number of decimal places we include indicates *the degree of precision with which the measurement has been made*, whereas the number of significant figures retained indicates *the degree of accuracy* that is sufficient for a given purpose.

Sometimes we are asked to record a value "correct to (so-many) decimal places"; and we should never confuse this familiar expression with the expression "correct to (so-many) significant figures."

Examples:

(1) If the value of *27.625918* is rounded off to *five decimal places,* it is written *27.62592;* but when rounded off to *five significant figures* it is written *27.626.*

(2) The value *54.326,* when rounded off to *54.3,* is precise to *one decimal place* but accurate to *three significant figures.*

Now, when we *calculate* with denominate—that is, with approximate— numbers, it is very easy to get results that are invalid *because they pretend to a greater accuracy or precision than is supplied in the data.*

To emphasize and clarify this often-ignored point, every uncertain figure included in the following discussion is identified by a slanting line indicating that its value is not absolute.

Invalid results are commonly met with in division. Forgetting that the *last* figure in a denominate number is always *uncertain,* we add a succession of zeros to the dividend and drive our quotient into the meaningless darkness of *too many decimal places,* perhaps in the hope that it will "come out even." (By definition, a denominate quotient is *never* "even" in the absolute sense: if you divide approximately *8* fluidounces by 2, no matter how close the approximation is, you get approximately *4* fluidounces.)

Example:

Divide 3.9*1* grains by 8.
    8)3.9*1000*
    0.488*73* grain, *invalid answer.*

Since the *1* of 3.9*1* grains is uncertain, when we divide the next figure beyond it by 8 the quotient will be uncertain, and it is sheer waste of time to proceed any farther than one more place in order to get a rough approximation to guide us in rounding off the result to 0.48*9* grain, with only one uncertain figure.

It is equally tempting, and equally foolish, to retain meaningless figures in the product of multiplication.

Example:

Multiply 0.0056*3* grain by 7.

       0.0056*3*
    ×   7
    ――――――
          2*1*
         42
         35
    ――――――
    0.0394*1* grain, *invalid answer.*

Since the 3 of 0.00563 *grain* is uncertain, the product of 7×3 will be 21. The final product should be rounded off to 0.0394 *grain*, again with only one uncertain figure.

The *principle* that *the result of any calculation involving an approximate number should be rounded off so as to contain only one uncertain figure* holds as well for sums and differences as for quotients and products.

With this principle in mind, we can get valid results, and save a good deal of time, by obeying the following rules for (a) recording measurements, (b) calculating with approximate numbers, and (c) recording the results of such calculations.

Rule 1. When recording a measurement, retain as many figures as will give only one uncertain figure.

The uncertain figure will sometimes represent an estimate between graduations on a scale. Thus, if you use a ruler calibrated in centimeters, you might record a measurement as approximately 11.3 *centimeters*, but not as approximately 11.32 *centimeters*. Since the 3 is uncertain, no other figure should follow it.

Rule 2. When rejecting superfluous figures in the result of a calculation, add 1 to the last figure retained if the following figure is 5 or more.

Thus, 2.443 may be rounded off to 2.4, but 2.448 should be rounded off to 2.5. Note that if a number like 2.597 is rounded off to three significant figures, the 1 added to the 9 makes 10, and the 0 should be recorded, for it is significant: 2.60.

Rule 3. Since you cannot increase the precision of the *least* precise number, therefore *before adding or subtracting approximate numbers, you may save time by rounding off each component so that it will contain one more decimal place than is contained in the component having the fewest decimal places. The result should always be rounded off to the same number of decimal places as are contained in that component.*

Example:

Add these approximate weights: 162.3 *grams,* 0.569 *gram,* 0.0373 *gram, and* 120.58 *grams.*

If the last figure in each of the given numbers is uncertain, the *total* should be rounded off to the one decimal place. Note that the shorter method (b) gives the same result as the longer method (a):

(a) 162.3
    0.560
    0.0373
  120.58
  283.0803 or
  283.7 grams, *answer.*

(b) 162.3
    0.57
    0.04
  120.58
  283.69 or
  283.7 grams, *answer.*

It is important to note that in filling a prescription, the pharmacist *must* assume that the physician means each quantity to be measured with *the same degree of precision.* Hence, if we add these quantities taken from a prescription:

$$5.5 \quad grams$$
$$0.01 \quad gram$$
$$0.005 \; gram$$

we must *not* round off the total to one decimal place. Rather we must retain at least *three* decimal places in the total by interpreting the given quantities to mean 5.500 *grams*, 0.010 *gram*, and 0.005 *gram*. Where greater precision is required, we may interpret the given quantities to mean 5.5000, 0.0100, and 0.0050, etc.

> *Rule 4.* Since you cannot increase the accuracy of the *least* accurate number, therefore, *before multiplying or dividing one approximate number by another approximate number, you may save time by rounding off the component with the greater number of significant figures to one more than are contained in the component having fewer significant figures. The result should be rounded off to the same number of significant figures as are contained in the latter component.*

Example:

Multiply 1.65370 *grams by* 0.20.

If the last figure in each number is uncertain, each of these methods gives the same result:

(a) 1.65370 grams
  × 0.20
    0002220
    330740
  0.4200020 or
  0.42 gram, *answer.*

(b) 1.63 grams
  ×0.20
    000
    330
  0.4200 or
  0.42 gram, *answer.*

Here again, when calculating with denominate numbers taken from a prescription or official formula, since we must assume that each quantity is meant to be measured with the same degree of accuracy, we must interpret each quantity as having at least as many significant figures as appear in the quantity containing the greatest number of significant figures. So, if the quantities 0.25 *gram*, 0.5 *gram*, and 5 *grams* are included in a prescription, they should be interpreted as 0.2*5* gram, 0.5*0* gram, and 5.*0* grams for purposes of multiplication or division (as when we enlarge or reduce a formula); and results should be rounded off to contain two significant figures. Where greater accuracy is required, we may interpret the given quantities to mean 0.250*0*, 0.500*0*, and 5.00*0*, etc.[1]

> *Rule 5. After* <u>*multiplying*</u> *or dividing an approximate number by an absolute number,* <u>*round off the result to*</u> *the same number of* <u>*significant figures*</u> *as are contained in the approximate number.*

This is consistent with Rule 4, for the denominate number contains fewer significant figures if the absolute number is interpreted as being followed by significant zeros to an infinite number of decimal places.

Example:

> *If a patient has taken 96 doses, each containing 2.5*4 *milligrams of active ingredient, how much of the active ingredient has he taken in all?*

    2.5*4* milligrams
    × 96
    ‾‾‾‾‾‾
    15 *24*
    228 *0*
    ‾‾‾‾‾‾
    24*3*.*84* or
    24*4* milligrams, *answer.*

Practice Problems

1. State the number of significant figures in each of the *italicized* quantities:

   (a) One gram equals *15.4324* grains.
   (b) One liter equals *1000* milliliters.

[1] When converting from one system of measurement to another, we are expressly ordered by the *United States Pharmacopeia* as follows: "For the conversion of specific quantities in converting pharmaceutical formulas, use the exact equivalents. For prescription compounding, use the exact equivalents rounded to three significant figures." However, it is interesting to note that the "exact" equivalents as they are given in the *Pharmacopeia* show a variation of from one-figure to six-figure accuracy.

(c) One inch equals *2.54* centimeters.
(d) The chemical costs *$1.05* a pound.
(e) One gram equals *1,000,000* micrograms.
(f) One microgram equals *0.001* milligram.

2. Assuming these numbers to be denominate, how many significant figures has each?

(a) 35.
(b) 609.
(c) 2.7.
(d) 9004.
(e) 506.03.
(f) 0.0047.
(g) 40.07.
(h) 350 (to nearest 1).
(i) 350 (to the nearest 10).
(j) 5000 (to the nearest 100).

3. Round off each of the following to three significant figures:

(a) 32.75.   (f) 1.0751.
(b) 200.39.   (g) 27.052.
(c) 0.03629.   (h) 0.86249.
(d) 21.635.   (i) 3.14159.
(e) 0.00944.   (j) 1.00595632

4. Round off each of the following to three decimal places:

(a) 0.00083.   (d) 6.12963.
(b) 34.79502.   (e) 14.8997.
(c) 0.00494.   (f) 1.00595632.

5. If a mixture of seven ingredients contains the following approximate weights, what can you validly record as the approximate total combined weight of the ingredients?

26.8*3* grains, 275.*3* grains, 2.75*6* grains, 4.0*0* grains, 5.19*7* grains, 16.*0* grains, and 0.00*1* grain.

6. You have 420.*3* grams of a chemical weighed on a balance sensitive to 0.*1* gram. After taking from this 0.01*0* gram weighed on a balance sensitive to 0.00*1* gram, what can you validly record to be the weight of what is left of the chemical?

7. If each of a batch of tablets contains 0.05Ø grain of active ingredient, what approximate weight of active ingredient will be contained in 750 tablets?

8. If each tablet contains 0.0Ƶ grain of active ingredient, what will be in the approximate weight of active ingredient in 750 tablets?

9. Perform the following computations and retain only significant figures in the results:

(a) 6.3Ø — 0.00Ƶ.

(b) 7.0Ӿ — 6.Ø.

(c) 97.Ӿ — 6.936Ƶ.

(d) 5.Ø × 48.Ƶ grains.

(e) 24 × 0.2Ƶ gram

(f) 350 × 0.6015Ø gram

(g) 0.72Ø × 0.09Ƶ grain

(h) 0.05Ø × 0.962Ø gram.

(i) 56.82Ӿ ÷ 0.09Ø.

(j) 25Ø ÷ 1.Ӿ.

(k) 5.000Ӿ ÷ 1.Ø.

(l) 0.0072Ø ÷ 0.273Ƶ.

(m) 71.42Ƶ ÷ 0.51Ƶ.

(n) 71.42Ƶ ÷ 3.

10. What is the difference in meaning between a volume recorded as 473 milliliters and one that is recorded as 473.0 milliliters?

11. What is the difference in meaning between a weight recorded as 0.65 gram and one that is recorded as 0.6500 gram?

12. The answers in the following computations are arithmetically correct. In each case, if the answer does not contain the proper number of significant figures, rewrite it so that all the figures retained are significant.

(a) 15.432 grains × 0.26 = 4.01232 grains

(b) 0.2350 grain ÷ 0.55 = 0.42727 grain

(c) 1.25500 grams + 0.650 gram + 0.125 gram
          + 12.78900 grams = 14.81900 grams

(d) 16.23 minims × 0.75 = 12.1725 minims

(e) 437.5 grains ÷ 1.25 = 350.000 grains

ESTIMATION

One of the best checks of the reasonableness of a numerical computation is an estimation of the answer. If we have arrived at a wrong answer by use of a wrong method, a thoughtless, mechanical final verification of our figuring may not show up the error. But an absurd result, such as occurs when the decimal point is put in the wrong place, will not likely slip past if we check it against a preliminary estimation of what the result should be.

Since it is imperative that the pharmacist insure the accuracy of his calculations by every means at his disposal, the student of pharmacy is urged to adopt estimation as one of those means; and since proficiency in estimating comes only from constant practice, he is urged to acquire the habit of estimating the answer to every problem he encounters before attempting to solve it. If so, he will discover, too, that his estimate not only will serve as a means for judging the reasonableness of the final result but also will very often serve as a guide in the solution of the problem.

Checking the accuracy of every calculation, of course, such as by adding a column first upwards and then downwards, is very important. Hence the student should follow this invariable procedure: (1) *estimate*, (2) *compute*, (3) *check*.

The estimating process is basically very simple. First the numbers given in a problem are mentally rounded off to slightly larger or smaller numbers containing fewer significant figures. So, the number *59* would be rounded off to *60*, and the number *732* to *700*. Then the required computations are performed, as far as possible mentally, and the result, although known to be somewhat greater or smaller than the exact answer, is close enough to serve as an estimate.

No set rules for estimating can be given to cover all the computations in arithmetic. But examples can illustrate some of the methods that can be used.

In *addition*, one way to obtain a reasonable estimate of the total is first to add the figures in the leftmost column. But the neglected remaining figures of each number are equally likely to express more or less than one-half the value of a unit of the order we have just added, and hence to the sum of the leftmost column should be added $\frac{1}{2}$ for every number—or *1* for every two numbers—in the column.

Examples:

    Add the following numbers: 7428, 3652, 1327, 4605, 2791, and 4490.

Estimation:	*Calculation:*
The figures in the thousands column add up to 21000, and with each number on the average contributing 500 more, or every pair 1000 more, we get 21000 + 3000 = 24000, *estimated answer.*	7428 3652 1327 4605 2791 4490 ——— 24293, *answer.*

Add the following numbers: 2556, 449, 337, 1572.

Estimation:	Calculation:

The figures of the thousands column add up to 3000, and with each pair of numbers contributing approximately another 1000, we get 3000 + 2000 = 5000, *estimated answer.*

2556
449
337
1572
———
4914, *answer.*

In *multiplication,* the product of the two leftmost digits plus a sufficient number of *zeros* to give the right place value will serve as a fair estimate. The number of *zeros* supplied must equal the total number of all discarded figures to the left of the decimal point. A closer approximation to the correct answer will result if the discarded figures are used to round off the value of those retained.

Examples:

Multiply 612 by 413.

Estimation:

Calculation:

4 × 6 = 24, and since we have discarded four figures, four zeros must be supplied, giving 240,000, *estimated answer.*

612
× 413
———
1836
612
2448
———
252756, *answer.*

Multiply 2889 by 209.

Estimation:

Calculation:

The given numbers round off to 3000 and 200. 3 × 2 = 6, and supplying five zeros we get 600,000, *estimated answer.*

2889
× 209
———
26001
5778
———
603801, *answer.*

The correct place value is easier to keep track of if relatively insignificant decimal fractions are ignored. When the multiplier is a decimal fraction, the possibility of error is reduced if we first convert it to a common fraction of approximately the same value.

Examples:

> *Multiply 41.76 by 20.3.*
> Estimate: $42 \times 20 = 840$.
>
> *Multiply 730.5 by 321.*
> Estimate: $700 \times 300 = 210,000$.
>
> *Multiply 314.2 by 0.18*
> Estimate: Since 0.18 or $\frac{18}{100}$ lies between $\frac{1}{6}$ and $\frac{1}{5}$, the answer will lie between 50 and 60.
>
> *Multiply 48.16 by 0.072.*
> Estimate: $\frac{7}{100}$ equals about $\frac{1}{15}$, and $\frac{1}{15}$ of 48 is about 3.

In *division*, the given numbers may be rounded off to convenient approximations, but here again care must be exercised to preserve correct place values.

Example:

> *Divide 2456 by 5.91.*
>
> Estimate: The numbers may be rounded off to 2400 and 6. We may divide 24 by 6 mentally; but we must not forget the two zeros substituted for the given 56 in 2456, and our estimated answer will be 400.

The use of short cuts and variations in arithmetical computations contributes to both speed and accuracy in mental calculation. Facility in the use of short cuts can be developed only if we select or devise variations that appeal to us and practice them constantly. Here are some short cuts that may suggest other possibilities:

(1) To multiply by 10, 100, 1000, etc., move the decimal place one, two, three places to the right, etc. To divide by 10, 100, 1000, etc., move the decimal place one, two, three places to the left, etc.

(2) To multiply by 200, 300, 500, etc., multiply by 2, 3, 5, etc., and then multiply by 100. To divide by the same numbers, divide by 2, 3, 5, etc., and divide by 100.

(3) To multiply by 2000, 4000, 6000, etc., multiply by 2, 4, 6, etc., and then multiply by 1000. To divide by these numbers, divide by 2, 4, 6, etc., and divide by 1000.

(4) To multiply by $87\frac{1}{2}$, which is $\frac{7}{8}$ of a hundred, multiply by 700 and divide by 8. To divide by $87\frac{1}{2}$, multiply by 8 and divide by 700.

(5) To multiply by $83\frac{1}{3}$, which is $\frac{5}{6}$ of a hundred, multiply by 500 and divide by 6. To divide by $83\frac{1}{3}$, multiply by 6 and divide by 500.

(6) To multiply by 75, which is $\frac{3}{4}$ of a hundred, multiply by 300 and divide by 4. To divide by 75, multiply by 4 and divide by 300.

(7) To multiply by $66\frac{2}{3}$, which is $\frac{2}{3}$ of a hundred, multiply by 200 and divide by 3. To divide by $66\frac{2}{3}$, multiply by 3 and divide by 200.

(8) To multiply by $62\frac{1}{2}$, which is $\frac{5}{8}$ of a hundred, multiply by 500 and divide by 8. To divide by $62\frac{1}{2}$, multiply by 8 and divide by 500.

(9) To multiply by 50, which is $\frac{1}{2}$ of a hundred, multiply by 100 and divide by 2. To divide by 50, multiply by 2 and divide by 100.

(10) To multiply by $37\frac{1}{2}$, which is $\frac{3}{8}$ of a hundred, multiply by 300 and divide by 8. To divide by $37\frac{1}{2}$, multiply by 8 and divide by 300.

(11) To multiply by $33\frac{1}{3}$, which is $\frac{1}{3}$ of a hundred, multiply by 100 and divide by 3. To divide by $33\frac{1}{3}$, multiply by 3 and divide by 100.

(12) To multiply by 25, which is $\frac{1}{4}$ of a hundred, multiply by 100 and divide by 4. To divide by 25, multiply by 4 and divide by 100.

(13) To multiply by $16\frac{2}{3}$, which is $\frac{1}{6}$ of a hundred, multiply by 100 and divide by 6. To divide by $16\frac{2}{3}$, multiply by 6 and divide by 100.

(14) To multiply by 15, multiply by 10 and add half the product. To divide by 15, divide $\frac{2}{3}$ of the dividend by 10 (or divide by 10 and multiply by $\frac{2}{3}$).

(15) To multiply by $12\frac{1}{2}$, which is $\frac{1}{8}$ of a hundred, multiply by 100 and divide by 8. To divide by $12\frac{1}{2}$, multiply by 8 and divide by 100.

(16) To multiply any *two-digit* number by 11, first add the two digits. If the sum is less than ten, place it between the digits; if the sum is ten or more, place the unit figure between the digits and add 1 to the left digit.

$$11 \times 43: \quad 4 + 3 = 7, \text{ hence } 473$$
$$11 \times 83: \quad 8 + 3 = 11, \text{ hence } 913$$

To multiply *any* number by eleven, multiply by 10 and add the multiplicand.

(17) To multiply by 0.25 and 0.50, divide by 4 and 2. To divide by 0.25 and 0.50, multiply by 4 and 2.

$$6947 \times 0.25 = 6947 \div 4$$
$$6947 \div 0.50 = 6947 \times 2$$

(18) Reduce inconvenient multipliers to their more convenient factors.

$$16 \times 55 = 8 \times 2 \times 55 = 8 \times 110 = 880$$

Practice Problems

1. In estimating the result of multiplying 8,329 by 7,242, how many zeros will follow 56?

2. In estimating the result of dividing 811500 by 16.23, how many zeros will follow 5?

3. How many terminal zeros are there in the product obtained by multiplying 5.100 by 90,000?

4. How many terminal zeros are there in the quotient obtained by dividing 8.100 by 0.009?

Estimate the sums:

5.	5641	7.	3298	9.	$ 75.82
	2177		368		37.92
	294		5192		14.69
	8266		627		45.98
	3503		4835		28.91
					49.87

6.	9874	8.	7466	10.	$ 49.55
	6018		5288		9.75
	459		9013		12.98
	1297		8462		53.36
	3361		716		29.79
	396		4369		14.56

Estimate the products:

11. 17 × 22 =
12. 28 × 31 =
13. 8 × 48 =
14. 19 × 38 =
15. 28 × 62 =
16. 39 × 77 =
17. 42 × 39 =
18. 125 × 92 =
19. 365 × 98 =
20. 473 × 102 =
21. 596 × 204 =
22. 604 × 122 =
23. 675 × 19 =
24. 998 × 13 =
25. 6549 × 830 =
26. 1073 × 972 =

27. 8431 × 9760 =
28. 7183 × 19 =
29. 5106 × 963 =
30. 2349 × 5907 =
31. $2\frac{1}{2}$ × $14\frac{1}{2}$
32. $\frac{2}{3}$ × 400 =
33. $21\frac{1}{3}$ × $6\frac{2}{3}$ =
34. $\frac{3}{4}$ × 816 =
35. $\frac{2}{3}$ × 425.65 =
36. 5.8 × 7165 =
37. 2.04 × 705.3 =
38. 0.016 × 589.4 =
39. 0.0726 × 6951 =
40. 98 × 0.0031 =
41. 6.1 × 67.39 =
42. 7569 × 0.0963 =

Estimate the quotients:

43. 171 ÷ 19 =
44. 165 ÷ 15 =
45. 184 ÷ 2300 =
46. 3080 ÷ 144 =
47. 160 ÷ 3200 =
48. 36900 ÷ 41 =
49. 86450 ÷ 72 =
50. 1078 ÷ 98 =

51. 98000 ÷ 49 =
52. 17015 ÷ 57 =
53. 1.0745 ÷ 500 =
54. 18.954 ÷ 0.39 =
55. 1.9214 ÷ 0.026 =
56. 19.223 ÷ 47 =
57. 458.4 ÷ 8 =
58. 448.32 ÷ 0.048 =

Estimate the final results:

59. $$\frac{272103 \times 300}{901} =$$

60. $$\frac{750 \times 300 \times 380.5}{760 \times 375} =$$

61. $$\frac{270\,(15 - 10)}{91 \times 5} =$$

62. $\frac{1}{120}$ × $\frac{1}{16}$ × 11.95 =

63. $$\frac{437.5}{8.05} \times \frac{1}{16} =$$

64. $$\frac{809 \times (35 - 25)}{4.01 \times 20} =$$

65. $$\frac{\frac{1}{100}}{\frac{1}{2}} \times 5123 =$$

66. $$\frac{627 \times (25 - 10)}{30 \times 15} =$$

67. $$\frac{750 \times 380 \times 319.53}{760 \times 750} =$$

68. What should be the approximate total cost of 625,250 tablets at $\frac{1}{5}$ cent each?

69. Estimate the approximate cost of 32,560 capsules at $12.50 per M.

70. Estimate the approximate cost of 30,125 capsules at 75 cents per hundred.

71. What should be the approximate cost of 120,050 tablets at $33\frac{1}{3}$ cents per C?

72. A formula for 1,250 capsules contains 3.635 grams of a medicament. Estimate the amount of medicament that should be used in preparing 325 capsules.

73. Approximately how many teaspoonful- (5 milliliter-) doses can be obtained from 1 gallon (3,784 milliliters) of a liquid?

74. The cost of 1000 capsules is $15.00. If they are sold at the rate of $1.50 for 48 capsules, estimate the profit that can be realized from the sale of 1000 capsules.

75. The cost of 5000 capsules is $50.00. If they are sold at the rate of 75 cents for 24 capsules, estimate the profit that can be realized from the sale of 500 capsules.

PERCENTAGE OF ERROR

Since measurements are never absolutely accurate, it is important for the pharmacist to recognize the limitations of his measuring instruments and to know the magnitude of the errors that may be incurred when he uses them.

When he weighs a substance on a torsion prescription balance, for instance, he may record the weight as a single quantity, such as *80 milligrams;* but he should be aware that a truer record of the weight should include two quantities, expressing (1) the apparent weight and (2) the possible excess or deficiency calculated from the known *sensitivity* or from the *sensitivity requirement* of the balance.[1] The second quantity is called the *maximum potential error*. So, if the pharmacist weighs *"80 milligrams"* on a torsion prescription balance having a *sensitivity requirement* of *4 milligrams,* he has actually weighed something between *76* and *84 milligrams,* for the maximum potential error is ± *4 milligrams.* This potential error may be used to calculate the percentage of possible error in order to determine whether an error of this magnitude may be allowed.

Percentage of error may be defined as *the maximum potential error multiplied by 100 and divided by the quantity desired.* The calculation may be formulated as follows:

$$\frac{\text{Error} \times 100\%}{\text{Quantity desired}} = \text{Percentage of error}$$

This formula is valid only if the error and the quantity desired are expressed in the same denomination.

Example:

When the maximum potential error is ± *4 milligrams in a total of 100 milligrams, what is the percentage of error?*

$$\frac{4 \times 100\%}{100} = 4\%, \text{ answer.}$$

[1] The *sensitivity* of a balance may be defined in several ways. Balance manufacturers use the term to designate the smallest weight that will just cause a perceptible movement of the balance indicator. Chemists define the *sensitivity* of an analytical balance as (1) the number of indicator scale divisions by which the zero point is displaced by a weight of 1 milligram or (2) the fraction of a milligram (expressed in tenths) necessary to produce a deflection of one scale division.

The term *sensitivity* as it applies to a prescription balance may be defined as the smallest weight that will disturb its equilibrium. This designation of the *sensitivity* of a prescription balance is not to be confused with the term *sensitivity requirement* (*SR*) which is defined in the National Formulary as "the maximum change in load that will cause a specified change in the position of rest of the indicating element or elements of the balance."

In view of the fact that the term *sensitivity* has been variously interpreted, the National Formulary has adopted the term *sensitivity requirement* to designate the sensitiveness of a balance. In accordance with this adoption the designation *sensitivity requirement* will be used herein when reference is made to the sensitiveness of a prescription balance.

The *sensitivity requirement* may be determined by the following procedure:
1. Level the balance.
2. Determine the rest point of the balance.
3. Determine the smallest weight which causes the rest point to shift one division on the index plate.

NOTE: The smaller the weight which is required to move the indicating element one division, the more sensitive is the balance.

Now, if the sensitivity of an instrument of dubious accuracy is not known, its performance may be checked with that of an instrument of known high accuracy. If the two intruments are used to measure the same thing, the difference between the two results will not be a potential error but a close approximation of an actual error; and given this, we may calculate the percentage of error actually committed by the less accurate instrument.

Example:

> *A prescription calls for 800 milligrams of a substance. After weighing this amount on a balance, the pharmacist decides to check by weighing it again on a much more sensitive balance. Now he finds that he has only 750 milligrams. Since the first weighing was 50 milligrams short of the desired amount, what was the percentage of error?*

$$\frac{50 \times 100\%}{800} = 6.25\%, \text{ answer.}$$

Finally, if a certain percentage of error is not to be exceeded, and the maximum potential error of an instrument is known, it is possible to calculate the smallest quantity that can be measured within the desired accuracy. Here is a convenient formula:

$$\frac{100 \times \text{maximum potential error}}{\text{Permissible percentage of error}} = \text{Smallest quantity}$$

Example:

> *What is the smallest quantity that can be weighed with a potential error of not more than 5% on a balance sensitive to 4 milligrams?*

$$\frac{100 \times 4 \text{ milligrams}}{5} = 80 \text{ milligrams, } answer.$$

Practice Problems

1. A pharmacist attempts to weigh 120 milligrams of atropine sulfate on a balance having a sensitivity requirement of 6 milligrams. Calculate the maximum potential error in terms of percentage.

2. In compounding a prescription, a pharmacist weighed 0.050 gram of a substance on a balance insensitive to quantities smaller than 0.004 gram. What was the maximum potential error in terms of percentage?

3. A pharmacist wants to weigh 5 grains of a substance on a balance having a sensitivity requirement of ¼ grain. Calculate the maximum potential error in terms of percentage.

4. A pharmacist weighed 825 milligrams of a substance. When checked on another balance, the weight was found to be 805 milligrams. Calculate the deviation from the original weighing in terms of percentage.

5. A pharmacist weighed 475 milligrams of a substance on a balance of dubious accuracy. When checked on a balance of high accuracy, the weight was found to be 445 milligrams. Calculate the percentage of error in the first weighing.

6. A 10-milliliter graduate weighs 42.745 grams. When 5 milliliters of distilled water are measured in it, the combined weight of graduate and water is 47.675 grams. By definition, 5 milliliters of water should weigh 5 grams. Calculate the weight of the measured water and express any deviation from 5 grams as percentage of error.

7. A graduate weighs 35.825 grams. When 10 milliliters of water are measured in it, the weight of the graduate and water is 45.835 grams. Calculate the weight of the water and express any deviation from 10 grams as percentage of error.

8. In preparing a certain ointment, a pharmacist used 45.5 grains of zinc oxide instead of the 48 grains called for. Calculate the percentage of error on the basis of the desired quantity.

9. A pharmacist attempts to weigh 0.375 gram of amaranth on a balance of dubious accuracy. When checked on a highly accurate balance, the weight is found to be 0.400 gram. Calculate the percentage of error in the first weighing.

10. On a prescription balance having a sensitivity requirement of 0.012 gram, what is the smallest amount that can be weighed with a maximum potential error of not more than 5%?

11. On a torsion prescription balance having a sensitivity requirement of $\frac{1}{16}$ grain, what is the smallest amount that can be weighed with a potential error of not more than 2%?

12. If an accuracy of 2% is desired, what is the minimum amount that should be weighed on a torsion prescription balance having a sensitivity requirement of 0.004 gram?

13. A pharmacist measured 60 milliliters of glycerin by difference, starting with 100 milliliters. After completing the measurement, he noted that the graduate which he used contained 45 milliliters of glycerin. Calculate the percentage of error that was incurred in the measurement.

14. A pharmacist failed to place the balance in equilibrium before weighing three grains of codeine. Later, he discovered that the balance was out of equilibrium and that a 20% error was incurred. If the balance pan on which he placed the codeine was heavy, how many grains of codeine did he actually weigh?

15. In compounding a prescription for a nasal spray, a pharmacist weighed $\frac{1}{2}$ grain of menthol on a balance having a sensitivity requirement of $\frac{1}{20}$ grain. Calculate the percentage of error that he may have incurred.

16. Assuming a torsion balance having a sensitivity requirement of 4 milligrams (or $\frac{1}{16}$ grain) and a rider beam calibrated in units of 10 milligrams and $\frac{1}{8}$ grain, state which of the following weights could be made on it with a dispensing error not greater than plus or minus 5 per cent:

(a) $\frac{5}{8}$ grain
(b) 0.085 gram
(c) $1\frac{1}{2}$ grains
(d) 50,000 micrograms
    (1 microgram = 0.001 milligram)
(e) 65 milligrams
(f) $1\frac{1}{4}$ grains

17. A Class B prescription balance is not to be used in weighing loads of less than 648 milligrams. Assuming that its sensitivity requirement is 30 milligrams, calculate the percentage of error that might be incurred in weighing the minimum specified load.

18. The sensitivity requirement of a Class A prescription balance is 0.006 gram. Calculate the percentage of error that might be incurred in weighing 0.1 gram on this balance.

19. A pharmacist measures 900 milliliters in a 1000-milliliter cylindrical graduate calibrated in units of 10 milliliters. Calculate the percentage of error that might be incurred in the measurement.

20. When substances are to be "accurately weighed" in an assay or a test, the *United States Pharmacopeia* directs that a quantity of 50 milligrams is to be weighed to the nearest 0.05 milligram. Calculate the percentage of error in the weighing.

21. You are directed to weigh 10 grams of a substance so as to limit the error to 0.2%. Calculate the maximum potential error, in terms of grams, that you would not be permitted to exceed.

22. In a certain assay, 100 milligrams of a substance are to be weighed so as to limit the error to 0.1%. Calculate the maximum potential error, in terms of milligrams, which the analyst must not exceed.

ALIQUOT METHOD OF MEASURING

When a degree of precision in measurement is required that is beyond the capacity of the instrument at hand, the pharmacist may achieve the desired precision by measuring and calculating in terms of aliquot parts.

An *aliquot part* may be defined as any part that is contained a whole number of times in a quantity. Thus, *2* is an aliquot part of *10;* and since *10 ÷ 2 = 5, 2* is called the *fifth aliquot* of *10.* Again, *4* is an aliquot part of *16;* and since *16 ÷ 4 = 4, 4* is the *fourth aliquot* of *16.*

To weigh by the Aliquot Method:

The aliquot method of weighing is a method by which small quantities of a substance may be obtained within the degree of accuracy desired. The procedure may be summed up as follows:

Step 1. Select some multiple of the desired quantity that can be weighed with the required precision. Weigh this multiple.

Step 2. Using an inert substance that is compatible with the given preparation, dilute the multiple quantity.

Step 3. Weigh the aliquot part of the dilution that contains the desired quantity.

To select the multiple quantity in Step 1, first calculate the smallest quantity of the substance that can be weighed with the required precision (see Percentage of Error, p. 29). To insure an error no greater than *5%,* for instance, a quantity at least twenty times the sensitivity requirement of the balance must be weighed; and hence, if the sensitivity requirement of a balance is *4 milligrams, 20 × 4 milligrams,* or *80 milligrams,* is the smallest amount that can be weighed. If *50 milligrams* were weighed on such a balance, the maximum potential error would be *8%* (see p. 30). Convenience in multiplying, availability of weights, and the cost of the substance are other factors that help determine the choice of the multiple quantity.

The amount of inert diluent used in Step 2 is determined by the fact that the aliquot part of the dilution to be weighed in *Step 3* must be a quantity large enough to be weighed within the desired degree of accuracy. In *Step 1* we have already calculated the minimum quantity that satisfies this condition. The aliquot must weigh at least as much as the multiple quantity weighed in *Step 1;* and to reduce the potential error its weight should usually be somewhat greater. So, if the multiple quantity weighs *80 milligrams,* the aliquot must weigh at least *80 milligrams,* but preferably *100 milligrams* or more. When we multiply the chosen aliquot by the multiple selected in *Step 1,* we get the quantity of the dilution, and have only to add sufficient diluent to the multiple quantity to equal this weight of dilution.

The aliquot weighed in Step 3 will contain the quantity originally desired, for if, say, *20* times the original quantity is diluted, $\frac{1}{20}$ of the dilution will contain the original quantity. And by arbitrarily selecting a sufficiently large multiple quantity and a sufficiently large dilution, we can be sure that we have measured within the required degree of precision.

Example:

> *A torsion prescription balance has a sensitivity requirement of 4 milligrams. Explain how you would weigh 5 milligrams of atropine sulfate with an accuracy of* ± *5%, using lactose as the diluent.*

Since 4 milligrams (mg.) is the potential balance error, 80 milligrams is the smallest amount that should be weighed to achieve the required precision.

If 100 milligrams, or 20 times the desired amount of atropine sulfate, is chosen as the multiple quantity to be weighed in Step 1, and if 150 milligrams is set as the aliquot to be weighed in Step 3, then—

(1) Weigh 20 × 5 mg., or   100 mg. of atropine sulfate
(2) Dilute with   2900 mg. of lactose
    to get   3000 mg. of dilution
(3) Weigh $\frac{1}{20}$ of dilution, or 150 mg. of dilution, which contain 5 milligrams of atropine sulfate, *answer.*

In this example the weight of the aliquot was arbitrarily set as *150 milligrams* which exceeds the weight of the multiple quantity, as it preferably should. If *100 milligrams* had been set as the aliquot, the multiple quantity should have been diluted with *1900 milligrams* of lactose to get *2000 milligrams* of dilution, and its twentieth aliquot, or *100 milligrams,* would have contained *5 milligrams* of atropine sulfate. On the other hand, if *200 milli-*

grams had been set as the aliquot, the multiple quantity of atropine sulfate should have been diluted with *3800 milligrams* of lactose to get *4000 milligrams* of dilution.

Another example:

> *A torsion prescription balance has a sensitivity requirement of $\frac{1}{10}$ grain. Explain how you would weigh $\frac{1}{4}$ grain of atropine sulfate with an accuracy of $\pm$ 5%, using lactose as the diluent.*

Since $\frac{1}{10}$ grain (gr.) is the potential balance error, 2 grains is the smallest amount that should be weighed to achieve the required precision.

If 12 is chosen as the multiple, and if 3 grains is set as the weight of the aliquot, then—

(1) Weigh 12 $\times$ $\frac{1}{4}$ gr., or   3 gr. of atropine sulfate
(2) Dilute with $\underline{33}$ gr. of lactose
     to get   36 gr. of dilution
(3) Weigh $\frac{1}{12}$ of dilution, or 3 gr. of dilution, which contain $\frac{1}{4}$ grain of atropine sulfate, *answer.*

To Measure Volume by the Aliquot Method:

The aliquot method of measuring volume, which is identical in principle to the aliquot method of weighing, may be used when relatively small volumes must be measured with great precision:

Step 1.   Select a multiple of the desired quantity that can be measured with the required precision.

Step 2.   Dilute the multiple quantity with a compatible diluent (usually a solvent for the liquid to be measured) to an amount evenly divisible by the multiple selected.

Step 3.   Measure the aliquot of the dilution that contains the quantity originally desired.

In conformity with the legal requirements for pharmaceutical graduates as stated in the National Bureau of Standards Handbook 44—Third Edition, it should be kept in mind that a graduate shall have an initial interval that is not subdivided, equal to not less than one-fifth and not more than one-fourth of the capacity of the graduate.

Examples:

A prescription calls for 0.5 milliliter of hydrochloric acid. Using a 10-milliliter graduate calibrated from 2 to 10 milliliters in 1 milliliter divisions, explain how you would obtain the desired quantity of hydrochloric acid by the aliquot method.

If 4 is chosen as the multiple, and if 2 milliliters is set as the volume of the aliquot, then—

(1) Measure 4 × 0.5 ml., or 2 ml. of the acid
(2) Dilute with   6 ml. of water
     to get   8 ml. of dilution
(3) Measure ¼ of dilution, or 2 ml. of dilution, which contain
     0.5 milliliter of hydrochloric acid, *answer.*

A prescription calls for 5 minims of clove oil. Using a 60-minim graduate calibrated from 15 to 60 minims in units of 5 minims, explain how you would obtain the clove oil by the aliquot method. Use alcohol as the diluent.

If 3 is chosen as the multiple, and if 20 minims is set as the volume of the aliquot, then—

(1) Measure 3 × 5 minims, or 15 minims of clove oil
(2) Dilute with   45 minims of alcohol
     to get   60 minims of dilution
(3) Measure ⅓ of dilution, or 20 minims of dilution, which
     contain 5 minims of clove oil, *answer.*

Practice Problems

1. If 1000 milliliters of a certain solution contain 30 milligrams of a dye, (a) what is the volume of the tenth aliquot and (b) how many milligrams of the dye will the tenth aliquot contain?

2. A prescription balance has a sensitivity requirement of 0.006 gram. Explain how you would weigh 0.012 gram of atropine sulfate with an error not greater than 5%, using lactose as the diluent.

3. A torsion prescription balance has a sensitivity requirement of 4 milligrams. Explain how you would weigh 5 milligrams of hydromorphone hydrochloride with an error not greater than 5%. Use lactose as the diluent.

4. The sensitivity requirement of a prescription balance is $\frac{1}{16}$ grain. Explain how you would weigh $\frac{1}{10}$ grain of atropine sulfate with an error not greater than 5%. Use milk sugar as the diluent.

5. A prescription balance has a sensitivity requirement of 6.5 milligrams. Explain how you would weigh 20 milligrams of a substance with an error not greater than 2%.

6. A prescription balance has a sensitivity requirement of $\frac{1}{6}$ grain. Explain how you would weigh 1 grain of a substance with an error not greater than 5%.

7. A torsion prescription balance has a sensitivity requirement of 0.004 gram. Explain how you would weigh 0.008 gram of a substance with an error not greater than 5%.

8. A prescription balance has a sensitivity requirement of $\frac{1}{8}$ grain. Explain how you would weigh $\frac{3}{4}$ grain of a substance with an error not greater than 5%.

9. A formula calls for 0.6 milliliter of a coloring solution. Using a 10-milliliter graduate calibrated from 2 to 10 milliliters in units of 1 milliliter, how could you obtain the desired quantity of the coloring solution by the aliquot method? Use water as the diluent.

10. In preparing 100 milliliters of a dilute solution of hydrochloric acid, 0.75 milliliter of hydrochloric acid is required. Using the graduate described in Problem 9, how could you obtain the desired 0.75 milliliter of the acid with satisfactory accuracy? Use water as the diluent.

11. A prescription calls for 0.8 milliliter of a stock solution of a chemical. Using the graduate described in Problem 9, how could you obtain the desired 0.8 milliliter of stock solution with satisfactory accuracy? Use water as the diluent.

12. Using the graduate described in Problem 9, explain how you would measure 1.25 milliliters of a dye solution by the aliquot method. Use water as the diluent.

13. A prescription calls for 6 minims of rose oil. Using a 60-minim graduate calibrated from 15 to 60 minims in units of 5 minims, explain how you would obtain the rose oil by the aliquot method. Use alcohol as the diluent.

14. Using a torsion prescription balance having a sensitivity requirement of $\frac{1}{10}$ grain, explain how you would obtain $\frac{3}{10}$ grain of menthol. Menthol is soluble in alcohol.

15. ℞ Sodium Citrate   5.0 g.
   Tartar Emetic   0.02 g.
   Cherry Syrup q.s. ad 120.0 ml.
   Sig. Use for cough.

Using a prescription balance having a sensitivity requirement of 0.004 gram (g.), state how you would obtain the correct quantity of tartar emetic. Use water as the solvent for tartar emetic.

COMMON AND DECIMAL FRACTIONS

Much of the arithmetic of pharmacy requires facility in the handling of common fractions and decimal fractions. Even if the student already has a good working knowledge of their use, the following brief review of certain principles and rules governing them should be helpful, and the practice problems should provide him with the means of gaining accuracy and speed in their manipulation.

COMMON FRACTIONS

A number in the form $\frac{1}{8}$, $\frac{3}{16}$, and so on, is called a *common fraction*, or very often simply a *fraction*. Its *denominator*, or second or lower figure, always indicates the number of aliquot parts into which *1* is divided; and its *numerator*, or first or upper figure, specifies the number of those parts with which we are concerned.

The *value* of a fraction is the quotient when its numerator is divided by its denominator. If the numerator is smaller than the denominator, the fraction is called *proper*, and its value is less than *1*. If the numerator and denominator are alike, its value is *1*. If the numerator is larger than the denominator, the fraction is called *improper*, and its value is greater than *1*.

Now, two principles must be understood by anyone attempting to calculate with common fractions.

First Principle. Multiplying the numerator increases the value of a fraction, and multiplying the denominator decreases the value; but *when both numerator and denominator are multiplied by the same number, the value does not change.*

$$\frac{2}{7} = \frac{3 \times 2}{3 \times 7} = \frac{6}{21}$$

This principle allows us to reduce two or more fractions to a common denomination when necessary. We usually want the *lowest common denominator*, which is the smallest number divisible by all the given denominators. It is most easily found by testing successive multiples of the largest given denominator until we reach a number divisible by all the other given denominators. Then we multiply both numerator and denominator of each fraction by the number of times its denominator is contained in the common denominator.

Example:

Reduce the fractions $\frac{3}{4}$, $\frac{4}{5}$, and $\frac{1}{3}$ to a common denomination.

By testing successive multiples of 5, we discover that 60 is the smallest number divisible by 4, 5, and 3.

4 is contained 15 times in 60; 5, 12 times; and 3, 20 times.

$$\left.\begin{array}{l}\dfrac{3}{4} = \dfrac{15 \times 3}{15 \times 4} = \dfrac{45}{60}\,, \\[2em] \dfrac{4}{5} = \dfrac{12 \times 4}{12 \times 5} = \dfrac{48}{60}\,, \\[2em] \dfrac{1}{3} = \dfrac{20 \times 1}{20 \times 3} = \dfrac{20}{60}\,, \end{array}\right\} answers.$$

Second Principle. Dividing the numerator decreases the value of a fraction, and dividing the denominator increases the value; but *when both numerator and denominator are divided by the same number, the value does not change.*

$$\frac{6}{21} = \frac{6 \div 3}{21 \div 3} = \frac{2}{7}$$

This principle allows us to reduce an unwieldy fraction to more convenient lower terms, either at any time during a series of calculations or when recording a final result. To reduce a fraction to its *lowest terms*, divide both the numerator and the denominator by the largest common divisor.

Example:

Reduce $\frac{36}{2880}$ to *its lowest terms.*

The largest common divisor is 36.

$$\frac{36}{2880} = \frac{36 \div 36}{2880 \div 36} = \frac{1}{80}, \text{ answer.}$$

These principles often suggest direct solutions to practical problems.

Examples:

A prescription calls for $\frac{3}{50}$ grain of atropine sulfate. How many $\frac{1}{200}$-grain tablets will supply the required amount?

50 is contained 4 times in 200.

$$\frac{3}{50} \text{ gr.} = \frac{4 \times 3}{4 \times 50} \text{ gr.} = \frac{12}{200} \text{ gr.}$$

Twelve $\frac{1}{200}$-grain tablets would supply $\frac{12}{200}$ gr. which equals the $\frac{3}{50}$ gr. required, *answer.*

Justify the assertion that nine $\frac{1}{150}$-grain tablets would supply the $\frac{3}{50}$ grain of atropine sulfate called for.

Nine $\frac{1}{150}$-grain tablets would supply $\frac{9}{150}$ gr.

50 is contained 3 times in 150.

$$\frac{9}{150} \text{ gr.} = \frac{9 \div 3}{150 \div 3} \text{ gr.} = \frac{3}{50} \text{ gr. required, } answer.$$

Besides developing a firm grasp of these two principles, the student should follow two rules before indulging in any short cuts.

Rule 1. Before performing any arithmetical operation involving fractions, *reduce every mixed number to an improper fraction.* To do so, multiply the integer, or whole number, by the denominator of the fractional remainder, add the numerator, and write the result over the denominator.

For example, before attempting to multiply $\frac{3}{4}$ by $1\frac{1}{5}$, first reduce the $1\frac{1}{5}$ to an improper fraction:

$$1\frac{1}{5} = \frac{(1 \times 5) + 1}{5} = \frac{6}{5}$$

If the final result of a calculation is an improper fraction, you may, if you like, reduce it to a mixed number. To do so, simply divide the numerator by the denominator and express the remainder as a common, not a decimal fraction:

$$\tfrac{6}{5} = 6 \div 5 = 1\tfrac{1}{5}$$

Rule 2. When performing an operation involving a fraction and a whole number, *express (or at least visualize) the whole number as a fraction having 1 for its denominator.*

Think of *3* as $\tfrac{3}{1}$, *42* as $\tfrac{42}{1}$, and so on.

As will be seen, this visualization is desirable when a fraction is subtracted from a whole number, and it is necessary when a fraction is divided by a whole number.

To add fractions :

To add common fractions, reduce them to a common denomination, add the numerators, and write the sum over the common denominator. If whole and mixed numbers are involved, the safest (though not the quickest) procedure is first to apply *Rules 1* and *2.* If the sum is an improper fraction, you may want to reduce it to a mixed number.

Examples:

A prescription for a capsule contains $\tfrac{3}{80}$ grain of ingredient A, $\tfrac{1}{200}$ grain of ingredient B, $\tfrac{1}{50}$ grain of ingredient C, and $\tfrac{3}{16}$ grain of ingredient D. What is the total weight of these four ingredients?

The lowest common denominator of the four fractions is 400.

Reducing to a common denomination:

$$\tfrac{3}{80} = \tfrac{15}{400},\ \tfrac{1}{200} = \tfrac{2}{400},\ \tfrac{1}{50} = \tfrac{8}{400},\ \text{and}\ \tfrac{3}{16} = \tfrac{75}{400}$$

Adding the numerators:

$$\frac{15 + 2 + 8 + 75}{400}\ \text{gr.} = \frac{100}{400}\ \text{gr.}$$

Reducing the sum to its simplest terms:

$$\tfrac{100}{400}\ \text{gr.} = \tfrac{1}{4}\ \text{gr., } answer.$$

A patient receives the following doses of a certain drug: $\frac{1}{4}$ *grain,* $\frac{1}{12}$ *grain,* $\frac{1}{8}$ *grain, and* $\frac{1}{6}$ *grain. Calculate the total amount of the drug received by the patient.*

The lowest common denominator of the fractions is 24.

$\frac{1}{4} = \frac{6}{24}, \frac{1}{12} = \frac{2}{24}, \frac{1}{8} = \frac{3}{24},$ and $\frac{1}{6} = \frac{4}{24}$

$$\frac{6 + 2 + 3 + 4}{24} \text{ gr.} = \frac{15}{24} \text{ gr.}$$

$\frac{15}{24}$ gr. $= \frac{5}{8}$ gr., *answer.*

To subtract fractions:

To subtract one fraction from another, reduce them to a common denomination, subtract, and write the difference over the common denominator. If a whole or mixed number is involved, first apply *Rule 1* or *2*. If the difference is an improper fraction, you may want to reduce it to a mixed number.

Examples:

A patient's medication chart shows that he has received a total of $\frac{7}{12}$ *grain of morphine sulfate. If he had not been given the last dose of* $\frac{1}{8}$ *grain, what quantity would he have received?*

The lowest common denominator is 24.

$\frac{7}{12} = \frac{14}{24}$ and $\frac{1}{8} = \frac{3}{24}.$

$$\frac{14 - 3}{24} \text{ gr.} = \frac{11}{24} \text{ gr., } \textit{answer.}$$

A capsule is to weigh 3 grains. If it contains $\frac{1}{24}$ *grain of ingredient A,* $\frac{1}{4}$ *grain of ingredient B, and* $\frac{1}{3}$ *grain of ingredient C, how much diluent should be added?*

The lowest common denominator of the fractions is 24.

$\frac{1}{24} = \frac{1}{24}, \frac{1}{4} = \frac{6}{24},$ and $\frac{1}{3} = \frac{8}{24}.$

$$\frac{1 + 6 + 8}{24} \text{ gr.} = \frac{15}{24} \text{ gr.} = \frac{5}{8} \text{ gr.}$$

Interpreting the given 3 grains as $\frac{3}{1}$ grains, and reducing it to a fraction with 8 for a denominator.

$\frac{3}{1}$ gr. $= \frac{24}{8}$ gr.

Subtracting:

$$\frac{24 - 5}{8} \text{ gr.} = \frac{19}{8} \text{ gr.}$$

Changing the difference to a mixed number:

$\frac{19}{8}$ gr. $= (19 \div 8)$ gr. $= 2\frac{3}{8}$ gr., *answer.*

To multiply fractions :

To multiply fractions, multiply the numerators and write the product over the product of the denominators. If either is a mixed number, first apply *Rule 1*. If the multiplier is a whole number, simply multiply the numerator of the fraction and write the product over the denominator.

Examples:

How much active ingredient is represented in 24 tablets each containing $\frac{1}{320}$ *grain of the ingredient?*

$$24 \times \frac{1}{320} \text{ gr.} = \frac{24 \times 1}{320} \text{ gr.} = \frac{24}{320} \text{ gr.} = \frac{3}{40} \text{ gr., } \textit{answer.}$$

The adult dose of a drug is $\frac{3}{20}$ *grain. Calculate the dose for a child if it is* $\frac{1}{12}$ *of the adult dose.*

$$\frac{1}{12} \times \frac{3}{20} \text{ gr.} = \frac{1 \times 3}{12 \times 20} \text{ gr.} = \frac{3}{240} \text{ gr.} = \frac{1}{80} \text{ gr., } \textit{answer.}$$

To divide fractions :

In the division of fractions, it is important for the student to grasp the meaning of *reciprocal*. By definition, the *reciprocal* of a number is *1* divided by the number. For example, the reciprocal of 3 is $\frac{1}{3}$. If you apply *Rule 2* above and regard 3 as the same as the fraction $\frac{3}{1}$, then its reciprocal equals the inversion of this fraction. In general, therefore, when a is a fraction, its reciprocal is $\frac{1}{a}$ and proves to have the same value as the fraction inverted. So, the reciprocal of $\frac{1}{4}$ is $\frac{4}{1}$ or 4, and the reciprocal of $2\frac{1}{2}$ or $\frac{5}{2}$ is $\frac{2}{5}$.

Now, if the fraction $\frac{3}{4}$ is interpreted as meaning 3 divided by 4, then it should be emphasized that dividing by 4 is exactly the same as multiplying by the reciprocal of 4, or $\frac{1}{4}$. This method of handling division when fractions are involved is called the *reciprocal method*, and it points out the reciprocal relation, or inverse relation, between multiplication and division.

To divide by a fraction, then, simply invert its terms and multiply. And when a fraction is to be divided by a whole number, first interpret the whole number as a fraction having 1 for its denominator, invert to get its reciprocal, and multiply.

Examples:

If $\frac{1}{2}$ ounce is divided into 4 equal parts, how much will each part contain?

Interpreting 4 as $\frac{4}{1}$:

$$\frac{1}{2} \text{ oz.} \div \frac{4}{1} = \frac{1}{2} \text{ oz.} \times \frac{1}{4} = \frac{1 \times 1}{2 \times 4} \text{ oz.} = \frac{1}{8} \text{ oz., } answer.$$

The dose of a drug is $\frac{1}{60}$ grain. How many doses can be made from $\frac{1}{5}$ grain?

$$\frac{1}{5} \div \frac{1}{60} = \frac{1}{5} \times \frac{60}{1} = \frac{1 \times 60}{5 \times 1} = 12 \text{ doses, } answer.$$

A child is given $\frac{5}{8}$ grain of a drug. If this represents $\frac{1}{16}$ of the adult dose, what is the adult dose?

If $\frac{1}{16}$ of (that is, *times*) the adult dose is $\frac{5}{8}$ grain, then $\frac{5}{8}$ grain divided by $\frac{1}{16}$ must equal the adult dose.

$$\frac{5}{8} \text{ gr.} \div \frac{1}{16} = \frac{5}{8} \text{ gr.} \times \frac{16}{1} = \frac{5 \times 16}{8 \times 1} \text{ gr.} = 10 \text{ gr., } answer.$$

DECIMAL FRACTIONS

A fraction whose denominator is 10 or any power of ten is called a *decimal fraction*, or simply a *decimal*. The denominator of a decimal fraction is never written, since the decimal point serves to indicate the place value of the numerals. The numerator and the decimal point are sufficient to express the fraction. So, $\frac{1}{10}$ is written 0.1, $\frac{45}{100}$ is written 0.45, and $\frac{65}{1000}$ is written 0.065.

All operations with decimal fractions are carried out in the same manner as with whole numbers, but care must be exercised in putting the decimal point in its proper place in the results.

Three familiar operations are worth recalling.

(1) As a direct consequence of the place value in the decimal notation, moving the decimal point one place to the right multiplies a number by 10, two places to the right multiplies it by 100, and so on. Likewise, moving the point one place to the left divides a number by 10, two places to the left divides it by 100, and so on.

(2) A decimal fraction may be changed to a common fraction by writing the numerator over the denominator and (if desired) reducing to lowest terms:

$$0.125 = \frac{125}{1000} = \frac{1}{8}$$

(3) A common fraction may be changed to a decimal by dividing the numerator by the denominator (note that the result may be a repeating or endless decimal fraction):

$$\frac{3}{8} = 3 \div 8 = 0.375$$

$$\frac{1}{3} = 1 \div 3 = 0.3333 \ldots$$

Practice Problems

1. Add each of the following:

(a) $\frac{5}{8}$ gr. $+ \frac{9}{32}$ gr. $+ \frac{1}{4}$ gr.
(b) $\frac{1}{150}$ gr. $+ \frac{1}{200}$ gr. $+ \frac{1}{100}$ gr.
(c) $\frac{1}{60}$ gr. $+ \frac{1}{20}$ gr. $+ \frac{1}{16}$ gr. $+ \frac{1}{32}$ gr.

2. Find the difference:

(a) $3\frac{1}{2}$ grain $- \frac{15}{64}$ grain.
(b) $\frac{1}{30}$ grain $- \frac{1}{40}$ grain.
(c) $2\frac{1}{3}$ grain $- 1\frac{1}{2}$ grain.

3. Find the product:

(a) $\frac{30}{75} \times \frac{15}{32} \times 25$.
(b) $2\frac{1}{2} \times 12 \times \frac{7}{8}$.
(c) $\frac{1}{125} \times \frac{9}{20}$.

4. What is the reciprocal of each of the following?

(a) $\frac{1}{10}$.   (d) $\frac{3}{2}$.
(b) $3\frac{1}{3}$.   (e) $1\frac{7}{8}$.
(c) $\frac{12}{1}$.   (f) $\frac{1}{64}$.

5. Find the quotient:

  (a) $\frac{2}{3} \div \frac{1}{24}$.
  (b) $\frac{1}{5000} \div 12$.
  (c) $6\frac{1}{4} \div \frac{1}{2}$.

6. Solve each of the following:

  (a) $(\frac{1}{120} \div \frac{1}{150}) \times 50 = ?$

  (b) $\dfrac{1\frac{1}{2}}{100} \times 1000 = ?$

  (c) $\frac{3}{4} \times ? = 48$.

  (d) $\dfrac{\frac{1}{500}}{5} \times ? = 5$.

7. What fractional part:

  (a) of 64 is 2?
  (b) of $\frac{1}{16}$ is $\frac{1}{20}$?
  (c) of $\frac{1}{32}$ is 2?

8. A prescription contains $\frac{5}{8}$ grain of ingredient A, $\frac{1}{4}$ grain of ingredient B, $\frac{1}{100}$ grain of ingredient C, and $\frac{3}{50}$ grain of ingredient D. Calculate the weight of the four ingredients in the prescription.

9. How many $\frac{1}{2000}$-grain doses can be obtained from $\frac{3}{80}$ grain of a certain drug?

10. A patient received the following doses of a drug:

  3 doses each containing $\frac{1}{20}$ grain
  3 doses each containing $\frac{1}{24}$ grain
  2 doses each containing $\frac{1}{32}$ grain
  2 doses each containing $\frac{1}{64}$ grain

Calculate the total amount of the drug received by the patient.

11. A capsule contains $\frac{1}{40}$ grain of ingredient A, $\frac{1}{4}$ grain of ingredient B, $\frac{1}{120}$ grain of ingredient C, and enough of ingredient D to make 4 grains. How many grains of ingredient D are in the capsule?

12. The adult dose of a certain drug is $\frac{1}{120}$ grain. If the child dose is $\frac{1}{6}$ of an adult dose, what fraction of a grain will be given if 8 doses are administered to a child?

13. Calculate the fractional difference between a $\frac{1}{100}$-grain tablet and a $\frac{1}{150}$-grain tablet of atropine sulfate.

14. The dose of a drug is $\frac{1}{120}$ grain. How many doses can be made from $\frac{2}{3}$ grain?

15. What decimal fraction:

    (a) of 18 is $2\frac{1}{4}$?
    (b) of 25 is 0.005?
    (c) of 7000 is 437.5?

16. Write the following as decimals and add:

$$\frac{3}{1000}, \frac{75}{100}, \frac{3}{20}, \frac{5}{8}, \frac{13}{25}$$

17. Write the following as decimals and add:

$$\frac{3}{5}, \frac{1}{20}, \frac{65}{1000}, \frac{19}{40}, \frac{3}{8}$$

18. How many 0.000065-gram doses can be made from 0.130 gram of a drug?

19. Calculate the fractional difference between a $\frac{1}{400}$-grain and a $\frac{1}{150}$-grain tablet of nitroglycerin.

20. Calculate the fractional difference between a $\frac{1}{24}$-grain and a $\frac{1}{32}$-grain tablet of hydromorphone hydrochloride.

21. A patient received the following doses of a drug:

    4 doses each containing $\frac{1}{120}$ grain
    4 doses each containing $\frac{1}{100}$ grain
    2 doses each containing $\frac{1}{150}$ grain
    4 doses each containing $\frac{1}{200}$ grain

Calculate the total amount of the drug received by the patient.

22. A pharmacist had three grains of hydromorphone hydrochloride. He used it in preparing the following:

    8 capsules each containing $\frac{1}{32}$ grain
    8 capsules each containing $\frac{1}{24}$ grain
    20 capsules each containing $\frac{1}{48}$ grain

How many grains of hydromorphone hydrochloride were left after he prepared the capsules?

23. A patient received the following doses of a drug:

6 doses each containing 0.0065 gram
6 doses each containing 0.00325 gram
4 doses each containing 0.005 gram

Calculate the total amount of the drug received by the patient.

24. A pharmacist had 5 grams of codeine phosphate. He used it in preparing the following:

6 capsules each containing 0.0325 gram
12 capsules each containing 0.015 gram
18 capsules each containing 0.008 gram

How many grams of codeine phosphate were left after he had prepared the capsules?

25. A child receives $\frac{1}{720}$ grain of a drug. This represents $\frac{1}{6}$ of the adult dose. Calculate the adult dose.

26. An ointment contains $\frac{1}{8}$ ounce of zinc oxide, $\frac{3}{8}$ ounce of starch, and $2\frac{1}{2}$ ounces of white petrolatum. What fraction of the ointment is represented by the zinc oxide?

RATIO, PROPORTION, VARIATION

RATIO

The relative magnitude of two like quantities is called their *ratio*. Ratio is sometimes defined as *the quotient of two like numbers*. But in order not to lose sight of the fact that *two* quantities are being *compared*, this quotient is always expressed as an *operation*, not as a *result:* in other words, it is expressed as a *fraction*, and the fraction is interpreted as indicating the operation of dividing the numerator by the denominator. Thus, a ratio presents us with the concept of a common fraction as expressing the relation of its two numbers.

The ratio of *20* and *10*, for example, is not expressed as *2* (that is, the quotient of *20* divided by *10*), but as the fraction $\frac{20}{10}$. And when this fraction is to be interpreted as a ratio, it is traditionally written *20:10* and always read *twenty to ten*. Similarly, when the fraction $\frac{1}{2}$ is to be interpreted as a ratio, it is traditionally written *1:2*, and it is read not as *one-half* but as *one to two*.

All the rules governing common fractions equally apply to a ratio. Of particular importance is the principle that *if the two terms of a ratio are multiplied or are divided by the same number, the value is unchanged*—the *value*, of course, being the quotient of the first term divided by the second.

For example, the ratio $20:4$ or $\frac{20}{4}$ has a value of 5. Now, if both terms are multiplied by 2, the ratio becomes $40:8$ or $\frac{40}{8}$, still with a value of $5;$ and if both terms are divided by 2, the ratio becomes $10:2$ or $\frac{10}{2}$, again with a value of 5.

The terms of a ratio must be of the same kind, for the *value* of a ratio is an abstract number expressing how many *times* greater or smaller the first term (or numerator) is than the second term (or denominator).[1] The terms may themselves be abstract numbers, or else they may be concrete numbers of the same denomination. Thus, we can have a ratio of 20 to 4 ($\frac{20}{4}$) or of *20 grains* to *4 grains* ($\frac{20\,\text{grains}}{4\,\text{grains}}$). To recognize this relationship clearly, it is useful to interpret a ratio as expressing in its *denominator* a number of parts that a certain quantity (used for comparison) is conveniently taken to contain, and in its *numerator* the number of *those parts* that the quantity we are measuring is found to contain.[2]

When two ratios have the same value they are *equivalent*. An interesting fact about equivalent ratios is this: *the product of the numerator of the one and the denominator of the other always equals the product of the denominator of the one and the numerator of the other*. That is to say, *the cross products are equal:*

Since $\frac{2}{4} = \frac{4}{8}$,

2×8 (or 16) $= 4 \times 4$ (or 16).

It is also true that *if two ratios are equal, their* reciprocals are equal:

Since $\frac{2}{4} = \frac{4}{8}$, then $\frac{4}{2} = \frac{8}{4}$.

We discover further that the *numerator of the one fraction equals the product of its denominator and the other fraction:*

If $\frac{6}{15} = \frac{2}{5}$,

then $6 = 15 \times \frac{2}{5}$ (or $\frac{15 \times 2}{5}$) $= 6$,

and $2 = 5 \times \frac{6}{15}$ (or $\frac{5 \times 6}{15}$) $= 2$.

[1] The ratio of *1* gallon to *3* pints is surely not *1:3*, for the gallon contains *8* pints, and the ratio therefore is *8:3*. To ignore this principle is to invite disaster in our calculations.

[2] Ratios are expressed or implied everywhere in mathematics, "the science of measure." A common fraction may always be understood to designate in its denominator the number of equal parts into which *1* is divided, and in its numerator the number of those parts we are concerned with. Decimal fractions are ratios with a fixed series of denominators: *10, 100, 1000*, and so on. We have observed that every whole number implies a ratio with *1*, our unit of counting. Percentage is a convenient ratio that expresses a number of parts in every hundred of the same kind.

And the denominator of the one equals the quotient of its numerator divided by the other fraction:

$$15 = 6 \div \tfrac{2}{5} \text{ (or } 6 \times \tfrac{5}{2}) = 15,$$

$$\text{and } 5 = 2 \div \tfrac{6}{15} \text{ (or } 2 \times \tfrac{15}{6}) = 5.$$

An extremely useful practical application of these facts is found in *proportion*.

PROPORTION

A *proportion* is the expression of the equality of two ratios. It may be written in any one of three standard forms:

(1) $a:b = c:d$

(2) $a:b :: c:d$

(3) $\dfrac{a}{b} = \dfrac{c}{d}$

Each of these expressions is read: *a is to b as c is to d,* and *a* and *d* are called the *extremes* (meaning "outer members") and *b* and *c* the *means* ("middle members").

In any proportion *the product of the extremes is equal to the product of the means.* This principle allows us to find the missing term of any proportion when the other three terms are known. If the missing term is a *mean,* it will be *the product of the extremes divided by the given mean:* and if it is an *extreme,* it will be *the product of the means divided by the given extreme.* And from this we may derive the following fractional equations:

If $\dfrac{a}{b} = \dfrac{c}{d}$, then

$$a = \frac{bc}{d}, \; b = \frac{ad}{c}, \; c = \frac{ad}{b}, \text{ and } d = \frac{bc}{a}.$$

Most experienced calculators are indifferent to the order of terms in the proportions they devise. For the sake of the greater mechanical accuracy gained by routine discipline, some teachers still prefer the old pattern of putting the unknown term in the fourth place—that is, in the denominator of the second fraction.

There are few arithmetic problems, save for the simplest, that cannot most directly be solved by proportion. Provided that we correctly interpret the relationships implied by the data, *given any three terms of a proportion, by appeal to the facts set forth above we may easily calculate the value of the fourth.* Since the missing fourth is usually the desired answer, proportion takes us to it without any intermediate steps.

Examples:

> *If 3 tablets contain 15 grains of aspirin, how many grains should be contained in 12 tablets?*

$$\frac{3 \text{ (tablets)}}{12 \text{ (tablets)}} = \frac{15 \text{ (grains)}}{x \text{ (grains)}}$$

$$x = \frac{12 \times 15}{3} \text{ grains} = 60 \text{ grains}, \textit{ answer.}$$

> *If 3 tablets contain 15 grains of aspirin, how many tablets should contain 60 grains?*

$$\frac{3 \text{ (tablets)}}{x \text{ (tablets)}} = \frac{15 \text{ (grains)}}{60 \text{ (grains)}}$$

$$x = \frac{3 \times 60}{15} \text{ tablets} = 12 \text{ tablets}, \textit{ answer.}$$

> *If 12 tablets contain 60 grains of aspirin, how many grains should 3 tablets contain?*

$$\frac{12 \text{ (tablets)}}{3 \text{ (tablets)}} = \frac{60 \text{ (grains)}}{x \text{ (grains)}}$$

$$x = \frac{3 \times 60}{12} \text{ grains} = 15 \text{ grains}, \textit{ answer.}$$

> *If 12 tablets contain 60 grains of aspirin, how many tablets should contain 15 grains?*

$$\frac{12 \text{ (tablets)}}{x \text{ (tablets)}} = \frac{60 \text{ (grains)}}{15 \text{ (grains)}}$$

$$x = \frac{12 \times 15}{60} \text{ tablets} = 3 \text{ tablets}, \textit{ answer.}$$

Some calculators will set up "mixed" ratios in their proportions, invoking the principle that if the ratios are regarded as abstract numbers *the means or the extremes may be interchanged without destroying the validity of the equation.*[1] However true this principle may be of abstract numbers, it is nevertheless illogical (and never necessary) to make a ratio between, say a number of tablets and a number of grains. It is very risky to ignore the rule that *ratios should express the relationship of denominate numbers of the same kind.* In many problems we find that the quantities given must be reduced or converted to a common denomination before we can proceed with the solution.

Proportions need not contain whole numbers. If common or decimal fractions are supplied in the data, they may be included in the proportion without changing the method.

But, since calculating with common fractions is more complicated than with whole numbers or decimal fractions, it is useful to know—and wherever possible to apply—these two facts:

(1) *Two fractions having a common denominator are directly proportional to their numerators.*

$$\frac{\frac{60}{100}}{\frac{50}{100}} = \frac{60}{50}$$

Proof: $\dfrac{60}{100} \div \dfrac{50}{100} = \dfrac{60}{100} \times \dfrac{100}{50} = \dfrac{60}{50}$

(2) *Two fractions having a common numerator are inversely proportional to their denominators.*

$$\frac{\frac{2}{3}}{\frac{2}{7}} = \frac{7}{3}$$

Proof. $\frac{2}{3} \div \frac{2}{7} = \frac{2}{3} \times \frac{7}{2} = \frac{7}{3}$

---

[1] So that if:

$$\frac{3 \text{ (tablets)}}{12 \text{ (tablets)}} = \frac{15 \text{ (grains)}}{60 \text{ (grains)}}$$

then:

$$\frac{3 \text{ (tablets)}}{15 \text{ (grains)}} = \frac{12 \text{ (tablets)}}{60 \text{ (grains)}}$$

and:

$$\frac{60 \text{ (grains)}}{12 \text{ (tablets)}} = \frac{15 \text{ (grains)}}{3 \text{ (tablets)}}$$

and:

$$\frac{60 \text{ (grains)}}{15 \text{ (grains)}} = \frac{12 \text{ (tablets)}}{3 \text{ (tablets)}}$$

Examples:

   If $1\frac{1}{2}$ grains of a drug represent 18 doses, how many doses are repre-sented in $\frac{1}{4}$ grain?

   $1\frac{1}{2}$ grains $= \frac{3}{2}$ grains $= \frac{6}{4}$ grains

   $$\frac{\frac{6}{4} \text{ (grains)}}{\frac{1}{4} \text{ (grain)}} = \frac{18 \text{ (doses)}}{x \text{ (doses)}}$$

   Or: $\dfrac{6}{1} = \dfrac{18}{x}$ (doses)

   $x = \dfrac{1 \times 18}{6}$ doses $= 3$ doses, *answer.*

   If 30 milliliters represent $\frac{1}{6}$ of the volume of a prescription, how many milliliters will represent $\frac{1}{4}$ of the volume?

   $$\frac{\frac{1}{6} \text{ (volume)}}{\frac{1}{4} \text{ (volume)}} = \frac{30 \text{ (ml.)}}{x \text{ (ml.)}}$$

   Or: $\dfrac{4}{6} = \dfrac{30}{x}$ (ml.)

   $x = \dfrac{6 \times 30}{4}$ ml. $= 45$ ml., *answer.*

VARIATION

In the examples above involving tablets and grains, the relationship was clearly *proportional*—that is, the variation between number of tablets and number of grains was known to be consistent and regular. In every pro-portion the "cause" must have a *constant rate* of "effect" if the equation is to be valid.

Most pharmaceutical calculations deal with simple, *direct* relationships: twice the cause, double the effect, and so on. Occasionally they deal with *inverse* relationships: twice the cause, half the effect, and so on—as when you *decrease* the strength of a solution by *increasing* the amount of diluent.[1]

---

[1] In expressing an inverse proportion we must not forget that *every* proportion asserts the equivalence of two fractions, and therefore the numerators must both be smaller or both larger than their respective denominators.

Here is a typical problem involving inverse proportion:

If 10 pints of a 5% solution are diluted to 40 pints, what is the percentage strength of the dilution?

$$\frac{10 \ (\text{pints})}{40 \ (\text{pints})} = \frac{\text{x} \ (\%)}{5 \ (\%)}$$

$$\text{x} = \frac{10 \times 5}{40}\% = 1.25\%, \ answer.$$

The use of proportion in pharmaceutical problems is abundantly illustrated in the text. The following miscellany reveals a variety of applications of the method.

Practice Problems

1. *Make valid ratios between these familiar quantities:*

   (a) 3 gallons and 2 quarts.

   (b) 1 yard and 2 feet.

   (c) ½ mile and 1760 feet.

   (d) 4 hours and 120 minutes.

   (e) 2 feet and 6 inches.

2. *Solve by proportion:*

   (a) If 250 pounds of a chemical cost $60.00, what will be the cost of 135 pounds?

   (b) If 75 pounds of a chemical cost $250, what will be the cost of 95 pounds?

   (c) A formula for 1250 capsules contains 3.25 grams of arsenic trioxide. How much arsenic trioxide should be used in preparing 350 capsules?

   (d) If 100 capsules contain ⅜ grain of an active ingredient, how much of the ingredient will 48 capsules contain?

   (e) If 450 pounds of Green Soap cost $103.50, what will be the cost of 33 pounds?

   (f) If 50 tablets contain 0.625 gram of an active ingredient, how many tablets can be prepared from 31.25 grams of the ingredient?

(g) If 24 pounds of a chemical cost \$15.60, how many pounds can be bought for \$26.00?

(h) If 15 gallons of a certain liquid cost \$7.25, how much will 4 gallons cost?

(i) If 125 gallons of a mouth rinse contain 20 grams of a coloring agent, how many grams will 160 gallons contain?

(j) If 50 tablets contain 1.5 grams of active ingredient, how much of the ingredient will 1,375 tablets contain?

(k) If 3 doses of a liquid preparation contain 7.5 grains of a substance, how many grains will 32 doses contain?

(l) If 1.625 grams of a coloring agent are used to color 250 liters of a certain solution, how many liters could be colored by using 0.750 gram?

(m) How many grains of a substance are needed for 350 tablets if 75 tablets contain 3 grains of the substance?

(n) If 48 pints of a preparation contain $2\frac{1}{2}$ grains of a certain substance, how much will 5 pints contain?

(o) If 12 pounds of a drug cost \$9.60, how many pounds can be bought for \$58.00?

(p) If 1000 grams of an ointment contain 0.875 gram of a certain ingredient, how much of the ingredient will 625 grams contain?

(q) If 50 grams of a 5% ointment are diluted to 125 grams, what is the percentage strength of the dilution?

(r) If a pharmacist can compound an average of 8 prescriptions per hour, how long should it take 2 pharmacists, working at the same rate, to compound 40 prescriptions?

(s) At a constant temperature, the volume of a gas varies inversely with the pressure. If a gas occupies a volume of 1000 milliliters at a pressure of 760 millimeters, what is its volume at a pressure of 570 millimeters?

(t) If 150 milliliters of a $\frac{1}{10}$% solution are diluted to 750 milliliters, what is the percentage strength of the resulting product?

(u) How many $\frac{1}{120}$ grain tablets will yield the same amount of atropine sulfate as 50 tablets each containing $\frac{1}{150}$ grain?

(v) A solution contains $\frac{1}{4}$ grain of morphine sulfate per 15 minims. How many minims will contain $\frac{1}{6}$ grain of morphine sulfate?

(w) How many milliliters of a 0.25% cresol solution can be prepared by diluting 250 milliliters of a 3% solution?

(x) A solution of digitoxin contains 0.2 milligram per milliliter. How many milliliters will contain 0.03 milligram of digitoxin?

(y) A pharmacist prepared a solution containing 5 million units of penicillin per 10 milliliters. How many units of penicillin will 0.25 milliliter contain?

Chapter 2

The Metric System

THE *measure* of a quantity is the number of times that it contains a standard quantity taken as a *unit*. A 5-pound weight, for instance, contains five times the weight of a standard 1-pound unit. Some kinds of quantities measured are temperature, length, area, volume, and time— respectively measured in such familiar units as degrees, feet, square miles, gallons, and hours.

The standard subdivisions and multiples of the unit in any system of measurement are called *denominations*, and we have seen that figures specifying their number are called *denominate numbers*. So, in the expression "ten cents" the term "cents" designates a denomination in our monetary system, and "ten" is a denominate number. We find it convenient, as a rule, to express large quantities in terms of large denominations, and small quantities in small—as great distances are measured by the common system in miles, short intervals in inches. Denominations are understood to stand in a fixed ratio with the unit upon which the system is based—as a cent has a fixed value of $\frac{1}{100}$ of a dollar—and therefore they have a fixed ratio with each other. A statement of the mutual relationships of denominations of the same kind is called a *table of measure*.

The *metric system* of measure was formulated in France in the late ·18th century. Its *use* in the United States was legalized in 1866. By act of Congress in 1893 it became our legal *standard* of measure, and all other systems are referred to it for official comparison.

Its acceptance by scientists the world over has resulted from these two merits: (1) its tables are simple, for they are based upon the decimal system of notation, and the greater of two consecutive denominations of the same kind is always ten times the less; (2) its tables of length, volume, and weight are conveniently correlated, for the meter is the fundamental unit of the system.

Each table of the metric system contains a definitive unit. The *meter* is the unit of length, the *liter* of volume, and the *gram* of weight.

Subdivisions and multiples of these principal units are indicated respectively by Latin and Greek prefixes:

(58)

Latin:

milli- to denote one-thousandth of the unit,
centi- to denote one-hundredth of the unit,
deci-   to denote one-tenth of the unit.

Greek:

deka-   to denote ten times the unit,
hekto- to denote one hundred times the unit,
kilo-   to denote one thousand times the unit,
myria- to denote ten thousand times the unit.

Anyone who wishes to become quickly used to the system should note that our money is "metrically" or decimally computed. The names of the chief fractions of the dollar unit are a clue to their value: a *mill* (for which we have no coin) is one-thousandth, a *cent* one-hundredth, and a *dime* one-tenth of the unit.

The italicized symbols in the tables of metric length, volume, and weight are those adopted by the National Bureau of Standards.

MEASURE OF LENGTH

The meter is the fundamental unit of this system. It has been determined as approximately one-ten-millionth part of the distance from the earth's equator to the North Pole, and is, in fact, a little over a yard long.

Table of metric length:

10 millimeters (mm. or *mm*) = 1 centimeter (cm. or *cm*)
10 centimeters = 1 decimeter (dm. or *dm*)
10 decimeters = 1 meter (M., m., or *m*)
10 meters = 1 dekameter (Dm. or *dam*)
10 dekameters = 1 hektometer (Hm. or *hm*)
10 hektometers = 1 kilometer (Km. or *km*)
10 kilometers = 1 myriameter (Mm.)

Further subdivisions of the unit are occasionally used. A millionth of a meter (a thousandth of a millimeter) is the *micron* (μ) used to express such small things as the diameter of a red blood corpuscle. A thousandth of a micron is the *millimicron* (mμ).

A very small unit equal to one ten-thousandth of a micron is the *angstrom* (Å) which is used in expressing the length of light waves.

The table may also be written:

$$1 \text{ meter} = 1000 \text{ millimeters}$$
$$= 100 \text{ centimeters}$$
$$= 10 \text{ decimeters}$$
$$= 0.1 \text{ dekameter}$$
$$= 0.01 \text{ hektometer}$$
$$= 0.001 \text{ kilometer}$$
$$= 0.0001 \text{ myriameter}$$

The most commonly used denominations are the millimeter, centimeter, and meter, as if the table were:

$$1000 \text{ millimeters (mm.)} = 100 \text{ centimeters (cm.)}$$
$$100 \text{ centimeters (cm.)} = 1 \text{ meter (m.)}$$

MEASURE OF VOLUME

The *liter* is the metric unit of volume. It represents the volume of the cube of one-tenth of a meter—that is, of one cubic decimeter.

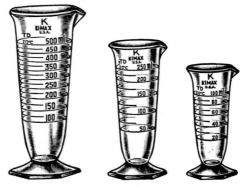

Metric Graduates.
(Courtesy of Kimble Glassware Co.)

Table of metric volume:

$$10 \text{ milliliters (ml. or } ml\text{)} = 1 \text{ centiliter (cl. or } cl\text{)}$$
$$10 \text{ centiliters} = 1 \text{ deciliter (dl. or } dl\text{)}$$
$$10 \text{ deciliters} = 1 \text{ liter (L. or l.)}$$
$$10 \text{ liters} = 1 \text{ dekaliter (Dl. or } dal\text{)}$$
$$10 \text{ dekaliters} = 1 \text{ hektoliter (Hl. or } hl\text{)}$$
$$10 \text{ hektoliters} = 1 \text{ kiloliter (Kl. or } kl\text{)}$$

This table may also be written:

$$1 \text{ liter} = 1000 \text{ milliliters}$$
$$= 100 \text{ centiliters}$$
$$= 10 \text{ deciliters}$$
$$= 0.1 \text{ dekaliter}$$
$$= 0.01 \text{ hektoliter}$$
$$= 0.001 \text{ kiloliter}$$

Although in theory the liter was meant to have the volume of one cubic decimeter, or a thousand cubic centimeters, precise modern measurement has discovered that the standard liter contains slightly less than this volume. But the discrepancy is insignificant for most practical purposes; and since the milliliter has so very nearly the volume of a cubic centimeter, the *United States Pharmacopeia* states: "One milliliter (ml.) is used herein as the equivalent of 1 cubic centimeter (cc.)."

A further subdivision of the unit is the *microliter* (μl) which is equal to one millionth of a liter or a thousandth part of a milliliter, used especially in microchemistry.

The most commonly used denominations are the milliliter and liter, as if the table were simply:

$$1000 \text{ milliliters (ml.)} = 1 \text{ liter (l.)}$$

MEASURE OF WEIGHT

The unit of weight in the metric system is the *gram*, which is the weight of 1 cubic centimeter of water at 4° centigrade, its temperature of greatest density.

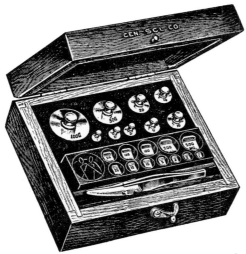

A set of Metric Weights.

Table of metric weight:

$$10 \text{ milligrams (mg. or } mg) = 1 \text{ centigram (cg. or } cg)$$
$$10 \text{ centigrams} = 1 \text{ decigram (dg. or } dg)$$
$$10 \text{ decigrams} = 1 \text{ gram (Gm., g., or } g)$$
$$10 \text{ grams} = 1 \text{ dekagram (Dg. or } dag)$$
$$10 \text{ dekagrams} = 1 \text{ hektogram (Hg. or } hg)$$
$$10 \text{ hektograms} = 1 \text{ kilogram (Kg., kg., or } kg)$$

This table may also be written:

$$1 \text{ gram} = 1000 \text{ milligrams}$$
$$= 100 \text{ centigrams}$$
$$= 10 \text{ decigrams}$$
$$= 0.1 \text{ dekagram}$$
$$= 0.01 \text{ hektogram}$$
$$= 0.001 \text{ kilogram}$$

The denominations most commonly used are the milligram, gram, and kilogram, as if the table were:

$$1000 \text{ milligrams (mg.)} = 1 \text{ gram (g.)}$$
$$1000 \text{ grams (g.)} = 1 \text{ kilogram (kg. or kilo)}$$

Metric weight also includes the *microgram*, which is one-thousandth of a milligram:

$$1 \text{ microgram (mcg.)} = 0.001 \text{ milligram (mg.)}$$
$$1000 \text{ micrograms (mcg.)} = 1 \text{ milligram (mg.)}$$

The abbreviation *mcg.* has come into general use in pharmaceutical literature and labeling. The term *gamma*, symbolized by γ, is customarily used for microgram in biochemical literature, while μg is generally accepted as the abbreviation in the literature of physics and physical chemistry.

When prescriptions are written in the metric system, arabic numerals are always used and are written *before* the abbreviations for the denominations, if such abbreviations are used. Quantities of weight are usually written as grams and *decimals* of a gram, and volumes as milliliters and *decimals* of a milliliter.

Example:

R̸   Codeine Phosphate   0.26 g.
     Ammonium Chloride   6.0 g.
     Cherry Syrup ad   120.0 ml.
     Sig. 5 ml. as directed.

FUNDAMENTAL COMPUTATIONS

To reduce to lower or higher denominations:

The restatement of a given quantity in terms of a higher or lower denomination is called *reduction*. "Thirty minutes" may equally be expressed as a "half hour" or, if occasion requires, as "1800 seconds." The process of changing from higher to lower denominations is known as *reduction descending;* from lower to higher, *reduction ascending.*

A length, a volume, or a weight expressed in one denomination of the metric system may be expressed in another denomination by simply moving the decimal point. In doing this, it is often best to reduce the given quantity first to the *unit* and then to the required denomination.

To change a metric denomination to the next smaller denomination, move the decimal point one place to the right. To change to the next larger denomination, move the decimal point one place to the left.

Examples:

Reduce 85 microns to centimeters.

85μ = 0.085 mm. = 0.0085 cm., *answer.*

Reduce 2.525 liters to milliliters.

2.525 l. = 2525 ml., *answer.*

Reduce 0.25 kilogram to milligrams.

0.25 kg. = 250 g. = 250000 mg., *answer.*

Reduce 250 micrograms to grams.

250 mcg. = 0.250 mg. = 0.000250 g., *answer.*

To add or subtract:

To add or subtract quantities in the metric system, we must reduce them to a *common denomination*—preferably the unit of the table—and arrange their denominate numbers for addition or subtraction as ordinary decimals.

Examples:

Add 1 kg., 250 mg., and 7.5 g. Express the total in grams.

1 kg.	=	1000. g.
250 mg.	=	0.250 g.
7.5 g.	=	7.5 g.

1007.750 g. or 1008 g., *answer.*

Add 4 l., 375 ml., and 0.75 l.   Express the total in milliliters.

$$\begin{array}{lll}
4 \text{ l.} & = & 4000 \text{ ml.} \\
375 \text{ ml.} & = & 375 \text{ ml.} \\
0.75 \text{ l.} & = & 750 \text{ ml.} \\
\hline
 & & 5125 \text{ ml., } answer.
\end{array}$$

A capsule contains the following amounts of medicinal substances: 0.075 g., 20 mg., 0.0005 g., 4 mg., and 500 mcg.   What is the total weight of the substances in the capsule?

$$\begin{array}{lll}
0.075 \text{ g.} & = & 0.075 \text{ g.} \\
20 \text{ mg.} & = & 0.020 \text{ g.} \\
0.0005 \text{ g.} & = & 0.0005 \text{ g.} \\
4 \text{ mg.} & = & 0.004 \text{ g.} \\
500 \text{ mcg.} & = & 0.0005 \text{ g.} \\
\hline
 & & 0.1000 \text{ g. or } 100 \text{ mg., } answer.
\end{array}$$

Subtract 2.5 mg. from 4.850 g.

$$\begin{array}{lll}
4.850 \text{ g.} & = & 4.850 \text{ g.} \\
2.5 \text{ mg.} & = & 0.0025 \text{ g.} \\
\hline
 & & 4.8475 \text{ g. or } 4.848 \text{ g., } answer.
\end{array}$$

A prescription calls for 0.060 g. of one ingredient, 2.5 mg. of another, and enough of a third to make 0.5 g.   How many milligrams of the third ingredient should be used?

Interpreting all quantities as accurate to the nearest tenth of a milligram—

$$\begin{array}{lll}
\text{1st ingredient: } 0.0600 \text{ g.} & = & 0.0600 \text{ g.} \\
\text{2nd ingredient: } 2.5 \text{ mg.} & = & 0.0025 \text{ g.} \\
\hline
 & & 0.0625 \text{ g.}
\end{array}$$

$$\begin{array}{ll}
\text{Total weight:} & 0.5000 \text{ g.} \\
\text{Weight of 1st and 2nd:} & 0.0625 \text{ g.} \\
\hline
\text{Weight of 3rd:} & 0.4375 \text{ g. or } 437.5 \text{ mg., } answer.
\end{array}$$

To multiply or divide :

Since every measurement in the metric system is expressed in a single given denomination, problems involving multiplication and division are solved by the methods used for any decimal numbers.

Examples:

Multiply 820 ml. by 12.5 and express the result in liters.

820 ml. $\times$ 12.5 = 10250 ml. = 10.25 l., *answer.*

Divide 0.465 g. by 15 and express the result in milligrams.

0.465 g. $\div$ 15 = 0.031 g. = 31 mg., *answer.*

Practice Problems

1. Add 0.5 kg., 50 mg., and 2.5 g. Reduce the result to grams.

2. Add 7.25 l. and 875 ml. Reduce the result to milliliters.

3. Reduce 25 mcg. to grams.

4. Divide 0.875 g. by 15 and reduce the result to milligrams.

5. Reduce 0.5 mg. to grams.

6. Multiply 30 mg. by 24 and reduce the result to grams.

7. How many 5-ml. doses may be obtained from 2 l. of a liquid?

8. Multiply 875 ml. by 12.5 and reduce the result to liters.

9. Multiply 0.00025 g. by $\frac{9}{20}$ and reduce the result to milligrams.

10. Multiply 0.4 mg. by 630 and reduce the result to grams.

11. Add 1 kg., 150 mg., and 6.5 g. Reduce the result to grams.

12. Reduce the tenth aliquot of 0.2 g. to milligrams.

13. Reduce the eighth aliquot of 2 l. to milliliters.

14. What fraction of 0.0002 g. is 0.5 mg.?

15. A capsule contains the following amounts of medicinal substances: 0.075 g., 20 mg., 0.0005 g., and 3 mg. What is the total amount of material in the capsule?

16. Add 0.040 g., and 0.5 mg., multiply the result by $\frac{2}{15}$, and reduce the result to milligrams.

17. A 1000-ml. solution contains 0.065 g. of active ingredient. What is the volume of the twelfth aliquot? How many milligrams of active ingredient will it contain?

18. Reduce the sixth aliquot of 4.55 g. to milligrams.

19. Reduce 1.256 g. to micrograms, to milligrams, and to kilograms.

20. How many 0.1-ml. doses may be obtained from 1 l. of a liquid?

21. Multiply 16.99 mg. by 75 and subtract the result from 3.968 g.

22. Divide 10.79 mg. by 100, multiply the result by 675, and reduce the result to grams.

23. Multiply 255 mg. by 380, divide the result by 0.85, and reduce the result to grams.

24. Divide 0.03 g. by 8000 and reduce the result to milligrams.

25. Multiply 0.003 g. by 500 and reduce the fiftieth aliquot of the result to milligrams.

26. Divide 8 g. by 3000 and reduce the result to milligrams.

27. Divide 4 g. by 8000, subtract the result from 4 g., and reduce the result to milligrams.

28. Divide 2 l. by 150 and reduce the result to milliliters.

29. Add 19 mg., 0.016 g., and 2.0 g.; multiply the result by 75; and express the result in grams.

30. Multiply 0.05 mg. by the quotient of 120 ÷ 0.5 and reduce the result to grams.

31. Subtract 250 mg. from 4.85 g.

32. What is the twelfth aliquot of 72 × 0.0006 mg.?

33. Multiply 50.32 mg. by 35, substract the result from 2 g., divide the result by 10, and express the result in milligrams.

34. Multiply 0.45 g. by 0.33 and reduce the result to milligrams.

35. Adhesive Plaster has a tensile strength of not less than 20.41 kg. per 2.54 cm. of width. Reduce these quantities to grams and millimeters.

36. Reduce 85 μ to millimeters.

37. Reduce 125 mcg. to milligrams.

38. Reduce 9520 μ to millimeters.

39. Subtract 245 mg. from 135.004 g.

40. Subtract 125 mg. from 10 g.

41. Divide 0.04 g. by 64 and express the result in milligrams.

42. A liquid contains 0.25 mg. of a substance per milliliter. How many milligrams of the substance will 3.5 l. contain?

43. Add 280 g. and 700 mg., divide by 8, and express the result in grams.

44. A prescription calls for 0.060 g. of one ingredient, 2.5 mg. of another, and enough of a third to make 2 g. How many milligrams of the third ingredient are required?

45. A tablet contains 45 mg. of one ingredient, 65 mg. of a second, and 1.3 mg. of a third. Express the amount, in grams, of each ingredient needed for 200 tablets.

46. Multiply 0.004603 g. by 48 and subtract the product from 1 g.

47. Multiply 0.005585 g. by 65 and reduce the product to milligrams.

48. The prophylactic dose of riboflavin is 2 mg. How many micrograms of riboflavin are in a multiple vitamin capsule containing $\frac{1}{5}$ the prophylactic dose?

49. A vitamin capsule contains 1.5 mg. of Ingredient A, 0.130 g. of Ingredient B, 250 mcg. of Ingredient C, and enough of Ingredient D to make 0.500 g. How many milligrams of Ingredient D are in the capsule?

50. If 480 ml. of a certain solution contain 0.24 g. of a chemical, (a) what is the volume of the thirtieth aliquot? (b) how many milligrams of the chemical will the thirtieth aliquot contain? (c) how many micrograms of the chemical are in this aliquot?

51. How many tablets, each containing 25 mcg., will furnish the equivalent of 0.5 mg. of sodium liothyronine?

52. How many grams of thiamine hydrochloride should be used to prepare 500 tablets each containing 200 mcg. of thiamine hydrochloride?

53. A prescription for a capsule specifies 0.05 mg. of Ingredient A, 50 mg. of Ingredient B, and 0.5 mg. of Ingredient C. How many grams of each ingredient are needed to make 250 capsules?

54. A certain formula specifies 0.625 g. of a substance in 2.5 l. How many milligrams of the substance are in each milliliter?

55. If 0.065 g. of thyroid extract represents 170 mcg. of thyroxin, how many micrograms of thyroxin are represented in 5 mg. of thyroid extract?

56. In compounding a prescription, a pharmacist used 15 mg. of atropine sulfate. How many 0.000075-g. doses were prescribed on the prescription?

57. One mg. of Streptomycin Sulfate contains the antibiotic activity of 650 mcg. of streptomycin base. How many grams of Streptomycin Sulfate would be the equivalent of 1 g. of streptomycin base?

Chapter 3

The Common Systems

In addition to the metric system, the avoirdupois and apothecaries' systems of measurement are used in the United States; and, in spite of the increasing use of the official metric system in pharmacy, some physicians continue to use the apothecaries' systems of measuring volume and weight in their prescriptions. The pharmacist, therefore, must have a practical knowledge of the so-called *common systems of measure.*

Table of apothecaries' fluid measure:

$$
\begin{aligned}
60 \text{ minims } (\mathfrak{M}) &= 1 \text{ fluidrachm (f$\mathfrak{Z}$ or $\mathfrak{Z}$)}^1 \\
8 \text{ fluidrachms (480 minims)} &= 1 \text{ fluidounce (f$\mathfrak{Z}$ or $\mathfrak{Z}$)}^1 \\
16 \text{ fluidounces} &= 1 \text{ pint (pt. or 0)} \\
2 \text{ pints (32 fluidounces)} &= 1 \text{ quart (qt.)} \\
4 \text{ quarts (8 pints)} &= 1 \text{ gallon (gal. or C)}
\end{aligned}
$$

This table may also be written:

gal.	*qt.*	*pt.*	f$\mathfrak{Z}$	f$\mathfrak{Z}$	$\mathfrak{M}$
1	4	8	128	1024	61440
	1	2	32	256	15360
		1	16	128	7680
			1	8	480
				1	60

Table of apothecaries' measure of weight:

$$
\begin{aligned}
20 \text{ grains (gr.)} &= 1 \text{ scruple } (\ni) \\
3 \text{ scruples (60 grains)} &= 1 \text{ drachm } (\mathfrak{Z}) \\
8 \text{ drachms (480 grains)} &= 1 \text{ ounce } (\mathfrak{Z}) \\
12 \text{ ounces (5760 grains)} &= 1 \text{ pound (℔)}
\end{aligned}
$$

[1] When there is no doubt that a liquid is to be measured, physicians commonly omit the *f* in this symbol.

(68)

This table may also be written:

℔	℥	ʒ	Ə	gr.
1	12	96	288	5760
	1	8	24	480
		1	3	60
			1	20

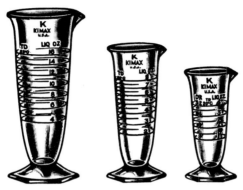

Apothecaries' Graduates.
(Courtesy of Kimble Glassware Co.)

A typical set of Apothecaries' Weights consists of the following units:

ʒii ʒi ʒss ʒii ʒi ʒss Əii Əi
5 grain, 4 grain, 3 grain, 2 grain, 1 grain, $\frac{1}{2}$ grain

Table of avoirdupois measure of weight:

$437\frac{1}{2}$ or 437.5 grains (gr.) = 1 ounce (oz.)
16 ounces (7000 grains) = 1 pound (lb.)

This table may also be written:

lb.	oz.	gr.
1	16	7000
	1	437.5

Only one denomination has a value common to the apothecaries' and avoirdupois systems of measuring weight, namely, the *grain*. The other denominations bearing the same name have quite different values.

The pharmacist buys by the avoirdupois system, for manufacturers and wholesalers customarily supply drugs and chemicals, when they are sold by weight, in avoirdupois units only. The pharmacist likewise sells in bulk "over the counter" by the avoirdupois system.

In contrast with the invariable use of *simple* quantities in the metric system, in the common systems measurements are recorded whenever possible in *compound quantities*—that is, quantities expressed in two or more denominations. So, *20 f℥* may be used during the process of calculating, but as a final result it should be recorded as *1 pt. 4 f℥*. The process of reducing a quantity to a compound quantity beginning with the highest possible denomination is called *simplification*. Decimal fractions may be used in calculation, but the subdivision of a minim or grain in a final result is recorded as a *common fraction*.

When prescriptions are written in the common system, the numbers are written in roman numerals and *follow* the abbreviations or symbols for the denominations.

Example:

℞	Codeine Phosphate	gr. iv
	Ammonium Chloride	ℨ iss
	Cherry Syrup ad	f℥ iv
	Sig. ℨi as directed.	

FUNDAMENTAL COMPUTATIONS

To reduce a compound quantity to a simple quantity :

Before a compound quantity can be used in a calculation it must usually be expressed in terms of a single denomination. To do so, reduce each of the denominations in the compound quantity to the required denomination and add the results.

Examples:

Reduce ℥ss ℨii ℈i to grains.

$$℥ss = \tfrac{1}{2} \times 480 \text{ gr.} = 240 \text{ gr.}$$
$$ℨ\text{ii} = 2 \times 60 \text{ gr.} = 120 \text{ gr.}$$
$$℈\text{i} = 1 \times 20 \text{ gr.} = \underline{20 \text{ gr.}}$$
$$380 \text{ gr., } \textit{answer.}$$

Reduce f℥ iv f℥ iiss to fluidrachms.

$$\text{f℥ iv} = 4 \times 8 \text{ f℥} = 32 \quad \text{f℥}$$
$$\text{f℥ iiss} = 2\tfrac{1}{2} \text{ f℥}$$
$$34\tfrac{1}{2} \text{ f℥}, \textit{answer.}$$

To reduce simple quantities to weighable or measurable denominations:

Before being weighed, a given quantity should be expressed in denominations equal to the actual weights on hand; and before a volume is measured, a given quantity should be expressed in denominations represented by the calibrations on the graduate.

Examples:

Change 165 grains to weighable apothecaries' units.

By selecting larger weight units to account for as many of the required grains as possible, beginning with the largest, we find that we may use the following weights:

℥ii, ℈ss, Ɔss, 5 gr., *answer.*

Check:
$$℥\text{ii} = 120 \text{ gr.}$$
$$℈\text{ss} = 30 \text{ gr.}$$
$$Ɔ\text{ss} = 10 \text{ gr.}$$
$$5 \text{ gr.} = 5 \text{ gr.}$$
$$165 \text{ gr.}, \textit{total.}$$

In enlarging a formula, we find that we are to measure 90 f℥ of a liquid. Using two graduates, if necessary, in what denominations may we measure this quantity?

11 f℥ and 2 f℥, *answer.*

Check:
$$11 \text{ f℥} = 88 \text{ f℥}$$
$$2 \text{ f℥} = 2 \text{ f℥}$$
$$90 \text{ f℥}, \textit{total.}$$

To add or subtract:

To add or subtract quantities in the common systems, reduce to a common denomination, add or subtract, and reduce the result (unless it is to be used in further calculation) to a compound quantity.

Examples:

A formula contains ℈ii of Ingredient A, ʒi of Ingredient B, ʒiv of Ingredient C, and gr. viiss of Ingredient D. Calculate the total weight of the ingredients.

$$℈ii = 2 \times 20 \text{ gr.} = 40 \text{ gr.}$$
$$ʒi = 1 \times 60 \text{ gr.} = 60 \text{ gr.}$$
$$ʒiv = 4 \times 60 \text{ gr.} = 240 \text{ gr.}$$
$$\text{gr. viiss} = 7\tfrac{1}{2} \text{ gr.}$$

$$347\tfrac{1}{2} \text{ gr.} = 5 \, ʒ \, 2 \, ℈ \, 7\tfrac{1}{2} \text{ gr., } answer.$$

A pharmacist had 1 gallon of alcohol. At different times he dispensed fʒiv, Oii, fʒviii, and fʒiv. What volume of alcohol was left?

$$fʒiv = 4 \text{ fʒ}$$
$$Oii = 2 \times 16 \text{ fʒ} = 32 \text{ fʒ}$$
$$fʒviii = 8 \text{ fʒ}$$
$$fʒiv = \tfrac{1}{2} \text{ fʒ}$$

$$44\tfrac{1}{2} \text{ fʒ, } total \; dispensed.$$

$$1 \text{ gal.} = 128 \text{ fʒ}$$
$$-44\tfrac{1}{2} \text{ fʒ}$$

$$83\tfrac{1}{2} \text{ fʒ} = 5 \text{ pt. } 3 \text{ fʒ } 4 \text{ fʒ, } answer.$$

To multiply or divide :

A *simple* quantity may be multiplied or divided by any *pure* number— as *12 × 10 oz. = 120 oz.* or *7 lb. 8 oz.*

But if *both* terms in division are derived from denominate numbers (as when we express one quantity as a fraction of another) they must be reduced to a *common* denomination before division can be performed.

A *compound* quantity is most easily multiplied or divided, and with least chance of careless error, if it is first reduced to a *simple* quantity: *2 × 8 fʒ 6 fʒ = 2 × 70 fʒ = 140 fʒ or 17 fʒ 4 fʒ.*

The *result* of multiplication should be (1) left as it is, if it is to be used in further calculations, (2) simplified, or (3) reduced to weighable or measurable denominations.

Examples:

A prescription for 24 powders calls for gr. ¼ of Ingredient A, ℈ss of Ingredient B, and gr. v of Ingredient C in each powder. How much of each ingredient should be used in compounding the prescription?

$24 \times$ gr.$\frac{1}{4}$ = 6 gr. of Ingredient A,
$24 \times \frac{1}{2}$ ℈ = 12 ℈, or 4 ʒ of Ingredient B,
$24 \times$ gr.v = 120 gr., or 2 ʒ of Ingredient C, *answers.*

A formula for 24 capsules contains ℈*ss of one ingredient,* ʒ*i of another, and* ʒ*iiss of a third. How many grains of each ingredient will be contained in each capsule?*

℈ss = 10 gr., and $\frac{10}{24}$ gr. = $\frac{5}{12}$ gr.,
ʒi = 60 gr., and $\frac{60}{24}$ gr. = $2\frac{1}{2}$ gr.,
ʒiiss = 150 gr., and $\frac{150}{24}$ gr. = $6\frac{1}{4}$ gr., *answers.*

How many 15-minim doses can be obtained from a mixture containing fʒ*iii of one ingredient and* fʒ*ii of another?*

fʒiii = 3 × 480 ℥   1440 ℥
fʒii = 2 × 60 ℥ =   120 ℥
_____
1560 ℥, *total.*

$\frac{1560}{15}$ doses = 104 doses, *answer.*

RELATIONSHIP OF AVOIRDUPOIS AND APOTHECARIES' WEIGHTS

As noted above, the *grain* is the same in both the avoirdupois and apothecaries' systems of weight, but other denominations with the same names are not equal.

To convert from either system to the other, first reduce the given quantity to grains in the one system, and then reduce the result to any desired denomination in the other system.

The custom of buying drugs by avoirdupois weight and dispensing them by apothecaries' weight leads to problems many of which can be most conveniently solved by proportion.

Examples:

Convert ʒ*ii* ℥*ii to avoirdupois weight.*

℥ii = 2 × 480 gr. = 960 gr.
℥ii = 2 × 60 gr. = 120 gr.
_____
Total: 1080 gr.

1 oz. = 437.5 gr.
$\frac{1080}{437.5}$ oz. = 2 oz. 205 gr., *answer.*

How many grains of a chemical are left in a 1-oz. bottle after ℥vii are dispensed from it?

$$1 \text{ oz.} = 1 \times 437.5 \text{ gr.} = 437.5 \text{ gr.}$$
$$℥\text{vii} = 7 \times 60 \text{ gr.} \quad = 420.0 \text{ gr.}$$

Difference: 17.5 gr., *answer.*

If a drug costs $1.75 per oz., what is the cost of 2 ℥?

$$1 \text{ oz.} = 437.5 \text{ gr., and } 2 ℥ = 120 \text{ gr.}$$

$$\frac{437.5 \text{ (gr.)}}{120 \text{ (gr.)}} = \frac{1.75 \text{ (\$)}}{x \text{ (\$)}}$$

$$x = \$0.48, \text{ } answer.$$

Practice Problems

1. Reduce each of the following quantities to grains:

    (*a*) ℥ii ℈iss.
    (*b*) ℥ii ℥iss.
    (*c*) ℥i ℥ss ℈i.
    (*d*) ℥i ℈i gr.x.

2. Reduce 0i ℥ii to fluidrachms.

3. Reduce each of the following quantities to weighable apothecaries' denominations:

    (*a*) 158 gr.
    (*b*) 175 gr.
    (*c*) 210 gr.
    (*d*) 75 gr.
    (*e*) 96 gr.

4. What is the weight, in grains, of a mixture containing ℥ii of one ingredient, ℥ii of another, and ℈i of a third?

5. A pharmacist had 1 gallon of phenobarbital elixir; at different times he dispensed 0i, f℥vi, f℥iv, 0ss, f℥iss, and f℥xii. What volume, in fluid-ounces, of the elixir was left?

6. How many dessertspoonful (2⅔f℥) doses can be obtained from f℥xii of the liquid medication?

7. How many 15-grain doses can be obtained from ℥ss of a powder?

8. How many f℥iv bottles of iodine tincture can be obtained from 2 pt. of iodine tincture?

9. How many f℥ii bottles of cough syrup can be obtained from 5 gal. of the cough syrup?

10. How many grains of a chemical are left in a 1-oz. package after ℥ii and Ði have been dispensed?

11. How many 5-grain capsules of aspirin can be made from a 4-oz. package of aspirin?

12. How many 10-grain capsules of reduced iron can be made from $\frac{1}{2}$ lb. of reduced iron?

13. How many $\frac{1}{4}$-gr. tablets of morphine sulfate can be made from $\frac{1}{8}$ oz. of morphine sulfate?

14. What is the volume, in fluidounces, of a mixture containing $\frac{1}{2}$ gal. of one liquid, 2 pt. of another, and 96 f℥ of a third?

15. What volume, in fluidounces, should a physician prescribe if he wishes to write a prescription for 48 teaspoonful ($1\frac{1}{3}$ f℥) doses?

16. A prescription contains gr.x of one ingredient, ℥i of a second, and Ðii of a third. How many 5-grain doses can be made from the mixture?

17. A formula for 40 powders contains Ði of one ingredient, ℥i of another, and ℥iv of a third. Express the amount, in grains, of each ingredient in each powder.

18. How many grains of a chemical are left in a 1-oz. bottle after enough of it has been used to make 2000 tablets each containing $\frac{1}{200}$ gr. of the chemical?

19. If a chemical costs $1.75 per oz., what is the cost of ℥iii?

20. A pharmacist compounded a prescription for 100 capsules each containing $\frac{1}{4}$ gr. of codeine phosphate. If 1 oz. of codeine phosphate costs $17.50, calculate the cost of the amount used in compounding the prescription.

21. How many $\frac{1}{120}$-gr. doses of atropine sulfate can be obtained from $\frac{1}{8}$-oz. bottle of atropine sulfate?

22. A cough syrup contains Ðss of ammonium chloride in f℥iv. How many grains should be used in preparing 1 gallon of the syrup?

23. How many $\frac{1}{32}$-gr. tablets can be made from $\frac{1}{8}$ oz. of hydromorphone hydrochloride?

24. If a chemical costs $2.50 per oz., what is the cost of ℥iv?

25. How many grains of a chemical are left in a ¼-oz. bottle after enough of it is used to make 5000 tablets each containing $\frac{1}{200}$ gr. of the chemical?

26. A pharmacist bought 2 oz. of a chemical from a wholesaler. At different times he dispensed ʒi, ℥ii, 15 gr., and ℥iv. How many grains of the chemical were left?

27. In checking a narcotic file, a pharmacist found that the following quantities of codeine phosphate had been used from a bottle originally containing 1 oz.:

         ℞1—gr.v
         ℞2—Ͽi
         ℞3—ʒss
         ℞4—Ͽss
         ℞5—gr.iiss

How many grains of codeine phosphate were left in the bottle?

Chapter 4

Conversion

WHEN we want to measure something, we are theoretically privileged to select any system of measure we please. But when we are required to measure a given quantity, in a formula, say, or in a prescription, the instrument at hand—the graduate or set of weights—may not happen to measure in the system specified. Consequently, a quantity called for in one system may have to be translated to its equivalent in the system of our available instrument. This translation is called *conversion*.

Conversion is frequently required in pharmacy, for the metric and common systems are sometimes jumbled together in every day experience. Pounds may not be added to grams, nor may scruples be subtracted from avoirdupois ounces, nor may a ratio be made between liters and fluidounces; and we must convert to a single system (as well as reduce to a common denomination) all miscellaneous quantities that are to be in any way compared.

Denominations in the metric system are incommensurate with those of the common systems. Hence there can be no *exact* equivalence. But the International Bureau of Standards has measured the meter in terms of inches and the kilogram in terms of pounds so precisely as to be able to express the linear equivalence with 7-figure accuracy and the weight equivalence with 9-figure accuracy. Such precision, of course, is not intended to have any ordinary practical application. From these figures the relationships of other denominations can be calculated as accurately as necessary for a given purpose.

The measurement of a denomination of one system in terms of another system is properly called a *conversion factor*. Any one conversion factor is sufficient to serve as a bridge between two systems; but in practice it is convenient to have a choice of several. We may use the equation *1 g. = 15.432 gr.*, for example, in converting a number of grams to grains; but in converting grains to grams, a more useful equation is *1 gr. = 0.065 g.* Again, it is convenient to have one equation for converting a large denomination directly to a large denomination, and another for converting a small denomination to a small denomination.

The question just how accurate our conversion factors should be has not been satisfactorily established. The *United States Pharmacopeia* allows very rough approximations when our calculations concern dosage (see Chapter 5), but insists that we use *"exact"* equivalents for the conversion of specific quantities in converting pharmaceutical formulas. Further, it directs that exact equivalents rounded to three significant figures be used for prescription compounding.

Ordinary pharmaceutical procedure actually seeks something between 2- and 3-figure accuracy in final results, and the following convenient figures, although not wholly consistent, are in widespread use and are more than sufficient for all practical purposes. *These should be memorized.*

SOME PRACTICAL EQUIVALENTS

1 M. = 39.37 in.
1 in. = 2.54 cm.

1 ml. = 16.23 ℳ
1 f℥ = 29.57 ml.
1 pt. = 473 ml.

1 g. = 15.432 gr.
1 kg. = 2.2 lb.[1]
1 gr. = 0.065 g. or 65 mg.
1 oz. = 28.35 g.
1 ℥ = 31.1 g.
1 lb. = 454 g.
1 oz. = 437.5 gr.
1 ℥ = 480 gr.

Note that such equivalents may be used in two ways. For example, to convert a number of fluidounces to milliliters, *multiply* by *29.57;* and to convert a number of milliliters to fluidounces, *divide* by *29.57.*

Note likewise that to the question: *Must we round off results so as to contain no more significant figures than are contained in the conversion factor?*—the answer is *Yes.* If we desire greater accuracy, we should use a more accurate conversion factor. But to the question: *If a formula includes the 1-figure quantity 5 g., and we convert it to grains, must we round off the result to 1 significant figure?*—the answer is decidedly *No.* We should interpret the quantity given in a formula as expressing the precision we are expected to achieve in compounding—usually not less than 3-figure accuracy. Hence, *5 g.* in a formula or prescription should be interpreted as meaning at least *5.00 g.*

[1] Since this conversion factor is an abbreviation of 2.20, it is really accurate to 3 figures.

CONVERSION OF LINEAR QUANTITIES

To convert metric lengths to common equivalents:

We may reduce any given metric length to meters—by moving the decimal point—and then multiply this quantity by *39.37* (the number of inches equivalent to each meter) to get inches. But if the metric quantity is small, it may be more convenient to reduce it to centimeters and divide by *2.54* to get inches.

Example:

The fiber length of a sample of purified cotton is 6.35 mm. Express the length in inches.

6.35 mm. = 0.635 cm.

$\frac{0.635}{2.54}$ in. = 0.250 in., or $\frac{1}{4}$ in., *answer*.

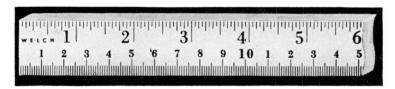

Portion of meter stick showing relation between centimeters and inches.
(Courtesy of W. M. Welch Scientific Co.)

To convert common lengths to metric equivalents:

If given a length of a yard or more, reduce it to inches and divide by *39.37* to get meters. If given a shorter length, reduce it to inches and multiply by *2.54* to get centimeters.

Example:

A medicinal plaster measures $4\frac{1}{2}$ in. by $6\frac{1}{2}$ in. What are its dimensions in centimeters?

Assuming 3-figure precision in the measurement,

$4\frac{1}{2}$ or 4.50 × 2.54 cm. = 11.4 cm. wide,

$6\frac{1}{2}$ or 6.50 × 2.54 cm. = 16.5 cm. long, *answers*.

CONVERSION OF LIQUID QUANTITIES

To convert metric volumes to apothecaries' fluid equivalents:

For small volumes, multiply the number of milliliters by *16.23* to get minims—and reduce the result to measurable units if necessary.

For larger volumes, reduce the given volume to milliliters and divide by *29.57* to get fluidounces or by *473* to get pints.

Examples:

Convert 0.4 ml. to minims.

To achieve 2-figure precision,

0.40×16.23 ℳ $= 6.492$ or 6.5 ℳ, *answer.*

Convert 2.5 l. to fluidounces.

2.5 l. $= 2500$ ml.

Assuming 3-figure precision,

$\frac{2500}{29.57} = 84.5$ f℥, *answer.*

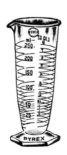
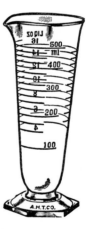

Dual scale graduates.
(Courtesy of Corning Glass Works and Arthur H. Thomas Co.)

To convert apothecaries' fluid volumes to metric equivalents:

For small volumes, reduce to minims and divide by *16.23* to get milliliters.

For larger volumes, reduce to fluidounces and multiply by *29.57* to get milliliters.

Examples:

Convert f℥iiss to milliliters.

f℥iiss = $2\frac{1}{2}$ × 60 ♍ = 150 ♍

$\frac{150}{16.23}$ ml. = 9.24 ml., *answer.*

Convert Oiiss to milliliters.

Oiiss = $2\frac{1}{2}$ × 16 f℥ = 40 f℥

40 × 29.57 ml. = 1182.8 or 1180 ml., *answer.*

CONVERSION OF WEIGHTS

To convert metric weights to common weights :

Reduce a given small quantity to grams and multiply by *15.432* or divide by *0.065* (whichever gives the answer more readily) to get grains, and reduce the quantity to any desired denomination.

For a larger quantity, divide the number of grams by *31.1* to get apothecaries' ounces, or by *28.35* to get ounces avoirdupois.

For a still larger quantity, divide the number of grams by *454* to get pounds avoirdupois.

Examples:

Convert 12.5 g. to grains.

12.5 × 15.432 gr. = 192.9 or 193 gr., *answer.*

Alternate solution (about 0.5% less accurate):

$\frac{12.5}{0.065}$ gr. = 192.3 or 192 gr., *answer.*

Convert 5 mg. to grains.

5 mg. = 0.005 g.

$\frac{0.005}{0.065}$ gr. = $\frac{1}{13}$ gr., *answer.*

Alternate solution, using a more convenient conversion factor:

Since 1 grain = 65 milligrams,

$\frac{5}{65}$ gr. = $\frac{1}{13}$ gr., *answer.*

Convert 15 kg. to pounds avoirdupois.

15 kg. = 15000 g.

$\frac{15000}{454}$ lb. = 33.0 lb., *answer.*

To convert common weights to metric equivalents :

Reduce a given small quantity to grains and multiply by *65* to get milligrams; or reduce the quantity to grains and multiply by *0.065* or divide by *15.432* (whichever gives the answer more readily) to get grams. Reduce the result to any required denomination.

For larger quantities, reduce to apothecaries' ounces and multiply by *31.1*, or to ounces avoirdupois and multiply by *28.35*, to get grams.

For still larger quantities, reduce to pounds avoirdupois and multiply by *454* to get grams, and then reduce, if required, to kilograms; or, more directly, reduce the given quantity to pounds avoirdupois and divide by 2.2 to get kilograms.

Examples:

Convert 6.2 gr. to milligrams.

6.2 × 65 mg. = 403 or 400 mg., *answer.*

How many grams are represented by 850 grains?

850 × 0.065 g. = 55.25 or 55 g., *answer.*

Convert 176 pounds avoirdupois to kilograms.

$\frac{176}{2.2}$ kg. = 80.0 kg., *answer.*

Practice Problems

1. Convert 8 cm. and 12 cm. to inches.

2. Convert 1.35 m. to inches.

3. How many inches are equivalent to 800 mm.?

4. Convert 250 ml. to fluidounces.

5. Convert f♌i ♍xx to milliliters.

6. Convert 4.5 l. to fluidounces.

7. Convert 2 gal. 20 f♌ to liters.

8. A medicinal plaster measures 12 cm. by 16 cm. What is its size in inches?

9. Express a micron as a fraction of an inch.

10. The average diameter of the oil globules in an emulsion is 2.5 microns. What is the average diameter in inches?

11. A pharmacist orders a 100-mm. funnel. What is its size in inches?

12. A mercury barometer reads 760 mm. Express this pressure reading in inches.

13. Convert 3 gal. 1 pt. 10 f℥ to milliliters.

14. A mercury barometer reads 29.2 in. Express this pressure in mm.

15. Urethral suppositories weighing about 2 g. should be 7 cm. in length. Express the weight in grains and the length in inches.

16. If a mixture weighing 30 g. is divided into 100 dosage forms, how many grains will each dose weigh?

17. How many $\frac{1}{2}$-gr. tablets can be made from 10 g. of a chemical?

18. Convert $\frac{1}{1000}$ gr. to milligrams, $2\frac{1}{2}$ gr. to grams, 5℩ to milliliters, and 2.4 ml. to minims.

19. Convert each of the following to the metric system:

   (a) $\frac{1}{60}$ gr.
   (b) f℥ii.
   (c) $\frac{3}{8}$ gr.
   (d) 30 ℩.
   (e) $\frac{1}{200}$ gr.

20. Convert each of the following to apothecaries' units:

   (a) 150 ml.
   (b) 0.3 ml.
   (c) 0.001 g.
   (d) 0.65 mg.

21. Adhesive Plaster has a tensile strength, determined warpwise, of not less than 20.41 kg. per 2.54 cm. of width. Convert these quantities to common equivalents.

22. A certain drug is available in 15-, 25-, and 30-mg. tablets. Express these amounts in the apothecaries' system.

23. Convert 50 micrograms to a fraction of a grain.

24. If 2 f℥ of a solution contain 7½ gr. of a chemical, how many grams would be contained in 125 ml. of the solution?

25. If a chemical costs $3.50 a pound, what is the cost of 15 g.?

26. If the cost of 1 oz. of merbromin is $2.75, what is the cost of 0.650 g.?

27. How many 6.5-mg. tablets can be obtained from ℥ss of a chemical?

28. If f℥i of a cough syrup contains 10 gr. of sodium citrate, how many grams are contained in 2500 ml.?

29. Convert $\frac{1}{1000}$ gr. to micrograms.

30. The dose of a drug is $\frac{1}{10}$ gr. per kg. of body weight. How many milligrams should be given to a person weighing 70 kg.?

31. A prescription calls for $\frac{4}{5}$ gr. of atropine sulfate to be divided into 80 doses. How many milligrams will each dose weigh?

32. A prescription calls for 20 grains of epinephrine bitartrate. If 10 g. of epinephrine bitartrate cost $7.50, what is the cost of the amount needed in the prescription?

33. In the compounding of a prescription, a pharmacist used $\frac{1}{4}$ grain of atropine sulfate. How many 0.000325-g. doses were prescribed on the prescription?

34. A certain elixir contains 0.325 g. of potassium thiocyanate per f℥i. At $6.20 per lb., what is the cost of the potassium thiocyanate required to make 1 gallon of the elixir?

35. A formula for a cough syrup calls for $\frac{1}{8}$ gr. of codeine phosphate per f℥i. How many g. of codeine phosphate should be used in preparing one pint of the cough syrup?

36. The standard width of Type I Absorbent Gauze is 96.5 cm., and that of all other types is 90.1 cm. Convert these widths to common equivalents.

37. In preparing talcum and face powders, the particles of the ingredients must be reduced to the order of less than 10 microns. Express 10 microns as a fraction of an inch.

38. The clearance between the rotor and stator of a colloid mill is set so that particles having a diameter of approximately 0.0005 in. will be produced. What is the size, in microns, of the dispersed particles?

Chapter 5

Calculation of Doses

ONE of the prime responsibilities of the pharmacist is the checking of doses specified in prescriptions against his knowledge of the usual and maximum dispensing doses of the medicines prescribed. If he should note an unusual dose, he would be ethically bound, if possible, to consult the physician, to make sure that the dosage as he reads it is correct.

For the patient, dosage is almost invariably measured in "household" terms—the teaspoonful, the tablespoonful, and sometimes even the wineglassful. In *calculating* doses, pharmacists and physicians traditionally accepted a capacity of 4 ml., or, if the apothecaries' system was used, f℥i for teaspoon dosages. It should be pointed out, however, that household teaspoons have capacities that vary from 3 to 7 ml., and the 5 ml.- rather than the 4 ml.-teaspoon represents a more realistic average. In view of these facts, pharmaceutical manufacturers have used the 5 ml.- teaspoon as a basis for the formulation of liquid preparations.

Agreement has not been reached on a standard official teaspoon, in spite of the need for such a standard measure in connection with compounding and labeling liquid medicines. According to the *United States Pharmacopeia,* "For household purposes, an American Standard Teaspoon has been established by the U.S.A. Standards Institute as containing 4.93 ± 0.24 ml. In view of the almost universal practice of employing teaspoons ordinarily available in the household for the administration of medicine, the teaspoon may be regarded as representing 5 ml. Preparations intended for administration by teaspoon preferably should be formulated on the basis of dosage in 5-ml. units." This statement gives support to the procedure of using the 5-ml. equivalent as the capacity of a teaspoon.

It should be noted, however, that certain factors such as viscosity and surface tension of a given liquid will influence the actual volume delivered by a teaspoon.

For calculation of dosage problems, the following Table is suggested:

TABLE OF APPROXIMATE EQUIVALENTS

"Household" measure:		Metric measure:		Apothecaries' measure:
1 teaspoonful	=	5 ml.	=	$1\frac{1}{3}$ f℥
1 dessertspoonful	=	10 ml.	=	$2\frac{2}{3}$ f℥
1 tablespoonful	=	15 ml.	=	4 f℥
1 wineglassful	=	60 ml.	=	2 f℥

In *judging the safety* of doses of potent substances that are prescribed in liquid form, where the liquid is to be administered in teaspoonful doses, the pharmacist should check the dosage on the basis of 6 doses per fluidounce.

Frequently, the "drop" is used as a measure for medicines. It does not represent a definite quantity, since drops of different liquids vary greatly. In an attempt to standardize the drop as a unit of volume, the *United States Pharmacopeia* defines the official medicine dropper as being constricted at the delivery end to a round opening having an external diameter of 3 mm. The dropper, when held vertically, delivers water in drops each of which weighs between 45 mg. and 55 mg. Accordingly, the official dropper is calibrated to deliver 20 drops of water per ml.

However, one should keep in mind that few medicinal liquids have the same surface and flow characteristics as water, and therefore the size of drops varies materially from one liquid to another. The "drop" should not be used as a measure until the volume that it represents has been determined for each specific liquid. This is done by *calibrating* the dispensing dropper. The calibrated dropper is the only one that should be used for the measurement of medicine.

CALIBRATION OF DROPPERS

A dropper may be calibrated by counting the drops of a liquid as they fall into a graduate until a measurable volume is obtained. The volume of the drop is then calculated in terms of a definite unit (ml. or ℳ).

It is common practice for pharmacists to employ calibrated droppers for measuring small volumes.

"APPROXIMATE" EQUIVALENTS vs "EXACT" EQUIVALENTS

All doses in the *United States Pharmacopeia* and *National Formulary* are given in the metric system. "Approximate" equivalents in the apothecaries' system may be calculated by reference to the "Table of Metric Doses with Approximate Apothecary Equivalents" in the *Pharmacopeia*. "These *approximate* dose equivalents represent the quantities usually prescribed, under identical conditions, by physicians using, respectively, the metric system and the apothecary system of weights and measures. . . .

"When prepared dosage forms such as tablets, capsules, pills, etc., are prescribed in the metric system, the pharmacist may dispense the corresponding *approximate* equivalent in the apothecary system, and vice versa. . . ."

The approximate dose equivalents cannot be used for the conversion of specific quantities in a prescription *which requires compounding* or in converting pharmaceutical formulas from one system of weights or measures to the other system. For such purposes *exact* equivalents must be used. However, for prescription compounding, these exact equivalents are to be rounded to three significant figures.

MISCELLANEOUS DOSAGE PROBLEMS

To calculate the number of doses in a specified amount of medicine:

$$\text{Number of doses} = \frac{\text{Total amount}}{\text{Size of dose}}$$

The *total* amount and the *dose* must be measured in a common denomination.

Examples:

If the dose of a drug is 200 milligrams, how many doses are contained in 10 grams?

10 g. = 10000 mg.

$$\text{Number of doses} = \frac{10000 \ (\text{mg.})}{200 \ (\text{mg.})} = 50 \text{ doses, } answer.$$

How many 20-minim doses are contained in 40 ml. of a liquid?

40 ml. = 40 × 16.23 $\mathfrak{m}$ = 649.2 $\mathfrak{m}$

$$\text{Number of doses} = \frac{649.2 \ (\mathfrak{m})}{20 \ (\mathfrak{m})} = 32 \text{ doses, } answer.$$

If the dose of a medicine is ⅕ grain, how many doses are contained in ½ drachm?

½ ℨ = ½ × 60 gr. = 30 gr.

$$\text{Number of doses} = \frac{30 \ (\text{gr.})}{\frac{1}{5} \ (\text{gr.})} = 30 \times \frac{5}{1} = 150 \text{ doses, } answer.$$

If 1 tablespoon is prescribed as the dose of a medicine, approximately how many doses will be contained in 12 fluidounces?

1 tablespoonful = 4 f℥
12 f℥ = 96 f℥

$$\text{Number of doses} = \frac{96 \ (\text{f℥})}{4 \ (\text{f℥})} = 24 \text{ doses, } answer.$$

If the dose of a drug is 50 micrograms, how many doses are contained in 0.020 gram?

0.020 g. = 20 mg.

50 mcg. = 0.05 mg.

$$\text{Number of doses} = \frac{20 \text{ (mg.)}}{0.05 \text{ (mg.)}} = 400 \text{ doses, } \textit{answer.}$$

To calculate the size of each dose, given a specified amount of medicine and the number of doses it contains:

$$\text{Size of dose} = \frac{\text{Total amount}}{\text{Number of doses}}$$

The *size of the dose* will be expressed in whatever denomination is chosen for measuring the given total amount.

Examples:

How many teaspoonfuls would be prescribed in each dose of a medicine if f℥ vi contained 18 doses?

f℥ vi = 48 f℥

1 teaspoonful = 1⅓ f℥

48 f℥ ÷ 1⅓ f℥ = 36 teaspoonfuls

$$\text{Size of dose} = \frac{36 \text{ (tsp.)}}{18} = 2 \text{ teaspoonfuls, } \textit{answer.}$$

How many drops would be prescribed in each dose of a medicine if 15 ml. contained 60 doses?   The dispensing dropper calibrates 32 drops per ml.

15 ml. = 15 × 32 drops = 480 drops

$$\text{Size of dose} = \frac{480 \text{ (drops)}}{60} = 8 \text{ drops, } \textit{answer.}$$

To calculate the amount of a medicine, given the number of doses it contains and the size of each dose:

Total amount = number of doses × size of dose

It is convenient first to convert the given dose to the denomination in which the total amount is to be expressed.

Examples:

How many ml. of a medicine would provide a patient with 2 tablespoonfuls twice a day for 8 days?

Number of doses = 16

Size of dose = 2 tablespoonfuls or 30 ml.

Total amount = 16 × 30 ml. = 480 ml., *answer.*

How many fluidounces of a mixture would provide a patient with a teaspoonful dose to be taken 3 times a day for 16 days?

Number of doses = 16 × 3 = 48

Size of dose = 1 teaspoonful = $1\frac{1}{3}$ f℥

Total amount = 48 × $1\frac{1}{3}$ f℥ = 64 f℥ = 8 f℥, *answer.*

How many milligrams of a drug will be needed to prepare 72 dosage forms if each is to contain $\frac{1}{12}$ grain?

Number of doses = 72

Size of dose = $\frac{1}{12}$ grain = 5.4 mg.

Total amount = 72 × 5.4 mg. = 390 mg., *answer.*

To calculate the quantity of an ingredient in each specified dose of a medicine, given the quantity in a total amount:

When the number of doses in the total amount is given or can be quickly calculated, this is a convenient equation:

$$\text{Quantity in each dose} = \frac{\text{Quantity in total amount}}{\text{Number of doses}}$$

The quantity of the ingredient in the total amount should first be reduced or converted to the denomination desired in the answer.

But when the number of doses is not given, it is sometimes more convenient to use this proportion:

$$\frac{\text{Total amount}}{\text{Size of dose}} = \frac{\text{Quantity of ingredient in total}}{x}$$

x = Quantity in each dose

Examples:

If 0.050 g. of a substance is used in preparing 125 tablets, how many micrograms are represented in each tablet?

0.050 g. = 50 mg. = 50000 mcg.

$$\frac{50000 \text{ (mcg.)}}{125} = 400 \text{ mcg.}, \textit{answer.}$$

If a preparation contains 5 g. of a drug in 500 ml., how many grams are contained in each tablespoonful dose?

1 tablespoonful = 15 ml.

$$\frac{500 \text{ (ml.)}}{15 \text{ (ml.)}} = \frac{5 \text{ (g.)}}{x}$$

x = 0.15 g., *answer.*

A cough mixture contains $\frac{3}{4}$ gr. of hydromorphone hydrochloride in f℥viii. How much hydromorphone hydrochloride is there in each dessertspoonful dose?

1 dessertspoonful = $2\frac{2}{3}$ fℨ

f℥viii = 64 fℨ

64 ÷ $2\frac{2}{3}$ = 24 doses

$\frac{3}{4}$ gr. ÷ 24 = $\frac{1}{32}$ gr., *answer.*

Or,

$$\frac{64 \text{ (fℨ)}}{2\frac{2}{3} \text{ (fℨ)}} = \frac{\frac{3}{4} \text{ (gr.)}}{x \text{ (gr.)}}$$

$$x = \frac{\frac{8}{3} \times \frac{3}{4}}{64} \text{ gr.} = \frac{1}{32} \text{ gr.}, \textit{answer.}$$

How much codeine sulfate and how much ammonium chloride will be contained in each dose of the following prescription?

R   Codeine Sulfate   gr. vi
     Ammonium Chloride   ℥iss
     Cherry Syrup ad   f℥ vi
     Sig. Teaspoonful for cough.

f℥ vi = 48 f℥

1 teaspoonful = 1⅓ f℥

48 ÷ 1⅓ = 36 doses

6 gr. ÷ 36 = ⅙ gr. of codeine phosphate, *and*

℥iss or 90 gr. ÷ 36 = 2½ gr. of ammonium chloride, *answers.*

Or,

$$\frac{48 \ (f℥)}{1\frac{1}{3} \ (f℥)} = \frac{6 \ (gr.)}{x \ (gr.)}$$

x = ⅙ gr. of codeine phosphate, *and*

$$\frac{48 \ (f℥)}{1\frac{1}{3} \ (f℥)} = \frac{90 \ (gr.)}{y \ (gr.)}$$

y = 2½ gr. of ammonium chloride, *answers.*

How much codeine phosphate and how much ammonium chloride will be contained in each dose of the following prescription?

R   Codeine Phosphate   0.6 g.
     Ammonium Chloride   6.0 g.
     Cherry Syrup ad   120.0 ml.
     Sig. Teaspoonful for cough.

1 teaspoonful = 5 ml.

120 ÷ 5 = 24 doses

0.6 g. ÷ 24 = 0.025 g. of codeine phosphate, *and*

6.0 g. ÷ 24 = 0.25 g. of ammonium chloride, *answers.*

Or,

$$\frac{120 \ (ml.)}{5 \ (ml.)} = \frac{0.6 \ (g.)}{x \ (g.)}$$

x = 0.025 g. of codeine phosphate, *and*

$$\frac{120 \ (ml.)}{5 \ (ml.)} = \frac{6 \ (g.)}{y \ (g.)}$$

y = 0.25 g. of ammonium chloride, *answers.*

To calculate the quantity of an ingredient in a specified total amount of of medicine, given the quantity of the ingredient in each specified dose:

As always, we can make a sound ratio of two amounts only by measuring them in a common denomination.

Here again, when the number of doses is known or can be quickly calculated, this equation is convenient:

Quantity in total = Quantity in dose × Number of doses

Otherwise this proportion may be used:

$$\frac{\text{Size of dose}}{\text{Total amount}} = \frac{\text{Quantity of ingredient in each dose}}{x}$$

x = Quantity in total amount

Examples:

How many grams of a chemical are required to make 120 ml. of a solution each teaspoonful of which will contain 3 mg. of the chemical?

1 teaspoonful = 5 ml.

$$\frac{5 \ \text{(ml.)}}{120 \ \text{(ml.)}} = \frac{3 \ \text{(mg.)}}{x \ \text{(mg.)}}$$

x = 72 mg. or 0.072 g., *answer.*

A six-fluidounce cough mixture is to contain, in each teaspoonful, ¼ gr. of codeine phosphate, ½ minim of chloroform, and 2½ gr. of sodium citrate. Calculate the quantity of each ingredient to be used in compounding.

f℥ vi = 48 f℈

1 teaspoonful = 1⅓ f℈

Number of doses = 48 ÷ 1⅓ = 36

36 × ¼ gr. = 9 gr. of codeine phosphate,

36 × ½ ℳ = 18 ℳ of chloroform,

36 × 2½ gr. = 90 gr. or ℥iss of sodium citrate, *answers.*

To calculate the dose of a drug, given the amount per kilo of body weight:

Example:

> *The dose of a drug is $\frac{1}{10}$ grain per kilo of body weight. How many milligrams should be given to a person weighing 154 lb.?*

$$\tfrac{1}{10} \text{ gr.} = 6.5 \text{ mg.}$$

$$1 \text{ kilo (kilogram)} = 2.2 \text{ lb.}$$

$$\frac{2.2 \text{ (lb.)}}{154 \text{ (lb.)}} = \frac{6.5 \text{ (mg.)}}{\text{x (mg.)}}$$

$$\text{x} = 455 \text{ mg., } answer.$$

CALCULATION OF DOSES FOR CHILDREN

To calculate doses for children on the basis of age:

The method that has long been most commonly used for calculating doses for children is known as *Young's Rule: Divide the age of the child by the age plus 12 and multiply by the adult dose.* The rule may bettter be expressed as a mathematical formula:

$$\frac{\text{Age}}{\text{Age} + 12} \times \text{Adult dose} = \text{Dose for child}$$

Examples:

> *If the adult dose of a drug is 5 mg., what is the dose for a child 8 years old?*

$$\frac{8}{8 + 12} \times 5 \text{ mg.} = \tfrac{2}{5} \times 5 \text{ mg.} = 2 \text{ mg., } answer.$$

> *If the adult dose of a drug is 3 grains, what is the dose for a child 6 years old?*

$$\frac{6}{6 + 12} \times 3 \text{ gr.} = \tfrac{1}{3} \times 3 \text{ gr.} = 1 \text{ gr., } answer.$$

If the adult dose of a drug is 0.1 ml., what is the dose for a child 12 years old?

$$\frac{12}{12 + 12} \times 0.1 \text{ ml.} = \tfrac{1}{2} \times 0.1 \text{ ml.} = 0.05 \text{ ml., } answer.$$

Other methods based on age or weight have required similar calculation.

Cowling's Rule:

$$\frac{\text{Age at next birthday (in years)} \times \text{Adult dose}}{24} = \text{Dose for child}$$

Fried's Rule for Infants:

$$\frac{\text{Age (in months)} \times \text{Adult dose}}{150} = \text{Dose for infant}$$

Clark's Rule:

$$\frac{\text{Weight (in pounds)} \times \text{Adult dose}}{150} = \text{Dose for child}$$

To calculate doses for children on a basis of surface area as related to weight:

Many physicians today believe that doses for children should be based upon body surface area, since the correct dosage of drugs seems more nearly proportional to the surface area.[1]

The accompanying Table shows the approximate relation between body weight and surface area of average body dimensions. It may be used in the calculation of pediatric doses which will usually be sufficiently accurate.

By reference to the Table, we find that the pediatric dose is expressed as a percent of the adult dose. This is based upon the relationship of the square meter area of a given weight and the adult normal (176 pounds, equivalent to an area of 2.0 square meters). Approximate doses for children may be calculated by multiplying the adult dose by this percentage. For more precise calculations of pediatric dosage based on the body surface

[1] See, for instance, Crawford, John D., Terry, Mary E., and Rourke, G. Margaret, Simplification of the Drug Dosage Calculation by Application of the Surface Area Principle, Pediatrics, *5*, 783, 1950.

area, one should refer to the standard nomograms that have been developed for this purpose.

TABLE OF THE APPROXIMATE RELATION OF SURFACE AREA AND WEIGHTS OF INDIVIDUALS OF AVERAGE BODY DIMENSIONS

Kilograms	Pounds	Square Meters	Per Cent of Adult Dose
2	4.4	0.12	6
3	6.6	0.20	10
4	8.8	0.23	12
5	11.0	0.25	13
6	13.0	0.29	15
7	15.0	0.33	17
8	18.0	0.36	18
9	20.0	0.40	20
10	22.0	0.44	22
15	33.0	0.62	31
20	44.0	0.79	40
25	55.0	0.93	42
30	66.0	1.07	51
35	77.0	1.20	60
40	88.0	1.32	65
45	99.0	1.43	70
50	110.0	1.53	75
55	121.0	1.62	80
60	132.0	1.70	85
65	143.0	1.78	90
70	154.0	1.84	92
75	165.0	1.95	95
80	176.0	2.00	100

Practice Problems

1. If the dose of a drug is 150 micrograms, how many doses are contained in 0.120 g.?

2. How many 15-minim doses are contained in 60 ml. of a tincture?

3. How many 6-grain doses are contained in 12 g. of a powder?

4. If the dose of a drug is $\frac{1}{16}$ gr., how many doses are contained in ℥i?

5. A medicine is to be taken in 5-minim doses. How many doses are contained in 15 ml. of the medicine?

6. If a medicine is to be taken three times daily, and if 180 ml. are to be taken in four days, how many tablespoonfuls should be prescribed for each dose?

7. What is the dosage in teaspoonfuls if 500 ml. of a medicine contain 50 doses?

8. How many teaspoonfuls per day must be taken if f℥ viii of a medicine are to be taken three times a day for eight days?

9. If a medicine is to be taken three times daily, and if 120 ml. are to be taken in four days, how many teaspoonfuls should be prescribed for each dose?

10. What is the dosage in teaspoonfuls if 240 ml. of a medicine contain 48 doses?

11. How many fluidounces of a mixture contain 48 dessertspoonful doses?

12. If a prescription contains 0.24 g. of codeine phosphate in 120 ml., how much is contained in each teaspoonful dose?

13. If a prescription contains 0.024 g. of atropine sulfate in 240 ml., what fraction of a grain is contained in 1 teaspoonful?

14. How many grains of a chemical are contained in each capsule if a mixture containing $1\frac{1}{4}$ grains of the chemical is divided into 30 capsules?

15. A powder contains $\frac{1}{20}$ gr. of atropine sulfate. If the powder is divided into 12 dosage forms, how much atropine sulfate will each dose contain?

16. If 180 ml. of a cough mixture contain $\frac{3}{4}$ gr. of hydromorphone hydrochloride, how much is contained in 1 teaspoonful of the mixture?

17. If f℥ iv of a mixture contain 6 gr. of phenobarbital, how much is contained in each teaspoonful dose?

18. If a solution of atropine sulfate contains 1 grain in each fluidounce, what volume will contain $\frac{1}{120}$ gr.?

19. If 240 ml. of a liquid contain 0.120 g. of a chemical and 2 teaspoonfuls are taken at a dose, what fraction of a grain will each dose contain?

20. If 500 ml. of a liquid contain 26.0 g. of a chemical and a teaspoonful is taken at a dose, how many grains will each dose contain?

21. A prescription for 250 ml. of a liquid contains 0.025 g. of atropine sulfate and specifies a dose of 5 ml. Calculate the fraction of a grain of atropine sulfate contained in each dose.

22. A physician prescribes Tetracycline Suspension for a patient to be taken in doses of two teaspoonfuls four times a day for 4 days, and then one teaspoonful four times a day for 2 days. How many milliliters of the suspension should be dispensed to provide the quantity for the prescribed dosage regimen?

23. ℞ Phenobarbital   0.6
        Belladonna Tincture   12.0
        Peppermint Water ad   120.0
        Sig. 5 ml. t.i.d.

How much phenobarbital and how much belladonna tincture will be contained in each dose?

24. Amobarbital Elixir contains 4.4 g. of amobarbital per liter. How many grains of amobarbital will be contained in a teaspoonful dose of the elixir?

25. One liter of Terpin Hydrate and Codeine Elixir contains 2 g. of codeine. The usual dose of the elixir is 5 ml. Calculate the quantity, in grains, of codeine in the usual dose.

26. A powder is divided into 36 capsules. If each capsule contains 0.5 mg. of one ingredient, 15 mg. of a second, and enough of a third to make 0.300 g., how much of each is there in the original powder?

27. ℞ Belladonna Tincture   ℥ iii
        Codeine Phosphate   gr. vi
        Phenobarbital Elixir ad   ℥ vi
        Sig. Teaspoonful ex aq.

How much belladonna tincture and how much codeine phosphate will be contained in each dose?

28. Lugol's Solution contains 5 g. of iodine per 100 ml. and its usual dose is 0.3 ml. three times a day. How many milligrams of iodine are represented in the daily dose of the solution?

29. How many grains of a chemical are required to make 3 fluidounces of a solution 1 fluidrachm of which is to contain $\frac{1}{30}$ gr.?

30. How many grams of a chemical are required to make 120 ml. of a mixture each teaspoonful of which is to contain 2.5 mg.?

31. A f℥ vi mixture is to contain, in each tablespoonful, 15 gr. of bismuth subcarbonate and f℥ ss of paregoric. Calculate the quantity of each that should be used in preparing the mixture.

32. A prescription for 240 ml. of a mixture calls for 4 mg. of one ingredient and 200 mg. of another in each teaspoonful dose. How much of each ingredient should be used in compounding the prescription?

33. A solution contains 1 g. of phenobarbital in 250 ml. How many milligrams of phenobarbital are contained in each dessertspoonful dose?

34. A solution contains 30 mg. of a chemical per 120 ml. and has a dose of 10 drops. If the dispensing dropper calibrates 25 drops per ml., how many mcg. of the chemical are contained in each dose?

35. How much of a solution containing 2 mg. of hyoscine per ml. should be used in preparing 120 ml. of a prescription each teaspoonful of which is to contain 0.5 mg. of hyoscine?

36. ℞   Sodium Bromide   gr. xv per tbsp.
        Compound Pepsin Elixir
        Aromatic Elixir aa ad   ℥ viii
        Sig. Tbsp. h.s.

How many grains of sodium bromide should be used in compounding the prescription?

37. ℞   Potassium Thiocyanate
        Aromatic Elixir   aa q.s.
        Make a solution to contain   0.2 g. per tsp.
        Dispense 180 ml.
        Sig. 5 ml. in water daily.

How much potassium thiocyanate should be used in compounding the prescription?

38. ℞   Dihydrocodeinone   gr. $\frac{1}{12}$ per tsp.
        Hydriodic Acid Syrup
        Cherry Syrup   aa   ℥ iii
        Sig. Tsp. every two hours for cough.

How many grains of dihydrocodeinone should be used in compounding the prescription?

39. The adult dose of a liquid medication is 1 ml. per 10 kilograms of body weight to be administered in a single dose. How many teaspoonfuls should be administered to a person weighing 220 lb.?

40. The dose of a drug is 5 mg. per kilogram of body weight. How many grams should be given to a child weighing 55 lb.?

41. The dose of a drug is 0.2 mg. per kilogram of body weight. How many grains should be given to a person weighing 209 lb.?

42. The usual rectal dose of tribromoethanol is 0.06 ml. for each kilogram of body weight. How many milliliters should be given to a person weighing 150 lb.?

43. The usual dose range of dimercaprol is 25 to 50 mg. per 10 kg. of body weight. What is the dose range for a person weighing 165 lb.?

44. If the usual adult dose of a drug is 324 mg., what is the dose for a child 6 years old?

45. If the usual adult dose of a drug is 0.10 g., what is the dose for a child 4 years old?

46. If the usual adult dose of a drug is 0.25 g., what is the dose for a child 9 years old?

47. If the usual adult dose of a drug is 8 grains, what is the dose for a child 4 years old?

48. If the usual adult dose of paregoric is 5 ml., what is the dose for a child 4 years old?

49. If the usual adult dose of atropine sulfate is 0.5 mg., what is the dose for a child 8 years old?

50. If the usual adult dose of a liquid preparation is a teaspoonful, how many minims should be prescribed for a child 4 years old?

51. The usual adult dose of a drug is 15 mg. Calculate the dose, in grains, for a child 6 years old.

52. The usual adult dose of hydromorphone hydrochloride is 2 mg. How much hydromorphone hydrochloride should be used in 120 ml. of a cough syrup so that each 5 ml. will contain the dose for a child 6 years old?

53. The usual adult dose of a drug is 0.0004 g. What is the dose, expressed in grains, for a child of five years?

54. The usual adult dose of tetracycline is 500 mg. What should be the dose for a child of twelve months?

55. The usual adult dose of atropine sulfate is 0.5 mg. Using Fried's Rule, calculate the dose for an infant of six months.

56. The usual adult dose of a drug is $\frac{1}{60}$ gr. Calculate (a) the dose for a 25-lb. child, (b) the dose for an infant of 7 months, and (c) the dose for a child of 6 years.

57. The usual adult dose of a certain solution is 0.5 ml. (a) What is the dose for a child 4 years old? (b) If the solution is to be dispensed in a dropper bottle, the dropper of which calibrates 24 drops per ml., how many drops should be given to obtain the correct dose for the child?

58. ℞ Atropine Sulfate   q.s.
       Phenobarbital   0.02 g.
       Water   ad   30.   ml.
       Sig. Ten (10) drops a.c.

The prescription is for a child of 15 months. Assuming that the dispensing dropper calibrates 20 drops per ml., how many grams of atropine sulfate should be used in compounding the prescription? The adult dose of atropine sulfate is 0.5 mg.

59. The dose of a certain drug is 20 mg. per kilogram of body weight per day. If a physician wishes to prescribe the drug for one week for a person weighing 165 lb., how many 250 mg. capsules of the drug should he order?

60. The usual adult dose of hydrocodone bitartrate is 5 to 10 mg. Calculate the dose for a child weighing 65 lb.

61. The usual adult dose of scopolamine hydrobromide is 0.6 mg. Calculate the dose, in micrograms, for a child weighing 45 lb.

Chapter 6

Reducing and Enlarging Formulas

IN dispensing, the pharmacist may have to reduce official formulas, and in manufacturing, he may be called upon to enlarge them to quantity production. Official formulas may be for quantities of 1000 ml. or 1000 g., whereas prescriptions may call for relatively small amounts such as 30 ml. or 30 g., and formulas for quantity manufacturing may call for relatively large amounts such as 5 gallons or 25 pounds.

When a formula specifies a *total amount,* we may determine how much of each ingredient is needed to obtain a desired total amount by this proportion:

$$\frac{\text{Total amount specified in formula}}{\text{Total amount desired}} = \frac{\text{Quantity of each ingredient in formula}}{x}$$

x = Quantity of each ingredient in amount desired

Although all problems specifying a total amount may be solved by this proportion, it is usually more convenient—particularly if the quantities are given in the metric system—to solve them by the use of short cuts. Thus, given a formula for 1000 ml. or 1000 g., we may divide or multiply the quantity of each ingredient by a power of 10 simply by moving the decimal point to the left or right the required number of places. Or, given a formula for the same amounts, we may reduce or enlarge it by using factors. For example, if we wish to prepare 1 gallon (3785 ml.) of a formula whose specified total amount is 1000 ml., we would multiply the quantity of each ingredient by the factor 3.785. And, if we were to prepare 50 g. of a formula whose specified total amount is 1000 g., we would multiply the quantity of each ingredient by $\frac{1}{20}$ (since 50 g. is $\frac{1}{20}$ of 1000 g.).

Some formulas, however, do not specify a total amount, instead indicating relative quantities of ingredients or *proportional parts* to be used in obtaining any desired total amount. Such problems may be solved by this proportion:

$$\frac{\text{Total number of parts in formula}}{\text{Number of parts of each ingredient}} = \frac{\text{Total amount desired}}{x}$$

x = Quantity of each ingredient in amount desired

In solving problems that involve reducing and enlarging formulas, these facts should be noted:

(1) To make a valid ratio, the total amounts compared must be expressed in a common denomination, whether in grams, fluidounces, pounds, or anything else. Consequently, if they are unlike to start with, one or the other must be reduced or converted. If, for example, the formula is given in the metric system and the required quantity is in the common system, it is generally best to convert the required quantity into the metric system. The answers may then be converted into weighable or measurable denominations in the common system or, if this is not indicated, the results may be left in the metric system.

(2) Since the quantity of each ingredient is calculated separately, it does not matter if the formula includes an assortment of terms (pounds and fluidounces, grams and milliliters, and so on).

FORMULAS THAT SPECIFY AMOUNTS OF INGREDIENTS

To calculate the quantities of ingredients to be used when reducing or enlarging a formula for a specified total amount:

Examples:

From the following formula, calculate the quantity of each ingredient required to make 240 ml. of Calamine Lotion.

Calamine	80 g.
Zinc Oxide	80 g.
Glycerin	20 ml.
Bentonite Magma	250 ml.
Lime Water, to make	1000 ml.

Using the factor 0.24 (since 240 ml. is 0.24 × 1000 ml.), the quantity of each ingredient is calculated as follows:

Calamine	=	80	×	0.24	=	19.2 g.
Zinc Oxide	=	80	×	0.24	=	19.2 g.
Glycerin	=	20	×	0.24	=	4.8 ml.
Bentonite Magma	=	250	×	0.24	=	60 ml.
Lime Water, to make						240 ml.,

answers.

If, in this problem, the required amount were *60 ml.*, we should *move the decimal point one place to the left and multiply by 0.6.* Or, if the required amount were *50 ml.*, we could either *divide by 20* or *move the decimal point one place to the left and divide by 2.* And, if the required amount were *125 ml.*, we should *multiply by the fraction ⅛* (since 125 ml. is ⅛ of 1000 ml.).

From the following formula, calculate the quantity of each ingredient required to make 1 gallon of Compound Benzoin Tincture.

Benzoin	100 g.
Aloe	20 g.
Storax	80 g.
Tolu Balsam	40 g.
Alcohol, to make	1000 ml.

1 gallon = 3785 ml.

Using the factor 3.785, the quantity of each ingredient is calculated as follows:

Benzoin	=	100	×	3.785	=	378.5 g.
Aloe	=	20	×	3.785	=	75.7 g.
Storax	=	80	×	3.785	=	302.8 g.
Tolu Balsam	=	40	×	3.785	=	151.4 g.
Alcohol, to make						3785 ml.

or 1 gal., *answers.*

From the following formula, calculate the quantity of each ingredient required to make 1 lb. of the ointment.

Coal Tar	50 g.
Starch	250 g.
Zinc Oxide	150 g.
Petrolatum	550 g.

1 lb. = 454 g.

Since the formula is for 1000 g., and using the factor 0.454, the quantity of each ingredient is calculated as follows:

Coal Tar	=	50	×	0.454	=	22.7 g.
Starch	=	250	×	0.454	=	113.5 g.
Zinc Oxide	=	150	×	0.454	=	68.1 g.
Petrolatum	=	550	×	0.454	=	249.7 g.

454.0 g.

or 1 lb., *answers.*

From the following formula for 100 capsules, calculate the quantity of each ingredient required to make 24 capsules.

Belladonna Extract	1.0 g.
Ephedrine Sulfate	1.6 g.
Phenobarbital	2.0 g.
Aspirin	32.0 g.

Using the factor 0.24 (since 24 capsules are represented by 0.24 × 100), the quantity of each ingredient is calculated as follows:

Belladonna Extract	=	1.0	×	0.24	=	0.24 g.
Ephedrine Sulfate	=	1.6	×	0.24	=	0.384 g.
Phenobarbital	=	2.0	×	0.24	=	0.48 g.
Aspirin	=	32.0	×	0.24	=	7.68 g.,

answers.

FORMULAS THAT SPECIFY PROPORTIONAL PARTS

To calculate the quantities of ingredients required to prepare a desired amount of a formula when it specifies proportional parts :

If a formula gives us quantities in terms of *proportional parts*, these facts should be noted:

(1) When parts by weight are specified, we can convert only to weights and not to volumes, whereas when parts by volume are specified, we can convert only to volumes.

(2) Just as the formula measures all quantities in a common denomination (namely, in terms of parts), so will our calculations result in a single denomination, and this will be the denomination we select at the outset for measuring the desired total amount.

Examples:

From the following formula, calculate the quantity of each ingredient required to make 1000 g. of the ointment.

Cade Oil	5 parts
Zinc Oxide	10 parts
Hydrophilic Ointment	50 parts

Total number of parts (by weight) = 65
1000 g. will contain 65 parts

$$\frac{65 \text{ (parts)}}{5 \text{ (parts)}} = \frac{1000 \text{ (g.)}}{x \text{ (g.)}}$$

x = 76.92 g. of Cade Oil,

and

$$\frac{65 \text{ (parts)}}{10 \text{ (parts)}} = \frac{1000 \text{ (g.)}}{\text{y (g.)}}$$

y = 153.85 g. of Zinc Oxide,

and

$$\frac{65 \text{ (parts)}}{50 \text{ (parts)}} = \frac{1000 \text{ (g.)}}{\text{z (g.)}}$$

z = 769.23 g. of Hydrophilic Ointment, *answers.*

(Check total: 1000 g.)

From the same formula, calculate the quantity of each ingredient required to make ℥i *of the ointment.*

Total number of parts (by weight) = 65

℥i or 480 grains will contain 65 parts

$$\frac{65 \text{ (parts)}}{5 \text{ (parts)}} = \frac{480 \text{ (gr.)}}{\text{x (gr.)}}$$

x = 36.9 gr. of Cade Oil,

and

$$\frac{65 \text{ (parts)}}{10 \text{ (parts)}} = \frac{480 \text{ (gr).}}{\text{y (gr.)}}$$

y = 73.9 gr. of Zinc Oxide,

and

$$\frac{65 \text{ (parts)}}{50 \text{ (parts)}} = \frac{480 \text{ (gr.)}}{\text{z (gr.)}}$$

z = 369.2 gr. of Hydrophilic Ointment, *answers.*

(Check total: 480 gr. or ℥i)

From the following formula, calculate the quantity of each ingredient required to make 5 lb. of the powder.

Bismuth Subcarbonate	8 parts
Kaolin	15 parts
Magnesium Oxide	2 parts
Total number of parts	25 parts

5 lb. (454 g. $\times$ 5) or 2270 g. will contain 25 parts

$$\frac{25 \text{ (parts)}}{8 \text{ (parts)}} = \frac{2270 \text{ (g.)}}{x \text{ (g.)}}$$

$x = 726.4$ g. of Bismuth Subcarbonate,

and

$$\frac{25 \text{ (parts)}}{15 \text{ (parts)}} = \frac{2270 \text{ (g.)}}{y \text{ (g.)}}$$

$y = 1362$ g. of Kaolin,

and

$$\frac{25 \text{ (parts)}}{2 \text{ (parts)}} = \frac{2270 \text{ (g.)}}{z \text{ (g.)}}$$

$z = 181.6$ g. of Magnesium Oxide, *answers.*

(Check total: 2270 g.)

To calculate the quantities of ingredients in a desired amount when proportional parts may be reckoned from the formula:

If the ingredients are all measured by weight, or all by volume, we may consider the sum of the weights (or volumes) when expressed in a common denomination as specifying a total number of parts.

Example:

From the following formula, calculate the quantity of each ingredient required to make 500 g. of the powder.

Boric Acid	5 g.
Starch	20 g.
Talc	50 g.

Total number of parts (by weight) = 75

500 g. will contain 75 parts

$$\frac{75 \text{ (parts)}}{5 \text{ (parts)}} = \frac{500 \text{ (g.)}}{x \text{ (g.)}}$$

x = 33.3 g. of Boric Acid,

and

$$\frac{75 \text{ (parts)}}{20 \text{ (parts)}} = \frac{500 \text{ (g.)}}{y \text{ (g.)}}$$

y = 133.3 g. of Starch,

and

$$\frac{75 \text{ (parts)}}{50 \text{ (parts)}} = \frac{500 \text{ (g.)}}{z \text{ (g.)}}$$

z = 333.3 g. of Talc, *answers.*

(Check total: 500 g.)

Practice Problems

1. From the following formula, calculate the quantities required to make 180 ml. of Benzyl Benzoate Lotion.

Benzyl Benzoate	250 ml.
Triethanolamine	5 g.
Oleic Acid	20 g.
Purified Water, to make	1000 ml.

2. From the following formula, calculate the quantities required to make 5 gallons of Camphor and Soap Liniment.

Green Soap	120 g.
Camphor	45 g.
Rosemary Oil	10 ml.
Alcohol	700 ml.
Purified Water, to make	1000 ml.

3. From the following formula, calculate the quantities required to make 5 lb. of Hydrophilic Ointment.

Methylparaben	0.25 g.
Propylparaben	0.15 g.
Sodium Lauryl Sulfate	10. g.
Propylene Glycol	120. g.
Stearyl Alcohol	250. g.
White Petrolatum	250. g.
Purified Water, to make	1000. g.

4. From the following formula, calculate the quantity of each ingredient required to prepare 1 gallon of Orange Syrup.

Sweet Orange Peel Tincture	50 ml.
Citric Acid (anhydrous)	5 g.
Talc	15 g.
Sucrose	820 g.
Purified Water, to make	1000 ml.

5. From the following formula, calculate the quantity of each ingredient required to prepare 10 lb. of Green Soap.

Vegetable Oil	380 g.
Oleic Acid	20 g.
Potassium Hydroxide	91.7 g.
Glycerin	50 ml.
Purified Water, to make	1000 g.

6. From the following formula for 100 capsules, calculate the quantity of each ingredient required to prepare 36 capsules.

Codeine Phosphate	1.6 g.
Acetophenetidin	4.0 g.
Acetylsalicylic Acid	16.0 g.
Atropine Sulfate	0.025 g.

7. From the following formula, calculate the quantity of each ingredient required to prepare one pint of a compound ephedrine solution.

Ephedrine Sulfate	0.30 g.
Chlorobutanol	0.15 g.
Menthol	0.15 g.
Alcohol	0.60 ml.
Sodium Chloride	0.15 g.
Dextrose	0.90 g.
Amaranth Solution	0.03 ml.
Water, to make	30.00 ml.

8. From the following formula, calculate the quantity of each ingredient required to make 1500 g. of the powder.

Calcium Carbonate	5 parts
Magnesium Oxide	1 part
Sodium Bicarbonate	4 parts
Bismuth Subcarbonate	3 parts

9. From the following formula, calculate the number of grams of each ingredient required to make 1 lb. of Zinc Oxide Paste.

Zinc Oxide	1 part
Starch	1 part
White Petrolatum	2 parts

10. From the following formula, calculate the quantity of each ingredient required to make ℥ii of the ointment.

Zinc Oxide	2 parts
Coal Tar	2 parts
Starch	15 parts
Petrolatum	25 parts

11. From the following formula, calculate the quantity of each ingredient required to make one liter of the lotion.

Witch Hazel	4 parts (by volume)
Glycerin	1 part
Boric Acid Solution	15 parts

12. From the following formula, calculate the quantity of each ingredient required to prepare 1 lb. of the ointment.

Bacitracin	500,000 U.S.P. units
Liquid Petrolatum	65 g.
White Petrolatum	925 g.
To make about	1000 g.

13. From the following formula, calculate the quantity of each ingredient required to prepare 5 pints of the liniment.

Arnica Tincture	10 parts (by volume)
Methyl Salicylate	20 parts
Isopropyl Alcohol	25 parts

14. How much of each ingredient should be used to prepare 5 gal. of Phenolated Calamine Lotion?

Liquefied Phenol	10 ml.
Calamine Lotion	990 ml.

15. From the following formula, calculate the quantity of each ingredient required to prepare 5 pints of the solution.

Resorcinol Monoacetate	50 ml.
Castor Oil	25 ml.
Chloral Hydrate	75 g.
Isopropyl Alcohol, to make	1000 ml.

16. How much of each ingredient should be used in preparing 1 lb. of the following ointment?

Benzoic Acid	6 parts
Salicylic Acid	3 parts
Polyethylene Glycol Ointment	91 parts

17. How much of each ingredient should be used to prepare 5 lb. of the following ointment base?

Stearic Acid	14.0 g.
Triethanolamine	1.0 g.
Cetyl Alcohol	4.0 g.
Glycerin	8.0 g.
Water	63.0 g.

18. From the following formula, calculate the quantity of each ingredient that should be used in preparing 2500 g. of the ointment.

Resorcinol	0.6 g.
Zinc Oxide	3.0 g.
Starch	4.0 g.
White Petrolatum, to make	30.0 g.

19. Calculate the quantity of each ingredient required to make ℥iv of Aluminum Paste.

Aluminum	1.0 parts
Liquid Petrolatum	0.5 part
Zinc Oxide Ointment	8.5 parts

20. From the following formula, calculate the quantity of each ingredient that should be used in preparing ℥ii of the ointment.

Crude Coal Tar	5.0 g.
Diglycol Stearate	10.0 g.
Petrolatum, to make	100.0 g.

21. A formula for 500 capsules contains 2.5 g. of amphetamine, 32.5 g. of thyroid, 0.5 g. of thiamine hydrochloride, 4.0 g. of phenobarbital, and enough lactose to make 50 g. How much of each ingredient should be used in preparing 36 capsules?

22. From the following formula, calculate the quantity of each ingredient required to prepare 1 gallon of the mixture.

Potassium Citrate	30.0 g.
Hyoscyamus Tincture	30.0 ml.
Tween 20	0.4 ml.
Distilled Water, to make	100.0 ml.

23. How much of each ingredient is required to prepare 5 gallons of Hydriodic Acid Syrup?

Diluted Hydriodic Acid	140 ml.
Dextrose	450 g.
Purified Water, to make	1000 ml.

24. How much of each ingredient is required to prepare one hundred 0.4-g. APC Capsules?

Acetylsalicylic Acid	250 mg.
Acetophenetidin	120 mg.
Caffeine	30 mg.

25. From the following formula, calculate the quantity of each ingredient required to prepare 25 lb. of the cream.

Stearic Acid	220 g.
Wool Fat	40 g.
Triethanolamine	15 g.
Carbitol	75 g.
Distilled Water, to make	1000 g.

26. From the following formula, calculate the quantity of each ingredient required to prepare 10 pints of the lotion.

Hexachlorophene	0.1 g.
Cetyl Alcohol	0.5 g.
Isopropyl Alcohol	70.0 ml.
Purified Water, to make	100.0 ml.

27. How much of each ingredient is required to prepare 240 ml. of preserved water?

Methylparaben	0.26 g.
Propylparaben	0.14 g.
Distilled Water, to make 1000.	ml.

28. From the following formula, calculate the quantity of each ingredient required to prepare 5 gallons of mouth wash.

Zinc Chloride	2.4 g.
Menthol	0.8 g.
Soluble Saccharin	0.4 g.
Formalin	0.4 ml.
Clove Oil	0.4 ml.
Cinnamon Oil	1.6 ml.
Alcohol	100.0 ml.
Distilled Water, to make 1000.	ml.

29. A formula for 30 suppositories contains the following:

Bismuth Subgallate	6.0 g.
Peruvian Balsam	2.5 g.
Zinc Oxide	4.5 g.
Cocoa Butter	50.0 g.

How much of each ingredient should be used to prepare 8 suppositories?

30. Calculate the quantity of each ingredient required to prepare 1 lb. of the following ointment base.

Cetyl Alcohol	22.5 g.
White Wax	1.5 g.
Glycerin	15.0 g.
Sodium Lauryl Sulfate	3.0 g.
Water	108.0 g.

31. From the following formula, calculate the quantity of each ingredient required to prepare 60 ml. of the buffer solution.

Boric Acid	12.4 g.
Potassium Chloride	7.4 g.
Distilled Water, to make	1000. ml.

32. From the following formula, calculate the quantity, in grams, of each ingredient required to prepare 1 lb. of the ointment.

Crude Coal Tar	5 parts
Zinc Oxide	5 parts
Hydrophilic Petrolatum	50 parts

33. Calculate the quantity of each ingredient required to prepare 1 gallon of Salicylic Acid Lotion.

Salicylic Acid	1.0 g.
Polysorbate 80	1.5 g.
2-propyl Palmitate	3.0 g.
Isopropyl Alcohol	70.0 ml.
Distilled Water, to make	100.0 ml.

34. From the following formula, calculate the quantity, in grams, of each ingredient required to prepare 5 lb. of Hydrated Petrolatum (MGH).

Sorbitan Sesquioleate	6.0 g.
White Petrolatum	54.0 g.
Methylparaben	0.1 g.
Distilled Water, to make	100.0 g.

35. Calculate the quantity of each ingredient required to prepare 1 pint of Scott's Solution.

Merbromin	2 g.
Water	35 ml.
Acetone	10 ml.
Neutralized Alcohol, to make	100 ml.

36. From the following formula, calculate the quantity of each ingredient required to prepare 1 lb. of Compound Iodochlorhydroxyquin Powder.

Iodochlorhydroxyquin	250 g.
Lactic Acid	25 g.
Zinc Stearate	200 g.
Lactose	525 g.

37. Calculate the quantity, in grams, of each ingredient required to prepare 10 lb. of the analgesic ointment.

Menthol	5 g.
Chloral Hydrate	95 g.
Camphor	85 g.
Wool Fat	815 g.

Chapter 7

Density, Specific Gravity, and Specific Volume

THE relative weights of equal volumes of substances are shown by their densities and their specific gravities.

DENSITY

Density is mass per unit volume of a substance, *e.g.*, the number of grams per cubic centimeter or milliliter, or the number of grains per fluidounce, or the number of pounds per gallon, and so on. It is *usually* expressed as *g. per cc.* Since the *gram* is defined as the mass of 1 cc. of water at 4° C., the density of water is *1 g. per cc.* Since the *Pharmacopeia* states that 1 ml. may be used as the equivalent of 1 cc., for our purposes the density of water may be expressed as *1 g. per ml.* One (1) ml. of mercury, on the other hand, weighs 13.6 g., hence its density is *13.6 g. per ml.*

Density may be calculated by dividing mass by volume. Thus, if 10 ml. of sulfuric acid weigh 18 g., its density is:

$$\frac{18 \ (g.)}{10 \ (ml.)} \ = \ \textit{1.8 g. per ml.}$$

SPECIFIC GRAVITY

Specific gravity is a ratio, *expressed decimally*, of the weight of a substance to the weight of an equal volume of a substance chosen as a standard, both substances having the same temperature or the temperature of each being definitely known. Water is used as the standard for the specific gravities of liquids and solids; the most useful standard for gases—which have little or no pharmaceutical significance—is hydrogen (although sometimes air is used).

Specific gravity may be calculated by dividing the weight of a given substance by the weight of an equal volume of water. Thus, if 10 ml. of sulfuric acid weigh 18 g., and 10 ml. of water, under similar conditions, weigh 10 g., the specific gravity of the acid is

$$\frac{\text{Weight of 10 ml. of sulfuric acid}}{\text{Weight of 10 ml. of water}} = \frac{18 \text{ (g.)}}{10 \text{ (g.)}} = 1.8$$

Specific gravities can be expressed decimally to as many places as the accuracy of their determination warrants. In pharmaceutical work this may be two, three, or four decimal places. Since substances expand or contract at different rates when their temperatures change, variations in the specific gravity of a substance must be carefully allowed for in accurate work. In the *United States Pharmacopeia* the standard temperature for specific gravities is 25° C., except for that of alcohol, which is 15.56° C. by government regulation.

DENSITY VS. SPECIFIC GRAVITY

The density of a substance is a concrete number (*1.8 g. per ml.* in the example), while specific gravity, being a ratio between like quantities, is an abstract number (*1.8* in the example). Whereas density must vary with the table of measure, specific gravity has no dimension and is, therefore, a constant value for each substance (when measured under controlled conditions). Thus, the density of water may be variously expressed as *1 g. per ml.*, or *455 gr. per f℥*, or *62½ lbs. per cu.ft;* but the specific gravity of water is always 1.

The specific gravity of a substance and its density in the metric system are numerically equal (as a result of the definition of the gram), but they are quite different when the density is expressed in the common system.

The factor *455* (rounded off from 454.57 or 454.6 gr., the weight of 1 f℥ of water at 25° C.) is useful for calculating the approximate weight of a small volume of water measured in the apothecaries' system. But if *455* is used, the result should be expressed in no more than three significant figures. When quantities greater than a pint are involved, it is usually more convenient to convert them to their metric equivalents before calculating.

SPECIFIC GRAVITY OF LIQUIDS

To calculate the specific gravity of a liquid when its weight and volume are known:

Examples:

    If 54.96 ml. of an oil weigh 52.78 g., what is the specific gravity of the oil?

54.96 ml. of water weigh 54.96 g.

Specific gravity of oil $= \dfrac{52.78 \text{ (g.)}}{54.96 \text{ (g.)}} = 0.9603$, *answer.*

If a pint of a certain liquid weighs 9250 grains, what is the specific gravity of the liquid?

1 pint = 16 f℥

16 f℥ of water weigh 7280 grains

Specific gravity of liquid $= \dfrac{9250 \text{ (gr.)}}{7280 \text{ (gr.)}} = 1.27$, *answer.*

To calculate the specific gravity of a liquid, determined with a specific gravity bottle :

In the determination of the specific gravity of a liquid by means of a *specific gravity bottle,*[1] the container is filled and weighed first with water and then with the liquid. By subtracting the weight of the empty container from the two weights, we have the *weights of equal volumes*—even though we may not know exactly what the volumes are.

Example:

A *specific gravity bottle weighs 23.66 g. When filled with water it weighs 72.95 g.; when filled with another liquid it weighs 73.56 g. What is the specific gravity of the liquid?*

73.56 g. − 23.66 g. = 49.90 g. of liquid

72.95 g. − 23.66 g. = 49.29 g. of water

Specific gravity of liquid $= \dfrac{49.90 \text{ (g.)}}{49.29 \text{ (g.)}} = 1.180$, *answer.*

To calculate the specific gravity of a liquid determined by the displacement or plummet method :

The basis for the determination of the specific gravity of a liquid by this method is *Archimedes' principle,* which states that a body immersed in a liquid displaces an amount of the liquid equal to its own volume and suffers

[1] A container intended to be used as a specific gravity bottle, with a known capacity (commonly 10, 25, or 100 ml.) so that the weight of water it will contain is already known, is called a *pycnometer.*

an apparent loss in weight equal to the weight of the displaced liquid. Thus, we can weigh a plummet when suspended in water and when suspended in a liquid whose specific gravity is to be determined, and by subtracting from these weights the weight of the plummet in air, we get the *weights of equal volumes of the liquids* needed in our calculation.

Example:

> *A glass plummet weights 12.64 g. in air, 8.57 g. when immersed in water, and 9.12 g. when immersed in an oil. Calculate the specific gravity of the oil.*
>
> 12.64 g. — 9.12 g. = 3.52 g. of displaced oil
>
> 12.64 g. — 8.57 g. = 4.07 g. of displaced water
>
> Specific gravity of oil $= \dfrac{3.52 \text{ (g.)}}{4.07 \text{ (g.)}} = 0.865$, *answer.*

SPECIFIC GRAVITY OF SOLIDS

To calculate the specific gravity of a solid heavier than and insoluble in water :

The specific gravity of a solid *heavier than* and *insoluble in water* may be calculated simply by dividing the weight of the solid in air by the weight of water that it displaces when immersed in it. The weight of water displaced (apparent loss of weight in water) is equal to the *weight of an equal volume of water.*

Example:

> *A piece of glass weighs 38.525 g. in air and 23.525 g. when immersed in water. What is its specific gravity?*
>
> 38.525 g. — 23.525 g. = 15.000 g. of displaced water
> *(weight of an equal volume of water)*
>
> Specific gravity of glass $= \dfrac{38.525 \text{ (g.)}}{15.000 \text{ (g.)}} = 2.5683$, *answer.*

To calculate the specific gravity of a solid heavier than and soluble in water :

The weights of equal volumes of any two substances are proportional to their specific gravities. Therefore, given a solid heavier than and soluble in water, we may use the method just discussed, but *substituting some liquid of known specific gravity* in which the solid is insoluble.

Example:

> *A crystal of a chemical salt weighs 6.423 g. in air and 2.873 g. when immersed in an oil having a specific gravity of 0.858. What is the specific gravity of the salt?*

> 6.423 g. − 2.873 g. = 3.550 g. of displaced oil

$$\frac{3.550 \text{ (g. of oil)}}{6.423 \text{ (g. of salt)}} = \frac{0.858 \text{ (sp. gr. of oil)}}{x \text{ (sp. gr. of salt)}}$$

> x = 1.55, *answer.*

To calculate the specific gravity of a solid lighter than and insoluble in water:

The determination of the specific gravity of a solid *lighter than* and *insoluble in water* involves the use of a sinker which is attached to the solid in order to prevent it from floating (and therefore having no apparent weight at all). The weight of the sinker in air is of no interest to us here, but its weight when immersed in water alone must be known so that the combined weight of the solid in air and the sinker in water may be calculated. By subtracting from this weight the weight of solid and sinker when immersed in water, the weight of the water displaced by the solid (and therefore the *weight of an equal volume of water*) is calculated.

Example:

> *A piece of wax weighs 16.35 g. in air, and a sinker weighs 32.84 g. immersed in water. When they are fastened together and immersed in water, their combined weight is 29.68 g. Calculate the specific gravity of the wax.*

> 32.84 g. + 16.35 g. = 49.19 g., combined weight of sinker in water and of wax in air

> 49.19 g. − 29.68 g. = 19.51 g., weight of water displaced by wax (*weight of equal volume of water*)

> Specific gravity of wax = $\dfrac{16.35 \text{ (g.)}}{19.51 \text{ (g.)}}$ = 0.8380, *answer.*

To calculate the specific gravity of granulated solids heavier than and insoluble in water:

A specific gravity bottle can be used with crystals, powders, and other forms of solids whose volume cannot be directly measured. If such a substance is *insoluble in water*, we may weigh a portion of it, introduce this amount into the bottle, fill up the bottle with water, and weigh the mixture. The solid will displace a *volume of water equal to its own volume*, and the weight of this displaced water can be calculated.

Example:

A bottle weighs 50.0 g. when empty and 96.8 g. when filled with water. If 28.8 g. of a granulated metal are placed in the bottle and the bottle is filled with water, the total weight is 118.4 g. What is the specific gravity of the metal?

96.8 g. — 50.0 g. = 46.8 g., weight of water filling the bottle

46.8 g. + 28.8 g. = 75.6 g., combined weight of water and metal

118.4 g. — 50.0 g. = 68.4 g., combined weight of water and metal in bottle

75.6 g. — 68.4 g. = 7.2 g., weight of water displaced by metal
(*weight of equal volume of water*)

$$\text{Specific gravity of metal} = \frac{28.8 \ (g.)}{7.2 \ (g.)} = 4.0, \textit{answer.}$$

SPECIFIC VOLUME

The volume of a unit weight of a substance may be expressed in any convenient denominations, such as so-many *cubic feet per lb.* or *gallons per lb.*, but more frequently as *ml. per g.*

Specific volume, in pharmaceutical practice, is usually defined as an abstract number representing the ratio, *expressed decimally*, of the volume of a substance to the volume of an equal weight of another substance taken as a standard, both having the same temperature. Water is the standard for liquids and solids.

Whereas specific gravity is a comparison of weights of equal volumes, specific volume is a comparison of volumes of equal weights. Because of this relationship, specific gravity and specific volume are *reciprocals* of each other—that is, if they are multiplied together the product is 1. Specific volume tells us how much greater (or smaller) in volume a mass is than the same weight of water. It may be calculated by dividing the volume of a given mass by the volume of an equal weight of water. Thus, if 25 g. of glycerin measure 20 ml., and 25 g. of water measure 25 ml. under the same conditions, the specific volume of the glycerin is

$$\frac{\text{Volume of 25 g. of glycerin}}{\text{Volume of 25 g. of water}} = \frac{20 \ (ml.)}{25 \ (ml.)} = \textit{0.8}$$

To calculate the specific volume of a liquid, given the volume of a specified weight:

Example:

Calculate the specific volume of a syrup, 91.0 ml. of which weigh 107.16 g.

107.16 g. of water measure 107.16 ml.

$$\text{Specific volume of syrup} = \frac{91.0 \text{ (ml.)}}{107.16 \text{ (ml.)}} = 0.850, \textit{answer.}$$

To calculate the specific volume of a liquid, given its specific gravity, and to calculate its specific gravity given its specific volume:

Since specific gravity and specific volume are reciprocals of each other, a substance that is heavier than water will have a higher specific gravity and a lower specific volume, whereas a substance that is lighter than water will have a lower specific gravity and a higher specific volume. It follows, therefore, that we may determine the specific volume of a substance by dividing 1 by its specific gravity; and we may determine the specific gravity of a substance by dividing 1 by its specific volume.

Examples:

What is the specific volume of phosphoric acid having a specific gravity of 1.71?

$$\frac{1}{1.71} = 0.585, \textit{answer.}$$

If a liquid has a specific volume of 1.396, what is its specific gravity?

$$\frac{1}{1.396} = 0.716, \textit{answer.}$$

Practice Problems

1. If 250 ml. of alcohol weigh 203 g., what is its density?

2. A piece of copper metal weighs 53.6 g. and has a volume of 6 ml. Calculate its density.

3. A 30 ml. sample of sulfuric acid weighs 55 g. Calculate its density.

4. If 125 ml. of a liquid weigh 160 g., what is its specific gravity?

5. If 1200 ml. of a liquid weigh 1125 g., what is its specific gravity?

6. If 500 ml. of ferric chloride solution weigh 650 g., what is its specific gravity?

7. If a liter of syrup weighs 1313 g., what is its specific gravity?

8. If 134 g. of a liquid measure 142.6 ml., what is its specific gravity?

9. One pint of hydrochloric acid weighs 558 g. Calculate its specific gravity.

10. If 2 f℥ of glycerin weigh 1140 grains, what is its specific gravity?

11. If 30 ml. of a certain liquid weigh 570 grains, what is its specific gravity?

12. If 46.63 g. of an oil measure 51.5 ml., what is its specific gravity?

13. A specific gravity bottle weighs 62.35 g. Filled with water it weighs 87.42 g.; filled with another liquid it weighs 91.68 g. What is the specific gravity of the liquid?

14. A pycnometer weighs 50.0 g. When filled with water, it weighs 100.0 g.; when filled with an oil, it weighs 94.0 g. Calculate the specific gravity of the oil.

15. A pycnometer weighs 21.62 g. Filled with water it weighs 46.71 g.; filled with another liquid it weighs 43.28 g. Calculate the specific gravity of the liquid.

16. A glass stopper weighs 39.625 g. in air, 24.625 g. in water, and 28.375 g. in ether. What is the specific gravity of the ether?

17. A glass plummet weighs 14.35 g. in air, 11.40 g. when immersed in water, and 8.95 g. when immersed in sulfuric acid. Calculate the specific gravity of the acid.

18. A piece of metal weighs 8.624 g. in air and 5.615 g. when immersed in water. What is its specific gravity?

19. If a solid weighs 84.62 g. in air and 58.48 g. when immersed in water, what is its specific gravity?

20. What is the specific gravity of a solid weighing 35.555 g. in air and 32.333 g. in water?

21. A crystal of a chemical salt weighs 19.705 g. in air and 13.270 g. when immersed in alcohol. If the alcohol has a specific gravity of 0.816, what is the specific gravity of the salt?

22. A chemical crystal weighs 3.630 g. in air and 1.820 g. when immersed in an oil. If the specific gravity of the oil is 0.837, what is the specific gravity of the chemical?

23. A piece of cork weighs 154 grains in air, and a sinker weighs 921 grains in water. Together they weigh 425 grains in water. What is the specific gravity of the cork?

24. A piece of wax weighs 42.65 g. in air, and a sinker weighs 38.42 g. in water. Together they weigh 33.18 g. in water. Calculate the specific gravity of the wax.

25. A bottle holds 115 g. of water. When 20 g. of an insoluble powder are introduced into the bottle and it is filled with water, the contents weigh 125 g. What is the specific gravity of the powder?

26. An insoluble powder weighs 12 g. A specific gravity bottle, weighing 21 g. when empty, weighs 121 g. when filled with water. When the powder is introduced into the bottle and the bottle is filled with water, the three together weigh 130 g. What is the specific gravity of the powder?

27. If 73.42 g. of a liquid measure 81.5 ml., what is its specific volume?

28. If 120 g. of acetone measure 150 ml., what is its specific volume?

29. If olive oil has a specific gravity of 0.912, what is its specific volume?

30. The specific gravity of alcohol is 0.815. What is its specific volume?

31. What is the specific volume of sulfuric acid having a specific gravity of 1.826?

32. If chloroform has a specific gravity of 1.476, what is its specific volume?

33. What is the specific gravity of a liquid having a specific volume of 0.825?

34. If a liquid has a specific volume of 1.316, what is its specific gravity?

Chapter 8

Weights and Volumes of Liquids

THE weights of equal volumes and the volumes of equal weights of liquids are proportional to their specific gravities. To calculate, therefore, the *weight of a given volume* or the *volume of a given weight* of a liquid, its specific gravity must be known.

When specific gravity is used as a factor in a calculation, the result should contain no more significant figures than the number in the factor.

Because of the simple relationship between the units in the metric system, such problems are simply and easily solved when only metric quantities are involved, but they become more complex when units of the common systems are used.

CALCULATIONS OF WEIGHT

To calculate the weight of a liquid when given its volume and specific gravity:

The *weight of any given volume* of a liquid of known specific gravity can be calculated by this proportion:

$$\frac{\text{Specific gravity of water}}{\text{Specific gravity of liquid}} = \frac{\text{Weight of equal volume of water}}{\text{x}}$$

x = Weight of liquid

And from this we may derive a useful equation:

Weight of liquid =

Weight of equal volume of water × Specific gravity of liquid

Examples:

What is the weight of 3620 ml. of alcohol having a specific gravity of 0.820?

3620 ml. of water weigh 3620 g.

3620 g. × 0.820 = 2968 g., *answer.*

(**124**)

What is the weight of 4 fʒ of paraldehyde having a specific gravity of 0.990?

4 fʒ of water weigh 455 gr. × 4 or 1820 gr.

1820 gr. × 0.990 = 1802 gr., or (retaining only significant figures)
1800 gr., *answer.*

What is the weight, in grams, of 2 fʒ of a liquid having a specific gravity of 1.118?

In this type of problem it is generally best to convert the given volume to its metric equivalent first and then to solve the problem in the metric system.

2 × 29.57 ml. = 59.14 ml.

59.14 ml. of water weigh 59.14 g.

59.14 g. × 1.118 = 66.12 g., *answer.*

What is the weight, in grains, of 50 ml. of ether having a specific gravity of 0.715?

In problems of this type it is generally best to solve the problem in the metric system and then to convert the weight to the common system.

50 ml. of water weigh 50 g.

50 g. × 0.715 = 35.75 g. = 551 gr., *answer.*

CALCULATIONS OF VOLUME

To calculate the volume of a liquid when given its weight and specific gravity:

The *volume of any given weight* of a liquid of known specific gravity can be calculated by this proportion:

$$\frac{\text{Specific gravity of liquid}}{\text{Specific gravity of water}} = \frac{\text{Volume of equal weight of water}}{x}$$

x = Volume of liquid

And the derived equation will be:

$$\text{Volume of liquid} = \frac{\text{Volume of equal weight of water}}{\text{Specific gravity of liquid}}$$

Examples:

  What is the volume of 492 g. of nitric acid with a specific gravity of 1.40?

  492 g. of water measure 492 ml.

  $$\frac{492 \text{ ml.}}{1.40} = 351 \text{ ml., } \textit{answer.}$$

  What is the volume, in minims, of 1 oz. of a perfume oil having a specific gravity of 0.850?

  1 oz. = 437.5 gr.

  437.5 gr. of water measure $\dfrac{437.5}{455}$ f℥ or 462 ℳ

  $$\frac{462 \text{ ℳ}}{0.850} = 544 \text{ or } 540 \text{ ℳ, } \textit{answer.}$$

Or:

  1 oz. = 28.35 g.

  28.35 g. of water measure 28.35 ml.

  $$\frac{28.35 \text{ ml.}}{0.850} = 33.25 \text{ ml.} = 541 \text{ or } 540 \text{ ℳ, } \textit{answer.}$$

  What is the volume, in f℥, of 1 lb. of methyl salicylate with a specific gravity of 1.185?

  1 lb. = 454 g.

  454 g. of water measure 454 ml.

  $$\frac{454 \text{ ml.}}{1.185} = 383.1 \text{ ml.} = 12.96 \text{ f℥, or (with 3-figure accuracy),}$$
  $$13.0 \text{ f℥, } \textit{answer.}$$

  What is the volume, in pints, of 50 lb. of glycerin having a specific gravity of 1.25?

  50 lb. = 454 × 50 = 22700 g.

  22700 g. of water measure 22700 ml.

  $$\frac{22700 \text{ ml.}}{1.25} = 18160 \text{ ml.} = 38.4 \text{ pints, } \textit{answer.}$$

To calculate the cost of a given volume of a liquid bought by weight:

Examples:

What is the cost of 1000 ml. of glycerin, specific gravity 1.25, bought at $1.00 per lb.?

1000 ml. of water weigh 1000 g.

Weight of 1000 ml. of glycerin = 1000 g. × 1.25 = 1250 g.

1 lb. = 454 g.

$$\frac{454 \ (g.)}{1250 \ (g.)} = \frac{(\$) \ 1.00}{(\$) \ x}$$

x = $2.75, *answer.*

What is the cost of 2 f℥ of cassia oil, specific gravity 1.055, bought at $9.00 per lb.?

2 f℥ = 59.14 ml.

59.14 ml. of water weigh 59.14 g.

Weight of 59.14 ml. of oil = 59.14 g. × 1.055 = 62.39 g.

1 lb. = 454 g.

$$\frac{454 \ (g.)}{62.39 \ (g.)} = \frac{(\$) \ 9.00}{(\$) \ x}$$

x = $1.24, *answer.*

What is the cost of 1 pint of chloroform, specific gravity 1.475, bought at $1.45 per lb.?

1 pint = 473 ml.

473 ml. of water weigh 473 g.

Weight of 473 ml. of chloroform = 473 g. × 1.475 = 697.7 g.

1 lb. = 454 g.

$$\frac{454 \ (g.)}{697.7 \ (g.)} = \frac{(\$) \ 1.45}{(\$) \ x}$$

x = $2.23, *answer.*

Practice Problems

1. What is the weight of 100 ml. of hydrochloric acid having a specific gravity of 1.16?

2. What is the weight of 300 ml. of glycerin having a specific gravity of 1.25?

3. What is the weight, in grams, of 14 ml. of mercury having a specific gravity of 13.6?

4. What is the weight, in grams, of 225 ml. of sulfuric acid having a specific gravity of 1.83?

5. What is the weight, in kilograms, of 5 liters of sulfuric acid with a specific gravity of 1.84?

6. What is the weight of 650 ml. of chloroform having a specific gravity of 1.475?

7. If the specific gravity of alcohol is 0.812, what is the weight, in kilograms, of 10 liters?

8. What is the weight, in grains, of 4 f℥ of glycerin having a specific gravity of 1.25?

9. What is the weight, in pounds, of 5 pints of nitric acid having a specific gravity of 1.42?

10. What is the weight, in grams, of 1 pint of chloroform having a specific gravity of 1.475?

11. What is the weight, in grams, of 8 f℥ of an oil with a specific gravity of 0.870?

12. Calculate the weight, in grams, of 10 pints of hydrochloric acid having a specific gravity of 1.155.

13. What is the weight, in kilograms, of 1 gallon of syrup having a specific gravity of 1.313?

14. What is the weight, in grams, of 1 pint of a mixture of equal parts of alcohol (specific gravity 0.812) and glycerin (specific gravity 1.25)?

15. What is the weight, in pounds, of 4370 ml. of a syrup with a specific gravity of 1.37?

16. What is the weight, in pounds, of 1 liter of glycerin having a specific gravity of 1.25?

17. What is the volume, in milliliters, of 100 g. of an acid having a specific gravity of 1.71?

18. What is the volume, in milliliters, of 227 g. of a liquid having a specific gravity of 1.230?

19. What is the volume, in milliliters, of 1 kg. of sulfuric acid with a specific gravity of 1.83?

20. What is the volume of 1000 g. of mercury having a specific gravity of 13.6?

21. A formula calls for 425 g. of hydrochloric acid with a specific gravity of 1.155. How many milliliters of the acid should be used?

22. What is the volume of 650 g. of ferric chloride solution with a specific gravity of 1.30?

23. A formula for 1000 ml. of a preparation calls for 800 g. of cottonseed oil with a specific gravity of 0.920. How many milliliters of cottonseed oil should be used in preparing 5 liters of the formula?

24. A formula for a vanishing cream contains 750 g. of glycerin. How many milliliters of glycerin (specific gravity 1.25) should be used?

25. What is the volume, in milliliters, of 1 kilogram of peppermint oil with a specific gravity of 0.908?

26. What is the volume, in milliliters, of a liniment containing 1 lb. of chloroform (specific gravity 1.475) and 5 lb. of methyl salicylate (specific gravity 1.180)?

27. What is the volume, in pints, of 9 lb. of sulfuric acid having a specific gravity of 1.83?

28. Calculate the volume, in fluidounces, of 1 lb. of an oil with a specific gravity of 0.90±?

29. What is the volume, in pints, of 40 lb. of a liquid with a specific gravity of 1.32?

30. What is the volume, in pints, of 10 lb. of peppermint oil having a specific gravity of 0.904?

31. What is the cost of 10 liters of a liquid (specific gravity 1.20) bought at 88 cents per lb.?

32. What is the cost of 3 liters of chloroform (specific gravity 1.475) bought at $1.45 per lb.?

33. What will 10 gallons of glycerin (specific gravity 1.25) cost at 96 cents per lb.?

34. A formula for a mouth rinse contains 1.6 ml. of cinnamon oil per 1000 ml. If the cinnamon oil (specific gravity 1.050) is bought at $9.00 per lb., calculate the cost of the oil required to prepare 5 gallons of the mouth rinse.

35. A perfume oil has a specific gravity of 0.960 and costs $5.75 per kg. What is the cost of 4 f℥?

36. A prescription calls for 0.3 g. of syrupy phosphoric acid (specific gravity 1.71). How many milliliters should be used in compounding the prescription?

37. A formula for 1000 g. of a soft soap contains 380 g. of a vegetable oil. If the oil has a specific gravity of 0.890, how many milliliters should be used in preparing 10 lb. of the soft soap?

38. A cosmetic formula calls for 500 g. of peach kernel oil (specific gravity 0.910) per 1000 g. of finished product. How many milliliters of the oil should be used in preparing 5000 g. of the formula?

39. A sunscreen lotion contains 5 g. of menthyl salicylate (specific gravity 1.045) per 100 ml. How many milliliters of menthyl salicylate should be used in preparing 1 gallon of the lotion?

40. The formula for 1000 g. of Polyethylene Glycol Ointment, U.S.P., calls for 600 g. of polyethylene glycol 400. At $1.50 per pint, what is the cost of the polyethylene glycol 400, specific gravity 1.140, needed to prepare 4000 g. of the ointment?

41.

Stearic Acid	14.0 g.
Triethanolamine	0.7 g.
Cetyl Alcohol	3.0 g.
Sodium Lauryl Sulfate	0.5 g.
Propylene Glycol	5.0 g.
Distilled Water	76.8 g.

How many milliliters of triethanolamine (specific gravity 1.125) and how many milliliters of propylene glycol (specific gravity 1.035) should be used in preparing 2500 g. of the above formula?

Chapter 9

Percentage Preparations

PERCENTAGE

THE term *percent* and its corresponding sign (%) mean "by the hundred" or "in a hundred," and *percentage* means "rate per hundred"; so *50 percent* (or *50%*) and *a percentage of 50* are equivalent expressions. A percent may also be expressed as a *ratio*, represented as a common or decimal fraction. For example, *50%* means *50 parts in 100* of the same kind, and may be expressed as $\frac{50}{100}$ or *0.50*. Percent, therefore, is simply another fraction of such frequent and familiar use that its numerator is expressed, but its denominator is left understood. It should be noted that percent is always an abstract quantity, and that, as such, it may be applied to anything.

For the purposes of computation, percents are usually changed to equivalent decimal fractions. This is done by dropping the % sign and dividing the expressed numerator by *100*. Thus, *12.5%* $= \frac{12.5}{100}$, or *0.125*; and *0.05%* $= \frac{0.05}{100}$, or *0.0005*. We must not forget that in the reverse process (changing a decimal to a percent) the decimal is multiplied by *100* and the % sign is affixed.

Percentage is an essential part of pharmaceutical calculations. The pharmacist encounters it frequently and uses it as a convenient means of expressing the concentration of a solute in a solution, of the amount of active material in a drug or preparation, or of the quantity of an ingredient in a mixture.

PERCENTAGE SOLUTIONS

Percentage, as it applies to solutions, has a very special meaning. It was pointed out above that percentage expresses *parts per 100 parts*. Obviously, then, in a *true percentage solution* the *parts* of the percentage would represent *grams* of a solute in *100 g.* of solution. In general practice, however, the pharmacist most frequently encounters a different kind of percentage solution, one in which the *parts* of the percentage represent *grams* of a solute in *100 ml.* of solution. In order to avoid the possibility of any misinterpretation of the meaning of the term "percentage solution," the *United States Pharmacopeia* states that:

"Percentage concentrations of solutions are expressed as follows:

"*Percent weight in weight*—(w/w) expresses the number of g. of a constituent in 100 g. of solution.

"*Percent weight in volume*—(w/v) expresses the number of g. of a constituent in 100 ml. of solution, and is used regardless of whether water or another liquid is the solvent.

"*Percent volume in volume*—(v/v) expresses the number of ml. of a constituent in 100 ml. of solution.

"The term *percent* used without qualification means, for mixtures of solids, percent weight in weight; for solutions or suspensions of solids in liquids, percent weight in volume; for solutions of liquids in liquids, percent volume in volume; and for solutions of gases in liquids, percent weight in volume. For example, a 1% solution is prepared by dissolving 1 g. of a solid or 1 ml. of a liquid in sufficient of the solvent to make 100 ml. of the solution.

"In the dispensing of prescription medications, slight changes in volume owing to variations in room temperatures may be disregarded."[1]

PERCENTAGE WEIGHT-IN-VOLUME

One way of making all weight-in-volume solutions conform to this official interpretation would be to convert all common and apothecaries' weights to grams and all volumes to milliliters before expressing percentage strength. But such a procedure is not required.

For, if *1 gram* in *100 milliliters of solution* is taken as the only "correct" strength of a 1% (w/v) solution, this means that 1 gram of solute is contained in a volume of solution *that would weigh 100 grams if, like water, the solution had a specific gravity of 1*—if, in other words, each milliliter of solution weighed *1 gram*. Hence, to make a solution of the same strength by any system of measure, we have only to dissolve *1* weight unit of solute in sufficient solvent to make a volume that would weigh *100* of those weight units if the solution were pure water.

A solution so compounded, then, would contain not only *1 g.* in every *100 ml.* (the volume of *100 g.* of water) but likewise approximately *4.55* grains[2] in every fluidounce (the volume of *455 grains* of water at 25° C.). Therefore, we may look upon a *weight-in-volume* solution as a kind of *weight-in-weight* solution in disguise: the percentage strength being based after all upon a comparison of parts by weight, but the weight of the solution being arbitrarily calculated from its designated volume as if it had a specific gravity of *1*.

---

[1] U.S.P. XVIII, 1970: General Notices, page 12.

[2] "Disregarding the difference between cubic centimeter and milliliter, which

To calculate the weight of the active ingredient in a specified volume of solution, given its percentage weight-in-volume :

Taking water to represent any solvent, we may prepare weight-in-volume percentage solutions which are equivalent in strength when calculated by either the metric or the apothecaries' system if we use the following rules:

---

is so small that it does not affect the equivalents used, this quantity was derived as follows:

> 1 cubic centimeter of water at 4° C. weighs 1 gram
> 1 fluidounce = 29.573 cubic centimeters
> 1 gram = 15.4324 grains

Using these equivalents

> 100 cc.   :   29.573 cc.   = 1 Gm.   : x
>   x = 0.29573 Gm.
> 1 Gm.   :   0.29573 Gm. = 15.4324 gr. : y
>   y = 4.5638 grains

"This would be the number of grains of a solid in 1 fluidounce of a 1 per cent solution if the liquid were measured at 4° C., but percentage solutions are generally prepared at or near the official temperature of 25° C., and any volume of a liquid weighs slightly less at 25° C. than it does at 4° C. The effect of this is that a theoretical 1% solution, containing 4.5638 grains of a chemical in 1 fluidounce at 4° C., will contain less than this weight in 1 fluidounce if it were prepared at 4° C. and the fluidounce is measured at 25° C. The quantities are approximately proportional to the quantities of water in fluidounces measured at each of the respective temperatures. The correction of this slight difference can be made by the following methods:

> 1 fluidounce of water weighs 456.38 grains in vacuum at 4° C.
> 1 fluidounce of water weighs 454.57 grains in air at 25° C.
> Using these numbers, we have this proportion:
> 456.38 : 454.57 = 4.5638 : z
>   z = 4.5457 grains in 1 fluidounce of a 1 per cent
>   solution at 25° C.

"In this correction, water is taken to represent any solvent, and the small amount of solvent displaced by the solid is disregarded. This can be done without introducing an appreciable error for any ordinary percentage solution, because the total difference is so small.

"The number of grains in one fluidounce of a 1 per cent weight-in-volume solution may be rounded off to 4.5, 4.55, or 4.546, to attain different degrees of accuracy in preparing such solutions."

(Quoted from "The Calculation of Percentage Solutions in the U.S.P. XI" by Dr. Theodore J. Bradley, *American Druggist*, July, 1936.)

Rule 1. In the metric system, multiply the required number of milliliters by the percentage strength, expressed as a decimal, to obtain the number of grams of solute in the solution. *The volume in milliliters represents the weight in grams of the solution if it were pure water.*

Vol. in ml. × % (expressed as a decimal) = g. of solute

Rule 2. In the apothecaries' system, multiply the *weight* of a fluidounce of water (455 grains) by the required number of fluidounces and by the percentage strength, expressed as a decimal, to obtain the number of grains of solute in the solution. *The volume in fluidounces times 455 grains represents the weight in grains of the solution if it were pure water.*

Vol. in f℥ × 455 gr. × % (expressed as a decimal) = gr. of solute

Examples:

How many grams of dextrose are required to prepare 4000 ml. of a 5% solution?

4000 ml. represent 4000 g. of solution

$$5\% = 0.05$$
$$4000 \text{ g.} \times 0.05 = 200 \text{ g., } answer.$$

How many grams of potassium permanganate should be used in compounding the following prescription?

> ℞ Potassium Permanganate   0.02%
>   Distilled Water   ad   250.0
>   Sig. As directed.

250 ml. represent 250 g. of solution

$$0.02\% = 0.0002$$
$$250 \text{ g.} \times 0.0002 = 0.05 \text{ g., } answer.$$

How many grains of mild silver protein should be used in preparing 4 f℥ of a 10% solution?

4 f℥ represent 4 × 455 gr. of solution

$$10\% = 0.10$$
$$4 \times 455 \text{ gr.} \times 0.10 = 182 \text{ gr., } answer.$$

How many grains of atropine sulfate should be used in compounding the following prescription?

R   Atropine Sulfate   2%
     Distilled Water   q.s.   ad   ℨiv
     Sig. Use in the eye.

$$\text{ℨiv} = \tfrac{1}{2}\ \text{f℥}$$

$\tfrac{1}{2}$ f℥ represents $\tfrac{1}{2}$ × 455 gr. of solution

$$2\% = 0.02$$

$\tfrac{1}{2}$ × 455 gr. × 0.02 = 4.55 gr., *answer.*

To calculate the percentage weight-in-volume of a solution, given the weight of the solute and the volume of the solution:

It should be remembered that the volume, in milliliters, of the solution represents the weight, in grams, of the solution if it were pure water.

Examples:

What is the percentage strength (w/v) of a solution of urea, if 80 ml. contain 12 g.?

80 ml. of water weigh 80 g.

$$\frac{80\ \text{(g.)}}{12\ \text{(g.)}} = \frac{100\ (\%)}{\text{x}\ (\%)}$$

x = 15%, *answer.*

What is the percentage strength (w/v) of a solution of boric acid if 45.5 grains are dissolved in enough water to make 8 f℥?

8 f℥ of water weigh 3640 gr.

$$\frac{3640\ \text{(gr.)}}{45.5\ \text{(gr.)}} = \frac{100\ (\%)}{\text{x}\ (\%)}$$

x = 1.25%, *answer.*

To calculate the volume of a solution, given its percentage strength weight-in-volume and the weight of the solute:

Examples:

> *How many milliliters of a 3% solution can be made from 27 g. of ephedrine sulfate?*

$$\frac{3\ (\%)}{100\ (\%)} = \frac{27\ (g.)}{x\ (g.)}$$

x = 900 g., weight of the solution if it were water

Volume in ml. = 900 ml., *answer.*

> *How many fluidounces of a 10% solution can be made from 182 grains of silver nitrate?*

$$\frac{10\ (\%)}{100\ (\%)} = \frac{182\ (gr.)}{x\ (gr.)}$$

x = 1820 gr., weight of solution if it were water

Volume in f℥ = $\frac{1820}{455}$ f℥ = 4 f℥, *answer.*

PERCENTAGE VOLUME-IN-VOLUME

Liquids are usually measured by volume, and the percentage strength indicates the number of parts by volume of the active ingredient that are contained in the total volume of the solution considered as 100 parts by volume. If there is any possibility of misinterpretation, this kind of percentage should be specified: *e.g., 10% (v/v).*

To calculate the volume of the active ingredient in a specified volume of a solution, given its percentage strength volume-in-volume:

Examples:

> *How many milliliters of liquefied phenol should be used in compounding the following prescription?*

℞	Liquefied Phenol	2.5%
	Boric Acid Solution ad	240.0 ml.
	Sig. For external use.	

Volume in ml. × % (expressed as a decimal) = ml. of active ingredient
240 ml. × 0.025 = 6 ml., *answer.*

How many minims of wintergreen oil should be used in compounding the following prescription?

R̠ Wintergreen Oil   5%
   Isopropyl Alcohol   ad   f℥iv
   Sig. Apply.

Vol. in m $\times$ % (expressed as a decimal) = vol. in m of active ingredient
    480 m $\times$ 4 $\times$ 0.05 = 96 m, *answer.*

To calculate the percentage volume-in-volume of a solution, given the volume of active ingredient and the volume of the solution:

The required volumes may have to be calculated from given weights and specific gravities.

Examples:

In preparing 250 ml. of a certain lotion, a pharmacist used 4 ml. of liquefied phenol. What was the percentage (v/v) of liquefied phenol in the lotion?

$$\frac{250 \ (ml.)}{4 \ (ml.)} = \frac{100 \ (\%)}{x \ (\%)}$$

x = 1.6%, *answer.*

A formula for 8 f℥ of a mouth rinse contains 10 m of a flavoring oil. What is the percentage (v/v) of the oil in the mouth rinse?

8 f℥ = 3840 m

$$\frac{3840 \ (m)}{10 \ (m)} = \frac{100 \ (\%)}{x \ (\%)}$$

x = 0.26%, *answer.*

What is the percentage strength (v/v) of a solution of 800 g. of a liquid with a specific gravity of 0.800 in enough water to make 4000 ml.?

800 g. of water measure 800 ml.

800 ml. ÷ 0.800 = 1000 ml. of active ingredient

$$\frac{4000 \ (ml.)}{1000 \ (ml.)} = \frac{1000 \ (\%)}{x \ (\%)}$$

x = 25%, *answer.*

To calculate the volume of a solution, given the volume of the active ingredient and its percentage strength (v/v):

The volume of the active ingredient may have to be first calculated from its weight and specific gravity.

Examples:

> *Peppermint spirit contains 10% (v/v) of peppermint oil. What volume of the spirit will contain 75 ml. of peppermint oil?*

$$\frac{10\ (\%)}{100\ (\%)} = \frac{75\ (ml.)}{x\ (ml.)}$$

x = 750 ml., *answer.*

> *Chloroform liniment contains 30% (v/v) of chloroform. How many milliliters of chloroform liniment can be prepared from 1 lb. of chloroform (sp. gr. 1.475)?*

1 lb. = 454 g.

454 g. of water measure 454 ml.

454 ml. ÷ 1.475 = 308 ml. of chloroform

$$\frac{30\ (\%)}{100\ (\%)} = \frac{308\ (ml.)}{x\ (ml.)}$$

x = 1027 or 1030 ml., *answer.*

PERCENTAGE WEIGHT-IN-WEIGHT

Percentage weight-in-weight (*true percentage* or *percentage by weight*) indicates the number of parts by weight of active ingredient that are contained in the total weight of the solution considered as 100 parts by weight.

Liquids are not customarily measured by weight, and therefore, a weight-in-weight solution of a solid or a liquid in a liquid should be so designated: *e.g., 10% (w/w).*

To calculate the weight of the active ingredient in a specified weight of the solution, given its weight-in-weight percentage strength:

Examples:

>   *How many grams of phenol should be used to prepare 240 g. of a 5%*
>   *(w/w) solution in water?*

Weight of solution in g. $\times$ % (expressed as a decimal) = g. of
solute

240 g. $\times$ 0.05 = 12 g., *answer.*

>   *How many g. of a chemical are required to make 120 ml. of a 20% (w/w)*
>   *solution having a specific gravity of 1.15?*

120 ml. of water weigh 120 g.

120 g. $\times$ 1.15 = 138 g., weight of 120 ml. of solution

138 g. $\times$ 0.20 = 27.6 g. plus enough water to make 120 ml., *answer.*

To calculate the weight of either active ingredient or diluent, given the weight of the other and the percentage strength (w/w) of the solution:

The weights of active ingredient and diluent are proportional to their
percentages.

Example:

>   *How many grams of a chemical should be dissolved in 240 ml. of water*
>   *to make a 4% (w/w) solution?*

100% − 4% = 96% (by weight) of water

240 ml. of water weigh 240 g.

$$\frac{96\ (\%)}{4\ (\%)} = \frac{240\ (g.)}{x\ (g.)}$$

x = 10 g., *answer.*

It is usually impossible to prepare a specified *volume* of a solution of given
weight-in-weight percentage strength, since the volume displaced by the
active ingredient cannot be known in advance. If an excess is not unde-
sirable, we may make a volume somewhat more than that specified by
taking the given volume to refer to the solvent and from this quantity
calculating the weight of the solvent (the specific gravity of the solvent
must be known). Using this weight, we may follow the method above to
calculate the corresponding weight of the active ingredient needed.

Examples:

> *How should you prepare 100 ml. of a 2% (w/w) solution of a chemical in a solvent having a specific gravity of 1.25?*

100 ml. of water weigh 100 g.

100 g. × 1.25 = 125 g., weight of 100 ml. of solvent

100% − 2% = 98% (by weight) of solvent

$$\frac{98\ (\%)}{2\ (\%)} = \frac{125\ (g.)}{x\ (g.)}$$

x = 2.55 g.

2.55 g. of chemical and 125 g. (or 100 ml.) of solvent, *answer.*

> *How should you prepare 6 f℥ of a 20% (w/w) solution of a chemical in water?*

6 f℥ of water weigh 2730 gr.

100% − 20% = 80% (by weight) of solvent

$$\frac{80\ (\%)}{20\ (\%)} \quad \frac{2730\ (gr.)}{x\ (gr.)}$$

x = 682 gr.

682 gr. of chemical plus 6 f℥ of water, *answer.*

To calculate the percentage strength (w/w) of a solution, given the weight of the active ingredient and the weight of the solution:

If the weight of the finished solution is not given, other data must be supplied from which it may be calculated: the weights of both ingredients, for instance, or the volume and the specific gravity of the solution.

Examples:

> *If 1500 g. of a solution contain 75 g. of a chemical, what is the percentage strength (w/w) of the solution?*

$$\frac{1500\ (g.)}{75\ (g.)} = \frac{100\ (\%)}{x\ (\%)}$$

x = 5%, *answer.*

If 5 g. of boric acid are dissolved in 100 ml. of water, what is the percentage strength (w/w) of the solution?

100 ml. of water weigh 100 g.

100 g. + 5 g. = 105 g., weight of solution

$$\frac{105 \ (g.)}{5 \ (g.)} = \frac{100 \ (\%)}{x \ (\%)}$$

x = 4.76%, *answer.*

If 1000 ml. of syrup with a specific gravity of 1.313 contain 850 g. of sucrose, what is its percentage strength (w/w)?

1000 ml. of water weigh 1000 g.

1000 g. × 1.313 = 1313 g., weight of 1000 ml. of syrup

$$\frac{1313 \ (g.)}{850 \ (g.)} = \frac{100 \ (\%)}{x \ (\%)}$$

x = 64.7%, *answer.*

To calculate the weight of a solution, given the weight of its active ingredient and its percentage strength (w/w):

Example:

What weight of a 5% (w/w) solution can be prepared from 2 g. of active ingredient?

$$\frac{5 \ (\%)}{100 \ (\%)} = \frac{2 \ (g.)}{x \ (g.)}$$

x = 40 g., *answer.*

WEIGHT-IN-WEIGHT MIXTURES OF SOLIDS

Solids are usually measured by weight, and the percentage strength of a mixture of solids indicates the number of parts by weight of the active ingredient that are contained in the total weight of the mixture considered as *100 parts* by weight.

To calculate the amount of active ingredient in a specified weight of a mixture of solids, given its percentage strength (w/w):

Examples:

How many milligrams of hydrocortisone should be used in compounding the following prescription?

  R Hydrocortisone $\frac{1}{8}$%
    Hydrophilic Ointment ad 10.0 g.
    Sig. Apply.

    $\frac{1}{8}$% = 0.125%

    10 g. × 0.00125 = 0.0125 g. or 12.5 mg., *answer.*

How many grains of ammoniated mercury should be used in compounding the following prescription?

  R Ammoniated Mercury   10%
    Hydrophilic Petrolatum ad ℨiv
    Sig. Apply to affected areas.

    ℨiv = 240 gr.

    240 gr. × 0.10 = 24 gr., *answer.*

How many grams of merbromin should be used in compounding the following prescription?

  R Merbromin   2%
    Polyethylene Glycol Base ad 2.0
    Make 24 such suppositories
    Sig. Insert one as directed.

    2 g. × 24 = 48 g., total weight of mixture

    48 g. × 0.02 = 0.96 g., *answer.*

How many grains of chlorophenothane should be used in compounding the following prescription?

  R Chlorophenothane   5%
    Talc   ad ℥iv
    Sig. Apply locally.

    ℥iv = 1920 gr.

    1920 gr. × 0.05 = 96 gr., *answer.*

RATIO STRENGTH

The concentrations of weak solutions are very frequently expressed in terms of ratio strength. Since all percentages are a ratio of parts per hundred, ratio strength is merely another way of expressing the percentage strength of solutions (and, less frequently, of mixtures of solids). For example, *5%* means *5 parts per 100* or *5:100*. Although *5 parts per 100* designates a ratio strength, it is customary to translate this designation into a ratio the first figure of which is *1;* thus, *5:100 = 1:20*.

When a ratio strength, for example *1:1000*, is used to designate a concentration, it is to be interpreted as follows:

For solids in liquids—*1 gram* of solute in *1000 milliliters* of solution or *1 grain* of solute in a volume of solution represented by that of *1000 grains* of water.

For liquids in liquids—*1 milliliter* of active ingredient in *1000 milliliters* of solution or *1 minim* of active ingredient in *1000 minims* of solution.

For solids in solids—*1 gram* of active ingredient in *1000 grams* of mixture or *1 grain* of active ingredient in *1000 grains* of mixture.

The ratio and percentage strengths of any solution or mixture of solids are proportional, and either is easily converted to the other by the use of proportion.

To calculate ratio strength, given the percentage strength:

Example:

Express 0.02% as a ratio strength.

$$\frac{0.02\ (\%)}{100\ (\%)} = \frac{1\ (\text{part})}{x\ (\text{parts})}$$

x = 5000

Ratio strength = 1:5000, *answer.*

To calculate percentage strength, given the ratio strength:

Example:

Express 1:4000 as a percentage strength.

$$\frac{4000 \ (parts)}{1 \ (part)} = \frac{100 \ (\%)}{x \ (\%)}$$

x = 0.025%, *answer.*

To calculate the ratio strength of a solution, given the weight of solute in a specified volume of solution:

Example:

A certain injectable contains 2 mg. of a drug per ml. of solution. What is the ratio strength (w/v) of the solution?

2 mg. = 0.002 g.

$$\frac{0.002 \ (g.)}{1 \ (g.)} = \frac{1 \ (ml.)}{x \ (ml.)}$$

x = 500 ml.

Ratio strength = 1:500, *answer.*

What is the ratio strength (w/v) of a solution made by dissolving two tablets, each containing 0.125 g. of mercury bichloride, in enough water to make 500 ml.?

0.125 g. × 2 = 0.250 g. of mercury bichloride

$$\frac{0.250 \ (g.)}{1 \ (g.)} = \frac{500 \ (ml.)}{x \ (ml.)}$$

x = 2000 ml.

Ratio strength = 1:2000, *answer.*

To solve problems involving ratio strength:

In solving problems in which the calculations are based on ratio strength, it is sometimes convenient to translate the problem into one based on percentage strength and to solve it according to the rules and methods discussed under percentage solutions and percentage mixtures of solids.

Examples:

How many grams of potassium permanganate should be used in preparing 500 ml. of a 1:2500 solution?

1:2500 = 0.04%

500 (g.) × 0.0004 = 0.2 g., *answer.*

Or,

1:2500 means 1 g. in 2500 ml. of solution

$$\frac{2500 \text{ (ml.)}}{500 \text{ (ml.)}} = \frac{1 \text{ (g.)}}{x \text{ (g.)}}$$

x = 0.2 g., *answer.*

How many milligrams of gentian violet should be used in preparing the following solution?

R Gentian Violet Solution   500 ml.
         1:10,000
     Sig. Instill as directed.

1:10,000 = 0.01%

500 (g.) × 0.001 = 0.050 g. or 50 mg., *answer.*

Or,

1:10,000 means 1 g. in 10,000 ml. of solution

$$\frac{10,000 \text{ (ml.)}}{500 \text{ (ml.)}} = \frac{1 \text{ (g.)}}{x \text{ (g.)}}$$

How many grains of mercuric chloride are required to prepare f℥viii of a 1:4000 solution?

1:4000 = 0.025%

455 (gr.) × 0.00025 × 8 = 0.91, or 0.9., *answer.*

Or,

1:4000 means 1 gr. in a volume of solution represented by that of 4000 gr. of water

8 f℥ of water weigh 3640 gr.

$$\frac{4000 \text{ (gr.)}}{3640 \text{ (gr.)}} = \frac{1 \text{ (gr.)}}{x \text{ (gr.)}}$$

x = 0.91, or 0.9 gr., *answer.*

How many milligrams of hexachlorophene should be used in compounding the following prescription?

℞ Hexachlorophene   1:400
    Hydrophilic Ointment   ad   10 g.
    Sig. Apply.

1:400 = 0.25%

10 g. × 0.0025 = 0.025 g. or 25 mg., *answer.*

Or,

1:400 means 1 g. in 400 g. of ointment

$$\frac{400 \text{ (g.)}}{10 \text{ (g.)}} = \frac{1 \text{ (g.)}}{x \text{ (g.)}}$$

x = 0.025 g. or 25 mg., *answer.*

How many grains of tetracaine should be used in compounding the following prescription?

℞ Tetracaine   1:200
    White Petrolatum   ad   ℥ii
    Sig. Apply to eye.

1:200 = 0.5%

℥ii = 120 gr.

120 gr. × 0.005 = 0.6 gr., *answer.*

Or,

1:200 means 1 gr. in 200 gr. of ointment

$$\frac{200 \text{ (gr.)}}{120 \text{ (gr.)}} = \frac{1 \text{ (gr.)}}{x \text{ (gr.)}}$$

x = 0.6 gr., *answer.*

Practice Problems

1. How many grams of mercuric chloride are required to prepare 250 ml. of a 5% (w/v) solution?

2. How many grams of boric acid are there in 30 ml. of a 2% (w/v) solution?

3. How many grams of phenol are required to prepare 480 ml. of a $\frac{1}{10}$% (w/v) solution?

4. ℞ Antipyrine   5%
       Glycerin   ad   60.0
       Sig. For the ear.

How many grams of antipyrine should be used in compounding the prescription?

5. ℞ Sol. Ephedrine Sulfate
          0.5%   60 ml.
       Sig. For the nose.

How many grams of ephedrine sulfate should be used in compounding the prescription?

6. How many milligrams of amaranth should be used in preparing 250 ml. of a 0.01% solution?

7. ℞ Resin of Podophyllum   25%
       Compound Benzoin Tincture ad 30.0
       Sig. Apply to warts.

How many grams of resin of podophyllum should be used in compounding the prescription?

8. ℞ Neo-Silvol Solution 10%
       Ephedrine Sulfate Solution 3%   aa   15.0 ml.
       Sig. For the nose.

How many grams of Neo-Silvol and how many milligrams of ephedrine sulfate should be used in compounding the prescription?

9. ℞ Atropine Sulfate Solution   30 ml.
                $\frac{1}{20}\%$
Sig.   Two drops in each feeding.

How many milligrams of atropine sulfate should be used in compounding the prescription?

10. ℞ Potassium Permanganate   0.01%
        Distilled Water   ad   250.0
        Sig. For irrigation.

How many milligrams of potassium permanganate should be used in compounding the prescription?

11. How many grains of silver nitrate should be used in preparing 1 pint of a 0.025% (w/v) solution?

12. How many grains of gentian violet should be used in preparing f℥ii of a ½% (w/v) solution?

13. ℞ Phenol   5%
        Glycerin   ad   ℥ii
        Sig.   Ear drops.

How many grains of phenol should be used in compounding the prescription?

14. ℞ Sol. Potassium Iodide
            100%   ℥i
        Sig. Ten drops in water a.c.

How many grains of potassium iodide should be used in compounding the prescription?

15. ℞ Cocaine   2%
        Mineral Oil   ad   ℥i
        Sig.   Nasal spray.

How many grains of cocaine should be used in compounding the prescription?

16. ℞ Argyrol   5%
        Distilled Water   ad   ℥iv
        Sig.   Swab as directed.

How many grains of Argyrol should be used in compounding the prescription?

17. ℞ Pilocarpine Nitrate   4%
        Phosphate Buffer Solution ad   ℥ ii
        Sig. For the eye.

How many grains of pilocarpine nitrate should be used in compounding the prescription?

18. ℞ Iodine   1%
        Potassium Iodide   2%
        Glycerin   ad   ℥ ii
        Sig. Use as a swab.

How many grains of iodine and of potassium iodide should be used in compounding the prescription?

19. A formula for a mouth rinse contains $\frac{1}{10}$% (w/v) of zinc chloride. How many grams of zinc chloride should be used in preparing 25 liters of the mouth rinse?

20. If 425 g. of sucrose are dissolved in enough water to make 500 ml., what is the percentage strength (w/v) of the solution?

21. If 2 liters of a solution of iodine in alcohol contain 7 g. of iodine, what is the percentage strength (w/v) of the solution?

22. If 0.25 g. of potassium permanganate is dissolved in enough distilled water to make a liter, what is the percentage strength of the solution?

23. If 60 mg. of phenacaine hydrochloride and 0.45 g. of boric acid are dissolved in enough distilled water to make 30 ml., what is the percentage of each in the solution?

24. If 1 gallon of a solution contains 18.2 gr. of potassium permanganate, what is the percentage strength of the solution?

25. A proprietary ophthalmic solution contains 2 gr. of zinc sulfate and 20 gr. of boric acid per fluidounce. Calculate the percentage of zinc sulfate and of boric acid in the solution.

26. How many milliliters of a $\frac{1}{10}$% (w/v) solution can be prepared from 1 g. of atropine sulfate?

27. How many liters of a 2% (w/v) iodine tincture can be made from 123 g. of iodine?

28. How many milliliters of a 10% (w/v) solution can be made from $\frac{1}{4}$ oz. of silver nucleinate?

29. How many milliliters of a 0.9% (w/v) sodium chloride solution can be made from 1 lb. of sodium chloride?

30. How many milliliters of a $\frac{1}{10}$% (w/v) solution of mercury bichloride can be prepared from 20 tablets, each containing 0.47 g.?

31. How many fluidounces of a $\frac{1}{2}$% solution can be prepared from 45 gr. of chlorobutanol?

32. A certain formula contains $\frac{1}{5}$% (v/v) of amaranth solution. How many milliliters of amaranth solution should be used in preparing 5 liters of the formula?

33. Peppermint Spirit contains 10% (v/v) of peppermint oil. How many milliliters of peppermint oil should be used in preparing 1 gallon of the spirit?

34. A sunscreen lotion contains 5% (v/v) of menthyl salicylate. How many milliliters of menthyl salicylate should be used in preparing 5 pints of the lotion?

35. A certain vehicle is to contain 15% (v/v) of glycerin. How many milliliters of glycerin should be used in preparing 5 gallons of the vehicle?

36. How many milliliters of wintergreen oil should be used to prepare 150 ml. of a 2.5% (v/v) solution in alcohol?

37. Chloroform liniment contains 30% (v/v) of chloroform. How many milliliters of chloroform should be used in preparing 5 pints of the liniment?

38. How many milliliters of liquefied phenol should be used in preparing 1 gallon of phenolated calamine lotion which contains 1% of liquefied phenol?

39. ℞ Mercury Bichloride   0.1%
        Resorcin Monoacetate   3.0%
        Isopropyl Alcohol   ad   250 ml.
        Sig. For the scalp.

How many milligrams of mercury bichloride and how many milliliters of resorcin monoacetate should be used in compounding the prescription?

40. ℞ Liquefied Phenol   0.5%
        Zinc Oxide   5.0%
        Lime Water   ad   ℥ viii
        Sig. Apply.

How many minims of liquefied phenol and how many grains of zinc oxide should be used in compounding the prescription?

41. ℞ Formic Acid Spirit   2.5%
        Isopropanol   ad   ℥ viii
        Sig. For the scalp.

How many minims of formic acid spirit should be used in compounding the prescription?

42. How many grains of zinc sulfate and how many minims of adrenalin solution should be used in preparing f℥ iv of an ophthalmic solution which is to contain $\frac{1}{10}$% of zinc sulfate and 2% of adrenalin solution?

43. If 1.32 ml. of liquefied phenol are dissolved in enough water to make 60 ml., what is the percentage strength (v/v) of the solution?

44. One gallon of a certain lotion contains 946 ml. of benzyl benzoate. Calculate the percentage (v/v) of benzyl benzoate in the lotion.

45. Lavender Spirit contains 12.5 ml. of lavender oil in 250 ml. Calculate the percentage strength (v/v) of the spirit.

46. A formula for 1 liter of an elixir contains 0.25 ml. of a flavoring oil. What is the percentage (v/v) of the flavoring oil in the elixir?

47. If f℥ iii of a solution contain 300 minims of an active ingredient, what is the percentage strength (v/v) of the solution?

48. Paregoric contains the equivalent of 0.4% of opium. How many milliliters of opium tincture (10% w/v) would contain the same equivalent as 100 ml. of paregoric?

49. Belladonna leaf contains 0.3% of alkaloids. How many milligrams of alkaloids are contained in 100 ml. of belladonna tincture (10%)?

50. ℞ Coal Tar Solution   15.0
        Glycerin   30.0
        Boric Acid Solution   ad   240.0
        Sig. Apply.

If coal tar solution contains the equivalent of 20% of active material, what percentage of the material is represented in the finished product?

51. ℞ Precipitated Sulfur   ℥i
       Alcohol   ℥iss
       Calamine Lotion   ad   ℥viii
       Sig. Apply locally.

Calculate the percentage (v/v) of alcohol in the finished product.

52. ℞ Zinc Sulfate   0.03
       Tetracaine Hydrochloride
          Solution 2%   5.0
       Boric Acid Solution   ad   30.0
       Sig. One drop o.d. as directed.

Calculate the percentage of tetracaine hydrochloride in the finished product.

53. A liniment contains 15% (v/v) of methyl salicylate. How many milliliters of the liniment can be made from 240 ml. of methyl salicylate?

54. How many milliliters of 6.5% (v/v) cinnamon spirit can be prepared from 50 ml. of cinnamon oil?

55. How many grams of a chemical are required to make 750 g. of a 0.25% (w/w) solution?

56. How many grams of tannic acid are required to prepare 375 g. of a 5% (w/w) solution in glycerin?

57. How many grams of sucrose must be dissolved in 475 ml. of water to make a 65% (w/w) solution?

58. How many grams of a chemical are required to prepare 1 liter of a 25% (w/w) solution having a specific gravity of 1.10%?

59. How many grams of tannic acid must be dissolved in 320 ml. of glycerin having a specific gravity of 1.25 to make a 20% (w/w) solution?

60. How should you prepare f℥ii of a 25% (w/w) solution of a chemical in water?

61. How many grams of a chemical should be dissolved in 180 ml. of water to make a 10% (w/w) solution?

62. If 3.1 g. of a chemical are dissolved in 13.9 ml. of water, what is the percentage strength (w/w) of the solution?

63. What is the percentage strength (w/w) of a solution made by dissolving 62.5 g. of potassium chloride in 187.5 ml. of water?

64. A ferric chloride solution has a specific gravity of 1.300 and contains the equivalent of 374 g. of iron in 2290 ml. Calculate the percentage strength (w/w) of the solution.

65. If 198 g. of dextrose are dissolved in 1000 ml. of water, what is the percentage strength (w/w) of the solution?

66. Twenty (20) g. of tannic acid are dissolved in 64 ml. of glycerin having a specific gravity of 1.25. Calculate the percentage (w/w) of tannic acid in the solution.

67. What weight of a 20% (w/w) solution can be made from 5 g. of a chemical?

68. How many grams of resorcinol and how many grams of hexachlorophene should be used in preparing 5 lb. of an acne ointment which is to contain 2% of resorcinol and 0.25% of hexachlorophene?

69. ℞   Basic Fuchsin   0.5%
      Hydrophilic Petrolatum   ad   ℥ i
      Sig.   Apply to affected area.

How many grains of basic fuchsin should be used in compounding the prescription?

70. ℞   Salicylic Acid   2%
      Menthol $\frac{1}{4}$%
      Talc   ad   60 g.
      Sig.   Dust on.

How many grams of salicylic acid and how many milligrams of menthol should be used in compounding the prescription?

71. One liter of purified water is mixed with 5 lb. of wool fat. Calculate the percentage (w/w) of purified water in the finished product.

72.   Sodium Borate   10.0%
       Sodium Perborate   5.0%
       Menthol   0.1%
       Camphor   0.1%
       Rose Soluble   0.2%
       Sodium Bicarbonate, to make   100.0%
       Label: Douche powder.

How many grams of each ingredient should be used in preparing 1 lb. of the powder?

73. How many milligrams of procaine hydrochloride should be used in preparing 120 suppositories each weighing 2 g. and containing ¼% of procaine hydrochloride?

74. How many milligrams of hydrocortisone acetate are contained in 5 g. of ⅛% hydrocortisone acetate ophthalmic ointment?

75. How many grains of ammoniated mercury and how many grains of an ophthalmic ointment base should be used in preparing ℥iv of a 3% ammoniated mercury ophthalmic ointment?

76. You are directed to mix an ounce of Whitfield's Ointment (6% salicylic acid) and two ounces of Lassar's Zinc Paste with Salicylic Acid (2% salicylic acid) with enough white petrolatum to make four ounces. What is the percentage of salicylic acid in the finished product?

77. ℞ Salicylic Acid   ℥ss
       Boric Acid Ointment
       Zinc Oxide Ointment   aa   ℥ss
       Sig. Apply.

Calculate the percentage of salicylic acid in the finished product.

78. ℞ Zinc Oxide
       Calamine
       Starch   aa   6.0
       Wool Fat
       Hydrophilic Petrolatum aa   60.0
       Sig. Apply.

What is the percentage of zinc oxide in the finished product?

79. A pharmacist incorporates 24 grains of ammoniated mercury into ℥i of a 5% ammoniated mercury ointment. Calculate the percentage strength of the finished product.

80. The formula for a fungicidal ointment calls for 9 g. of undecylenic acid and enough hydrophilic ointment base to make 1 lb. What is the percentage of undecylenic acid in the ointment?

81. ℞ Salicylic Acid
       Zinc Oxide   aa   ℥ss
       Lanolin   ℥iii
       Petrolatum   ℥vi
       Sig. Apply as directed.

Calculate the percentage of salicylic acid in the finished product.

82. Express each of the following as a percentage strength:

(a) 1:1500   (d) 1:400
(b) 1:10,000   (e) 1:3300
(c) 1:250   (f) 1:4000

83. Express each of the following as a ratio strength:

(a) 0.125%   (d) 0.6%
(b) 2.5%   (e) $\frac{1}{3}$%
(c) 0.80%   (f) $\frac{1}{20}$%

84. Express each of the following concentrations as a ratio strength:

(a) 2 mg. of active ingredient in 2 ml. of solution
(b) 0.275 mg. of active ingredient in 5 ml. of solution
(c) 2 g. of active ingredient in 250 ml of solution
(d) 1 mg. of active ingredient in 0.5 ml. of solution

85. A scopolamine hydrobromide injection contains 500 mcg. of scopolamine hydrobromide per ml. Express this concentration as a ratio strength.

86. One hundred (100) ml. of purified water yield a residue of 1 mg. in the pharmacopeial test for total solids. Express this amount of residue as a ratio strength.

87. Calcium Hydroxide Solution contains 170 mg. of calcium hydroxide per 100 ml. at 15° C. Express this concentration as a ratio strength.

88. A sample of white petrolatum contains 10 mg. of tocopherol per kg. as a preservative. Express the amount of tocopherol as a ratio strength.

89. R Potassium Permanganate Tablets #100
0.2 g.
Sig. Four tablets to a quart of water.

Express the concentration, as a ratio strength, of the solution prepared according to the directions given in the prescription.

90. Preserved water is prepared by dissolving 0.04% of a mixture of 65 parts of methylparaben and 35 parts of propylparaben in distilled water. Express the concentration of methylparaben as a ratio strength.

91. A solution of sodium fluoride contains 500 mcg. of sodium fluoride per half liter. Express this concentration as a ratio strength.

92. Given a solution of potassium permanganate prepared by dissolving four 0.325-g. tablets in enough distilled water to make 650 ml., calculate (a) the ratio strength and (b) the percentage strength of the solution.

93. How many grams of a chemical should be used to prepare 500 ml. of a 1:2000 (w/v) solution?

94. How many grains of a chemical are required to make 1 pint of a 1:400 (w/v) solution?

95. How many milligrams of potassium permanganate should be used in preparing 5 liters of a 1:8000 solution?

96. How many grams of mercuric chloride should be used in preparing 1 gallon of a 1:4000 solution?

97. ℞ Epinephrine Solution 1:1000   7.5 ml.
      Simple Syrup   ad   60.0 ml.
      Sig. Teaspoonful as directed.

What is the concentration of epinephrine in the prescription?

98. How many milliliters of a 1:4000 solution can be made from $\frac{1}{8}$ oz. of potassium permanganate?

99. ℞ Phenacaine Hydrochloride   1:100
      Mercury Bichloride   1:4000
      Ophthalmic Base   ad   10 g.
      Sig. Apply to right eye.

How many milligrams of phenacaine hydrochloride and of mercury bichloride should be used in compounding the prescription?

100. ℞ Atropine Base   1:200
      Castor Oil   ad   5 g.
      Sig. Apply topically to eye.

How many milligrams of atropine base should be used in compounding the prescription?

101. ℞ Menthol   1:500
      Hexachlorophene   1:800
      Hydrophilic Ointment Base   ad   30 g.
      Sig. Apply to hands.

How many milligrams of menthol and of hexachlorophene should be used in compounding the prescription?

102. How many milligrams of isoflurophate are contained in 15 g. of a 1:10,000 ophthalmic solution of isoflurophate in peanut oil?

Chapter 10

Dilution and Concentration

IN the previous chapter we have considered problems arising from the quantitative relationship, in given solutions or mixtures, between the active ingredients and the total amounts of solution or mixture, or between the ingredients themselves.

Problems of a slightly different character arise when given solutions or mixtures are *diluted* (by the addition of diluent, or by admixture with solutions or mixtures of lower strength) or are *concentrated* (by the addition of active ingredient, or by admixture with solutions or mixtures of greater strength, or by evaporation of the diluent).

Such problems sometimes seem complicated and difficult. But the complication proves to be nothing more than a series of steps required in the calculation, and the difficulty usually vanishes as each step, in itself, proves to be a simple matter.

Very often a problem can be solved in several ways. The best way is not necessarily the shortest: the best way is the one that clearly is grasped and that leads to the correct answer.

These two rules, wherever they may be applied, will greatly simplify the calculations:

(1) *When ratio strengths are given, convert them to percentage strengths before setting up a proportion.* It is very much more troublesome to calculate with a ratio like $\frac{1}{10} : \frac{1}{500}$ than with the equivalent *10 (%):0.2(%)*.

(2) *Whenever proportional parts enter into a calculation, reduce them to lowest terms.* Instead of calculating with a ratio like *75 (parts):25 (parts)*, simplify it to *3 (parts):1 (part)*.

RELATIONSHIP BETWEEN STRENGTH AND TOTAL QUANTITY

If a mixture of a given percentage or ratio strength is diluted to twice its original quantity, its active ingredient will be contained in twice as many parts of the whole, and its strength therefore will be reduced by one-half. Contrariwise, if a mixture is concentrated by evaporation to one-half its original quantity, the active ingredient (assuming that none was lost by evaporation) will be contained in one-half as many parts of the whole, and the strength will be doubled. So, if 50 ml. of a solution containing 10 g. of active ingredient with a strength of 20% or 1:5 (w/v) are diluted to 100 ml., the original volume is doubled, but the original strength is now reduced by one-half to 10% or 1:10 (w/v). And if by evaporation of the solvent the volume of the solution is reduced to 25 ml. or one-half the original quantity, the 10 g. of the active ingredient now indicate a strength of 40% or 1:2.5 (w/v).

It turns out, then, that *if the amount of active ingredient remains constant, any change in the quantity of a solution or mixture of solids is inversely proportional to the percentage or ratio strength;* that is, the percentage or ratio strength decreases as the quantity increases, and conversely.

This relationship is generally true for all mixtures except volume-in-volume and weight-in-volume solutions containing components that contract when mixed together.

DILUTION AND CONCENTRATION OF LIQUIDS

To calculate the percentage or ratio strength of a solution made by diluting or concentrating (by evaporation) a solution of given quantity and strength:

Examples:

> *If 500 ml. of a 15% (v/v) solution are diluted to 1500 ml., what will be the percentage strength (v/v)?*

$$\frac{1500 \ (ml.)}{500 \ (ml.)} = \frac{15 \ (\%)}{x \ (\%)}$$

x = 5%, *answer.*

Or,

> 500 ml. of 15% (v/v) solution contain 75 ml. of active ingredient

$$\frac{1500 \ (ml.)}{75 \ (ml.)} = \frac{100 \ (\%)}{x \ (\%)}$$

x = 5%, *answer.*

> *If 20 ml. of a 1:200 (w/v) solution of a chemical are diluted to 500 ml., what is the ratio strength (w/v)?*

1:200 = 0.5%

$$\frac{500 \ (ml.)}{20 \ (ml.)} = \frac{0.5 \ (\%)}{x \ (\%)}$$

x = 0.02% = 1:5000, *answer.*

Or,

$$\frac{500 \text{ (ml.)}}{20 \text{ (ml.)}} = \frac{\frac{1}{200}}{x}$$

$$x = \frac{1}{5000} = 1:5000, \textit{ answer.}$$

Or,

20 ml. of a 1:200 solution contain 0.1 g. of chemical

$$\frac{0.1 \text{ (g.)}}{1 \text{ (g.)}} = \frac{500 \text{ (ml.)}}{x \text{ (ml.)}}$$

$$x = 5000 \text{ ml.}$$

Ratio strength $= 1:5000, \textit{ answer.}$

If 8f℥ of a 1:2000 (w/v) solution of a chemical are diluted to 1 quart, what will be the ratio strength (w/v)?

1 quart $= 32$ f℥

$1:2000 = 0.05\%$

$$\frac{32 \text{ (f℥)}}{8 \text{ (f℥)}} = \frac{0.05 \text{ (\%)}}{x \text{ (\%)}}$$

$$x = 0.0125\% = 1:8000, \textit{ answer.}$$

Or,

$$\frac{32 \text{ (f℥)}}{8 \text{ (f℥)}} = \frac{\frac{1}{2000}}{x}$$

$$x = \frac{1}{8000} = 1:8000, \textit{ answer.}$$

If a syrup containing 65% (w/v) of sugar is evaporated to 85% of its volume, what percent (w/v) of sugar will it contain?

Any convenient amount of the syrup—say, 100 ml.—may be used in the calculation. If we evaporate 100 ml. of the syrup to 85% of its volume, we shall have 85 ml.

$$\frac{85 \text{ (ml.)}}{100 \text{ (ml.)}} = \frac{65 \text{ (\%)}}{x \text{ (\%)}}$$

$$x = 76.47\% \text{ or } 76\%, \textit{ answer.}$$

To calculate the amount of solution of desired strength that can be made by diluting or concentrating (by evaporation) a specified quantity of a solution of given strength:

Examples:

How many grams of 10% (w/w) ammonia water can be made from 1800 g. of 28% (w/w) ammonia water?

$$\frac{10\ (\%)}{28\ (\%)} = \frac{1800\ (g.)}{x\ (g.)}$$

x = 5040 g., *answer.*

Or,

1800 g. of 28% ammonia water contain 504 g. of ammonia (100%)

$$\frac{10\ (\%)}{100\ (\%)} = \frac{504\ (g.)}{x\ (g.)}$$

x = 5040 g., *answer.*

How many milliliters of a 1:5000 (w/v) solution of potassium permanganate can be made from 50 ml. of a 0.5% solution?

$$1:5000 = 0.02\%$$

$$\frac{0.02\ (\%)}{0.5\ (\%)} = \frac{50\ (ml.)}{x\ (ml.)}$$

x = 1250 ml., *answer.*

Or,

$$\frac{\frac{1}{5000}}{\frac{1}{200}} = \frac{50\ (ml.)}{x\ (ml.)}$$

x = 1250 ml., *answer.*

Or,

50 ml. of a 1:5000 solution contain 0.25 g. of potassium permanganate

$$\frac{1\ (g.)}{0.25\ (g.)} = \frac{5000\ (ml.)}{x\ (ml.)}$$

x = 1250 ml., *answer.*

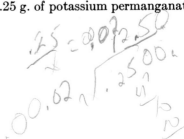

If 10 f℥ of a 30% (w/v) solution are to be evaporated so that the solution will have a strength of 50% (w/v), what will be its volume?

$$\frac{50\ (\%)}{30\ (\%)} = \frac{10\ (\text{f℥})}{\text{x}\ (\text{f℥})}$$

x = 6 f℥, *answer.*

STOCK SOLUTIONS

Stock solutions are solutions of known concentration that are frequently prepared by the pharmacist for convenience in dispensing. They are usually strong solutions from which weaker ones may be conveniently made; and, when correctly prepared, they enable the pharmacist to obtain small quantities of medicinal substances that are to be dispensed in solution.

Stock solutions are invariably prepared on a weight-in-volume basis, and their concentration is expressed as a ratio strength or, less frequently, as a percentage strength.

To calculate the amount of a solution of given strength that must be used to prepare a solution of desired amount and strength:

Examples:

How many milliliters of a 1:400 (w/v) stock solution should be used to make 4 liters of a 1:2000 (w/v) solution?

4 liters = 4000 ml.

1:400 = 0.25%   1:2000 = 0.05%

$$\frac{0.25\ (\%)}{0.05\ (\%)} = \frac{4000\ (\text{ml.})}{\text{x}\ (\text{ml.})}$$

x = 800 ml., *answer.*

Or,

$$\frac{\frac{1}{400}}{\frac{1}{2000}} = \frac{4000\ (\text{ml.})}{\text{x}\ (\text{ml.})}$$

x = 800 ml., *answer.*

How many fluidounces of a 1:400 (w/v) stock solution should be used in preparing 1 gallon of a 1:2000 (w/v) solution?

1 gallon = 128 f℥

1:400 = 0.25%   1:2000 = 0.05%

$$\frac{0.25\ (\%)}{0.05\ (\%)} = \frac{128\ (f℥)}{x\ (f℥)}$$

x = 25⅗ f℥, *answer.*

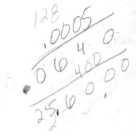

How many milliliters of a 2% stock solution of potassium permanganate should be used in compounding the following prescription?

℞   Sol. Potassium Permanganate
        1:5000   200 ml.
        Sig. Use as directed.

1:5000 = 0.02%

$$\frac{2\ (\%)}{0.02\ (\%)} = \frac{200\ (ml.)}{x\ (ml.)}$$

x = 2 ml., *answer.*

Check:

2% stock solution   1:5000 solution
   2 g. × 0.02 ⟶ 0.04 g. ⟵ 200 g. × 0.0002
                        potassium
                        permanganate

How many milliliters of a 1:400 stock solution of mercury bichloride should be used in compounding the following prescription?

℞   Solution Mercury Bichloride
        0.025%   250.0
        Sig. As directed.

1:400 = 0.25%

$$\frac{0.25\ (\%)}{0.025\ (\%)} = \frac{250\ (ml.)}{x\ (ml.)}$$

x = 25 ml., *answer.*

How many milliliters of a 1:50 stock solution of ephedrine sulfate should be used in compounding the following prescription?

R̸ Ephedrine Sulfate   0.25%
    Rose Water   ad   10.0 ml.
    Sig. For the nose.

    1:50 = 2%

$$\frac{2\ (\%)}{0.25\ (\%)} = \frac{10\ (ml.)}{x\ (ml.)}$$

    x = 1.25 ml., *answer.*

Or,

    10 (g.) × 0.0025 = 0.025 g. of ephedrine sulfate needed
    1:50 means 1 g. in 50 ml. of stock solution

$$\frac{1\ (g.)}{0.025\ (g.)} = \frac{50\ (ml.)}{x\ (ml.)}$$

    x = 1.25 ml., *answer.*

How many minims of a 1:50 stock solution of zinc sulfate should be used in compounding the following prescription?

R̸ Zinc Sulfate   gr. ¾
    Distilled Water   ad   ℥iv
    Sig. For the eye.

    1:50 = 2%

    1 f℥ (480 minims) of stock solution contains 1 × 455 gr. × 0.02 or 9.1 gr.

$$\frac{9.1\ (gr.)}{0.75\ (gr.)} = \frac{480\ (\mathfrak{m})}{x\ (\mathfrak{m})}$$

    x = 39.5 or 40 𝔪, *answer.*

A stock solution contains 3 gr. of ephedrine sulfate per fluidrachm. How many minims should be used in compounding the following prescription?

R̸ Ephedrine Sulfate   1%
    Rose Water   ad   ℥i
    Sig. For the nose.

1×455 gr. $\times 0.01 = 4.55$ gr. of ephedrine sulfate needed

The stock solution contains 3 gr. per f℥i (60 ℳ)

$$\frac{3 \text{ (gr.)}}{4.55 \text{ (gr.)}} = \frac{60 \text{ (ℳ)}}{x \text{ (ℳ)}}$$

$x = 91$ ℳ, *answer.*

To calculate the quantity of active ingredient in any specified amount of solution when given the strength of a diluted portion of the solution:

From the strength of the diluted portion we may calculate the *quantity of active ingredient* that the undiluted portion must have contained, and then by proportion we may calculate how much active ingredient must be present in any other amount of the stock solution.

Examples:

How much silver nitrate should be used in preparing 50 ml. of a solution such that 5 ml. diluted to 500 ml. will yield a 1:1000 solution?

1:1000 means 1 g. of silver nitrate in 1000 ml. of solution

$$\frac{1000 \text{ (ml.)}}{500 \text{ (ml.)}} = \frac{1 \text{ (g.)}}{x \text{ (g.)}}$$

$x = 0.5$ g. of silver nitrate in 500 ml. of diluted solution (1:1000) which is also the amount in 5 ml. of the stronger (stock) solution,

and,

$$\frac{5 \text{ (ml.)}}{50 \text{ (ml.)}} = \frac{0.5 \text{ (g.)}}{y \text{ (g.)}}$$

$y = 5$ g., *answer.*

The accompanying diagrammatic sketch should prove helpful in solving the problem.

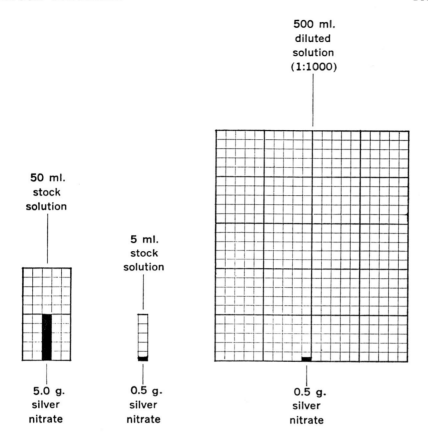

50 ml.
stock
solution

5.0 g.
silver
nitrate

5 ml.
stock
solution

0.5 g.
silver
nitrate

500 ml.
diluted
solution
(1:1000)

0.5 g.
silver
nitrate

How many grains of mercuric chloride should be used to prepare f℥ viii of a solution such that f℥i diluted to a pint will yield a 1:5000 solution?

1:5000 = 0.02%

1 pt. = 16 f℥

16 × 455 gr. × 0.0002 = 1.46 gr. of mercuric chloride in 1 pint of 1:5000 solution, which is also the amount in f℥i of stock solution.

f℥ viii = 64 f℥

$$\frac{1 \ (f℥)}{64 \ (f℥)} = \frac{1.46 \ (gr.)}{x \ (gr.)}$$

x = 93 gr., *answer.*

*How many grams of benzalkonium chloride should be used in com-
pounding the following prescription?*

℞ Benzalkonium Chloride Solution   500 ml.
   Make a solution such that 15 ml. diluted to
   a liter will equal a 1:5000 solution
   Sig. Dilute and use as directed.

   1:5000 means 1 g. in 5000 ml. of solution

$$\frac{5000 \ (ml.)}{1000 \ (ml.)} = \frac{1 \ (g.)}{x \ (g.)}$$

x = 0.2 g. of benzalkonium chloride in a liter of 1:5000 solution,
which is also the amount in 15 ml. of the stock solution.

and,

$$\frac{15 \ (ml.)}{500 \ (ml.)} = \frac{0.2 \ (g.)}{y \ (g.)}$$

y = 6.66 or 6.7 g., *answer.*

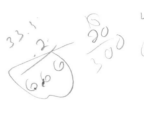

To calculate the amount of diluent that should be added to a solution of given strength and quantity to make a solution of specified lower strength :

When given the quantity and strength of a solution, we may easily
determine how much diluent should be added to reduce its strength as
desired by first calculating the quantity of weaker solution that can be
made and then subtracting from this the original quantity.

Examples:

*How much water should be added to 150 ml. of a 1:500 (w/v) stock
solution of a chemical to make a 1:2000 (w/v) solution?*

   1:500 = 0.2%   1:2000 = 0.05%

$$\frac{0.05 \ (\%)}{0.2 \ (\%)} = \frac{150 \ (ml.)}{x \ (ml.)}$$

   x = 600 ml. of 0.05% solution

   600 ml. − 150 ml. = 450 ml., *answer.*

How many fluidounces of water should be added to 6 f℥ of an 8% (w/v) solution to make a 3% (w/v) solution?

$$\frac{3\ (\%)}{8\ (\%)} = \frac{6\ (f℥)}{x\ (f℥)}$$

x = 16 f℥ of 3% solution

16 f℥ — 6 f℥ = 10 f℥, *answer.*

If we are not given the strength of the original solution, but the quantity of active ingredient it contains, the simplest procedure is to calculate directly what must be the amount of solution of the strength desired if it contains this quantity of active ingredient; then by subtraction of the given original amount, as above, we may determine the required amount of diluent.

Examples:

How many milliliters of water should be added to 250 ml. of a solution containing 0.35 g. of a chemical to make a 1:4000 (w/v) solution?

$$\frac{1\ (g.)}{0.35\ (g.)} = \frac{4000\ (ml.)}{x\ (ml.)}$$

x = 1400 ml. of 1:4000 (w/v) solution containing 0.35 g. of the chemical.

1400 ml. — 250 ml. = 1150 ml., *answer.*

How much water should be added to 250 ml. of a 5% (w/v) solution of potassium permanganate to make a solution such that 5 ml. diluted to 500 ml. will give a 1:5000 solution?

1:5000 means 1 g. in 5000 ml. of solution

$$\frac{5000\ (ml.)}{500\ (ml.)} = \frac{1\ (g.)}{x\ (g.)}$$

x = 0.1 g. of potassium permanganate in 500 ml. of 1:5000 solution, which is also the amount in 5 ml. of stock solution.

250 × 0.05 = 12.5 g. of potassium permanganate in 250 ml. of 5% solution,

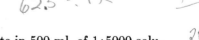

and,

$$\frac{0.1 \text{ (g.)}}{12.5 \text{ (g.)}} = \frac{5 \text{ (ml.)}}{y \text{ (ml.)}}$$

y = 625 ml.

625 ml. − 250 ml. = 375 ml., *answer.*

DILUTION OF ALCOHOL

Since there is a noticeable contraction in volume when alcohol and water are mixed, we cannot calculate the volume of water needed to dilute alcohol to a desired *volume-in-volume* strength. But this contraction does not affect the *weights* of the components, and hence the *weight of water* (and from this, the *volume*) needed to dilute alcohol to a desired *weight-in-weight* strength may be calculated.

To solve miscellaneous problems involving dilution of alcohol:

Examples:

 How much water should be mixed with 5000 ml. of 85% (v/v) alcohol to make 50% (v/v) alcohol?

$$\frac{50 \text{ (\%)}}{85 \text{ (\%)}} = \frac{5000 \text{ (ml.)}}{x \text{ (ml.)}}$$

x = 8500 ml.

Therefore, use 5000 ml. of 85% (v/v) alcohol and enough water to make 8500 ml., *answer.*

 How many milliliters of 95% (v/v) alcohol and how much water should be used in compounding the following prescription?

R   Boric Acid   1.0 g.
     Alcohol 70%   30.0 ml.
     Sig. Ear drops.

$$\frac{95 \text{ (\%)}}{70 \text{ (\%)}} = \frac{30 \text{ (ml.)}}{x \text{ (ml.)}}$$

x = 22 ml.

Therefore, use 22 ml. of 95% (v/v) alcohol and enough water to make 30 ml., *answer.*

How much water should be added to 4000 g. of 90% (w/w) alcohol to make 40% (w/w) alcohol?

$$\frac{40\ (\%)}{90\ (\%)} = \frac{4000\ (g.)}{x\ (g.)}$$

x = 9000 g., weight of 40% (w/w) alcohol equivalent to 4000 g. of 90% (w/w) alcohol

9000 g. — 4000 g. = 5000 g. or 5000 ml., *answer.*

DILUTION OF ACIDS

The strength of an official undiluted (*concentrated*) acid is expressed as percentage weight-in-weight. For example, Phosphoric Acid contains not less than 85.0 percent and not more than 88.0 percent, by weight, of H_3PO_4. But the strength of an official *diluted* acid is expressed as percentage weight-in-volume. For example, Diluted Phosphoric Acid contains, in each 100 ml., not less than 9.5 g. and not more than 10.5 g. of H_3PO_4.

It is necessary, therefore, to consider the specific gravity of concentrated acids in calculating the volume to be used in preparing a desired quantity of a diluted acid.

To calculate the volume of a concentrated acid required to prepare a desired quantity of a diluted acid:

Examples:

How many milliliters of 96% (w/w) sulfuric acid having a specific gravity of 1.84 are required to make 1000 ml. of diluted sulfuric acid 10% (w/v)?

1000 g. × 0.10 = 100 g. of H_2SO_4 (100%) in 1000 ml. of
10% (w/v) acid

$$\frac{96\ (\%)}{100\ (\%)} = \frac{100\ (g.)}{x\ (g.)}$$

x = 104 g. of 96% acid

104 g. of water measure 104 ml.

104 (ml.) ÷ 1.84 = 56.5 ml., *answer.*

How many milliliters of 85% (w/w) phosphoric acid having a specific gravity of 1.71 should be used in preparing 1 gallon of ¼% phosphoric acid solution which is to be used for bladder irrigation?

1 gallon = 3784 ml.

3784 (g.) × 0.0025 = 9.46 g. of H_3PO_4 (100%) in 3784 ml.
(1 gallon) of ¼% (w/v) solution

$$\frac{85\ (\%)}{100\ (\%)} = \frac{9.46\ (g.)}{x\ (g.)}$$

x = 11.13 g. of 85% phosphoric acid

11.13 g. of water measure 11.13 ml.

11.13 (ml.) ÷ 1.71 = 6.5 ml., *answer.*

DILUTION AND CONCENTRATION OF SOLIDS

To solve miscellaneous problems involving dilution and concentration of solids:

Examples:

How many grams of opium containing 15% (w/w) of morphine and how many grams of lactose should be used to prepare 150 g. of opium containing 10% (w/w) of morphine?

$$\frac{15\ (\%)}{10\ (\%)} = \frac{150\ (g.)}{x\ (g.)}$$

x = 100 g. of 15% opium, *and*

150 g. − 100 g. = 50 g. of lactose, *answers.*

If some moist crude drug contains 7.2% (w/w) of active ingredient and 21.6% of water, what will be the percentage (w/w) of active ingredient after the drug is dried?

100 g. of moist drug would contain 21.6 g. of water and would therefore weigh 78.4 g. after drying.

$$\frac{78.4\ (g.)}{100\ (g.)} = \frac{7.2\ (\%)}{x\ (\%)}$$

x = 9.2%, *answer.*

How many grams of 5% ammoniated mercury ointment and how many grams of white petrolatum (diluent) should be used in preparing 5 lb. of 2% ammoniated mercury ointment?

5 lb. = 454 g. × 5 = 2270 g.

$$\frac{5\ (\%)}{2\ (\%)} = \frac{2270\ (g.)}{x\ (g.)}$$

x = 908 g. of 5% ointment, *and*

2270 g. − 908 g. = 1362 g. of white petrolatum, *answers.*

How many grains of 20% zinc oxide ointment and how many grains of ophthalmic base should be used in compounding the following prescription?

℞   Ophthalmic Zinc Oxide Ointment   ℥ii
        3%
     Sig. Apply to lids.

     ℥ii = 120 gr.

$$\frac{20\ (\%)}{3\ (\%)} = \frac{120\ (gr.)}{x\ (gr.)}$$

x = 18 gr. of 20% ointment, *and*

120 gr. − 18 gr. = 102 gr. of ophthalmic base, *answers.*

How many grams of coal tar should be added to 3200 g. of 5% coal tar ointment to prepare an ointment containing 20% of coal tar?

3200 g. × 0.05 = 160 g. of coal tar in 3200 g. of 5% ointment

3200 g. − 160 g. = 3040 g. of base (diluent) in 3200 g. of 5% ointment

In the 20% ointment the diluent will represent 80% of the total weight.

$$\frac{80\ (\%)}{20\ (\%)} = \frac{3040\ (g.)}{x\ (g.)}$$

x = 760 g. of coal tar in the 20% ointment

But since the 5% ointment already contains 160 g. of coal tar, 760 g. − 160 g. = 600 g., *answer.*

A much simpler method of solving the problem above can be used if we mentally translate it to read:

How many grams of coal tar should be added to 3200 g. of coal tar ointment containing 95% diluent to prepare an ointment containing 80% diluent?

$$\frac{80 \ (\%)}{95 \ (\%)} = \frac{3200 \ (g.)}{x \ (g.)}$$

x = 3800 g. of ointment containing 80% diluent and 20% coal tar

3800 g. — 3200 g. = 600 g., *answer.*

For another simple method, using alligation alternate, see page 181.

How many milliliters of water should be added to 150 g. of wool fat to prepare hydrous wool fat containing 25% of water?

100% — 25% = 75% wool fat in hydrous wool fat

$$\frac{75 \ (\%)}{100 \ (\%)} = \frac{150 \ (g.)}{x \ (g.)}$$

x = 200 g. of hydrous wool fat

200 g. — 150 g. = 50 g. or ml. of water, *answer.*

A more direct solution:

$$\frac{75 \ (\%)}{25 \ (\%)} = \frac{150 \ (g.)}{x \ (g.)}$$

x = 50 g. or ml. of water, *answer.*

TRITURATIONS

Triturations are dilutions of potent medicinal substances. They were at one time official and were prepared by *diluting one part by weight of the finely powdered medicinal substance with nine parts by weight of finely powdered lactose.* They are, therefore, *10%* or *1:10 (w/w)* mixtures.

These dilutions offer a means of obtaining conveniently and accurately small quantities of potent medicaments.

To calculate the quantity of a trituration required to obtain a given amount of a medicinal substance :

Examples:

How many grams of a 1:10 trituration of atropine sulfate are required to obtain 25 mg. of atropine sulfate?

10 g. of trituration contain 1 g. of atropine sulfate

25 mg. = 0.025 g.

$$\frac{1 \ (g.)}{0.025 \ (g.)} = \frac{10 \ (g.)}{x \ (g.)}$$

x = 0.25 g., *answer.*

How many grains of a 1:10 trituration of colchicine are needed to obtain the amount needed for 100 capsules each containing $\frac{1}{120}$ gr. of colchicine and 5 gr. of aspirin?

$\frac{1}{120}$ gr. × 100 = $\frac{100}{120}$ gr. or $\frac{5}{6}$ gr. of colchicine needed

10 gr. of trituration contain 1 gr. of colchicine

$$\frac{1 \ (gr.)}{\frac{5}{6} \ (gr.)} = \frac{10 \ (gr.)}{x \ (gr.)}$$

x = $8\frac{1}{3}$ gr., *answer.*

How many milligrams of a 10% trituration of atropine sulfate should be used in preparing 500 ml. of a solution of atropine sulfate which is to contain $\frac{1}{400}$ gr. of atropine sulfate per teaspoonful?

1 teaspoonful = 5 ml.

500 ÷ 5 = 100 doses

$\frac{1}{400}$ gr. × 100 = $\frac{100}{400}$ or $\frac{1}{4}$ gr. of atropine sulfate needed

10% trituration contains 1 gr. of atropine sulfate in 10 gr.

$$\frac{1 \ (gr.)}{\frac{1}{4} \ (gr.)} = \frac{10 \ (gr.)}{x \ (gr.)}$$

x = $2\frac{1}{2}$ gr., *answer.*

ALLIGATION

Alligation is an arithmetical method of solving problems that involve the mixing of solutions or mixtures of solids possessing different percentage strengths.

ALLIGATION MEDIAL

Alligation medial is a method by which the "weighted average" percentage strength of a mixture of two or more substances whose quantities and concentrations are known may be quickly calculated. The percentage strength, expressed as a whole number, of each component of the mixture is multiplied by its corresponding quantity, and the sum of the products is divided by the sum of the quantities to give the percentage strength of the mixture—provided, of course, that the quantities have been expressed in a common denomination, whether of weight or of volume.

To calculate the percentage strength of a mixture that has been made by mixing two or more components of given percentage strengths:

Examples:

> *What is the percentage (v/v) of alcohol in a mixture of 3000 ml. of 40% (v/v) alcohol, 1000 ml. of 60% (v/v) alcohol, and 1000 ml. of 70% (v/v) alcohol?*

$$40 \times 3000 = 120000$$
$$60 \times 1000 = 60000$$
$$70 \times 1000 = 70000$$

Totals: 5000   250000

$$250000 \div 5000 = 50\%, answer.$$

> *What is the percentage of zinc oxide in an ointment prepared by mixing 200 g. of 10% ointment, 50 g. of 20% ointment, and 100 g. of 5% ointment?*

$$10 \times 200 = 2000$$
$$20 \times 50 = 1000$$
$$5 \times 100 = 500$$

Totals: 350   3500

$$3500 \div 350 = 10\%, answer.$$

In some problems the addition of a solvent or vehicle must be considered. It is generally best to consider the diluent as of zero percentage strength as in the following problem.

Example:

What is the percentage (v/v) of alcohol in a cough mixture containing 500 ml. of terpin hydrate elixir, 100 ml. of chloroform spirit, and enough hydriodic acid syrup to make 1000 ml.? Terpin hydrate elixir contains 40% (v/v) of alcohol, and chloroform spirit contains 90% (v/v) of alcohol.

$$40 \times 500 = 20000$$
$$90 \times 100 = 9000$$
$$0 \times 400 = 0$$

Totals: 1000   29000

29000 ÷ 1000   29%, *answer.*

ALLIGATION ALTERNATE

Alligation alternate is a method by which we may calculate the number of parts of two or more components of a given strength when they are to be mixed to prepare a mixture of desired strength. A final proportion permits us to translate relative parts to any specific denomination.

The strength of a mixture must lie somewhere between the strengths of its components—that is, the mixture must be somewhat stronger than its weakest component and somewhat weaker than its strongest; and, as already indicated, the strength of the mixture is always a "weighted" average: it lies nearer to that of its weaker or stronger components depending upon the relative amounts involved.

This "weighted" average can be found by means of an extremely simple scheme, as illustrated in the diagram on page 176.

To find the relative amounts of solutions or other substances of different strengths that should be used to make a mixture of required strength:

Examples:

In what proportion should alcohols of 95% and 50% strengths be mixed to make 70% alcohol?

Note that the difference between the *strength of the stronger component* (95%) and the *desired strength* (70%) indicates the *number of parts of the weaker* to be used (25 parts); and the difference between the *desired strength* (70%) and the *strength of the weaker component* (50%) indicates the *number of parts of the stronger* to be used (20 parts).

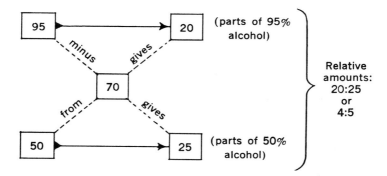

The mathematical validity of this relationship can be demonstrated.

Percent given	*Percent desired*	*Proportional parts required*
a		x
	c	
b		y

Given these data, the ratio of x to y may be derived algebraically as follows:

$$ax + by = c(x + y)$$
$$ax + by = cx + cy$$
$$ax - cx = cy - by$$
$$x(a - c) = y(c - b)$$

$$\frac{x}{y} = \frac{c - b}{a - c}$$

And given a = 95%, b = 50%, and c = 70%, we may therefore solve the problem as follows:

$$.95\,x + .50\,y = .70\,(x + y)$$

Or, $95 x + 50 y = 70 x + 70 y$

$95 x - 70 x = 70 y - 50 y$

$x(95 - 70) = y(70 - 50)$

$$\frac{x}{y} = \frac{70 - 50}{95 - 70} = \frac{20}{25} = \frac{4 \text{ (parts)}}{5 \text{ (parts)}}, \text{ answer.}$$

The result can be shown to be correct by *alligation medial:*

$$95 \times 4 = 380$$
$$50 \times 5 = 250$$
$$\text{Totals: } \overline{9} \qquad \overline{630}$$
$$630 \div 9 = 70\%$$

The customary layout of *alligation alternate,* used in the examples below, is a convenient simplification of the diagram above.

Examples:

In what proportion should 15% boric acid ointment be mixed with white petrolatum to produce a 2% boric acid ointment?

15%		2 parts of 15% ointment
	2%	
0%		13 parts of white petrolatum

Relative amounts: 2:13, *answer.*

$$\text{Check: } 15 \times 2 = 30$$
$$0 \times 13 = 0$$
$$\text{Totals: } \overline{15} \qquad \overline{30}$$
$$30 \div 15 = 2\%$$

A hospital pharmacist wants to use three lots of ichthammol ointment containing respectively 50%, 20%, and 5% of ichthammol. In what proportion should they be mixed to prepare a 10% ichthammol ointment?

Here the two lots containing *more* (50% and 20%) than the desired percentage may be separately linked to the lot containing *less* (5%) than the desired percentage:

```
┌─50%  │        │  5 parts of 50% ointment
│      │        │
│  ┌─20%  │ 10% │  5 parts of 20% ointment
│  │      │     │
└──└─5%   │     │  10 + 40 = 50 parts of 5% ointment
```

Relative amounts: 5:5:50, or 1:1:10, *answer.*

Check: $50 \times 1 = 50$

$20 \times 1 = 20$

$5 \times 10 = 50$

Totals: 12   120

$120 \div 12 = 10\%$

There are, of course, other answers, for the two stronger lots may be mixed first in any proportions desired, yielding a mixture that may then be mixed with the weakest lot in a proportion giving the desired strength.

In what proportions may a manufacturing pharmacist mix 20%, 15%, 5%, and 3% zinc oxide ointments to produce a 10% ointment?

Each of the weaker lots is paired with one of the stronger to give the desired strength; and since we may pair them in two ways, we may get two sets of correct answers.

```
┌─20%   │        │  7 parts of 20% ointment
│       │        │
│  ┌─15%  │ 10% │  5 parts of 15% ointment
│  │      │     │
│  └─5%   │     │  5 parts of 5% ointment
│         │     │
└──3%     │     │  10 parts of 3% ointment
```

Relative amounts: 7:5:5:10, *answer.*

Check: $20 \times 7 = 140$

$15 \times 5 = 75$

$5 \times 5 = 25$

$3 \times 10 = 30$

Totals: 27   270

$270 \div 27 = 10\%$

Or,

┌─20% │	5 parts of 20% ointment
├─15% │ 10%	7 parts of 15% ointment
└─5% │	10 parts of 5% ointment
└─3% │	5 parts of 3% ointment

Relative amounts: 5:7:10:5, *answer.*

Check:

$$20 \times 5 = 100$$
$$15 \times 7 = 105$$
$$5 \times 10 = 50$$
$$3 \times 5 = 15$$

Totals: 27   270

$$270 \div 27 = 10\%$$

How many milliliters of 50% (w/v) dextrose solution and how many milliliters of 5% (w/v) dextrose solution are required to prepare 4500 ml. of a 10% (w/v) solution?

50% │	5 parts of 50% solution
│ 10%	
5% │	40 parts of 5% solution

Relative amounts: 5:40, or 1:8, with a total of 9 parts

$$\frac{9 \text{ (parts)}}{1 \text{ (part)}} = \frac{4500 \text{ (ml.)}}{x \text{ (ml.)}}$$

$x = 500$ ml. of 50% solution, *and*

$$\frac{9 \text{ (parts)}}{8 \text{ (parts)}} = \frac{4500 \text{ (ml.)}}{y \text{ (ml.)}}$$

$y = 4000$ ml. of 5% solution, *answers.*

A concentration of 30% alcohol is required to keep the phenobarbital of the following prescription in solution. How many milliliters of high alcoholic elixir (78%) and how many milliliters of low alcoholic elixir (10%) should be used in compounding the prescription?

R̞   Phenobarbital   2.5
     Iso-Alcoholic Elixir   480.0
     Sig. 5 ml. at bedtime.

78%		20 parts of high alcoholic elixir
	30%	
10%		48 parts of low alcoholic elixir

Relative amounts: 20:48, or 5:12 with a total of 17 parts

$$\frac{17 \text{ (parts)}}{5 \text{ (parts)}} = \frac{480 \text{ (ml.)}}{x \text{ (ml.)}}$$

x = 141 ml. of high alcoholic elixir, *and*

$$\frac{17 \text{ (parts)}}{12 \text{ (parts)}} = \frac{480 \text{ (ml.)}}{y \text{ (ml.)}}$$

y = 339 ml. of low alcoholic elixir, *answers.*

To calculate the quantity of a solution or mixture of given strength that should be mixed with a specified quantity of another solution or mixture of given strength to make a solution or mixture of desired strength:

Examples:

How many grams of 10% ammoniated mercury ointment should be mixed with 450 g. of 3% ointment to make a 5% ammoniated mercury ointment?

10%		2 parts of 10% ointment
	5%	
3%		5 parts of 3% ointment

Relative amounts: 2:5

$$\frac{5 \text{ (parts)}}{2 \text{ (parts)}} = \frac{450 \text{ (g.)}}{x \text{ (g.)}}$$

x = 180 g., *answer.*

Alternate (algebraic) solution of the same problem:

$$.1(x) + .03(450) = .05(450 + x)$$

Or, $10(x) + 3(450) = 5(450 + x)$

$$10x + 1350 = 2250 + 5x$$

$$5x = 900 \text{ g.}$$

$$x = 180 \text{ g., } answer.$$

How many grams of petrolatum should be mixed with 250 g. of 10% and 750 g. of 20% tannic acid ointments to prepare a 5% ointment?

$$
\begin{array}{rr}
10 \times 250 = & 2500 \\
20 \times 750 = & 15000 \\
\hline
\text{Totals:} \quad 1000 & 17500
\end{array}
$$

$17500 \div 1000 = 17.5\%$ of tannic acid in 1000 g. of a mixture of 10% and 20% ointments.

17.5%		5 parts of 17.5% mixture
	5%	
0%		12.5 parts of petrolatum

Relative amounts: 5:12.5, or 2:5

$$\frac{2 \text{ (parts)}}{5 \text{ (parts)}} = \frac{1000 \text{ (g.)}}{x \text{ (g.)}}$$

$$x = 2500 \text{ g., } answer.$$

Check:
$$
\begin{array}{rr}
17.5 \times 1000 = & 17500 \\
0 \times 2500 = & 0 \\
\hline
\text{Totals:} \quad 3500 & 17500
\end{array}
$$

$$17500 \div 3500 = 5\%$$

To calculate the amount of active ingredient that must be added to increase the strength of a mixture of given amount and strength:

Example:

How many grams of coal tar should be added to 3200 g. of 5% coal tar ointment to prepare an ointment containing 20% of coal tar?

Coal tar (active ingredient) = 100%

$$
\begin{array}{c|c|l}
100\% & & 15 \text{ parts of } 100\% \text{ coal tar} \\
& 20\% & \\
5\% & & 80 \text{ parts of } 5\% \text{ ointment}
\end{array}
$$

Relative amounts: 15:80, or 3:16

$$
\frac{16 \text{ (parts)}}{3 \text{ (parts)}} = \frac{3200 \text{ (g.)}}{x \text{ (g.)}}
$$

x = 600 g., *answer.*

Check:
$$
\begin{array}{rl}
100 \times 600 = & 60000 \\
5 \times 3200 = & 16000 \\
\hline
\text{Totals:} \quad 3800 & 76000
\end{array}
$$

$$76000 \div 3800 = 20\%$$

Compare the solution of the problem above by use of alligation alternate with other methods on pp. 171–172.

SPECIFIC GRAVITY OF MIXTURES

The methods of alligation medial and alligation alternate may be used in solving problems involving the specific gravities of different quantities of liquids of known specific gravities—provided that there is no change in volume when the liquids are mixed, and that they are measured in a common denomination of *volume*.

To calculate the specific gravity of a mixture given the specific gravities of its ingredients:

Example:

What is the specific gravity of a mixture of 1000 ml. of syrup with a specific gravity of 1.300, 400 ml. of glycerin with a specific gravity of 1.250, and 1000 ml. of an elixir with a specific gravity of 0.950?

$$
\begin{array}{rll}
1.300 \times 1000 = & 1300 \\
1.250 \times 400 = & 500 \\
0.950 \times 1000 = & 950 \\
\hline
\text{Totals:} \quad 2400 & 2750
\end{array}
$$

$$2750 \div 2400 = 1.146, \ answer.$$

To calculate the relative or specific amounts of ingredients of given specific gravities required to make a mixture of desired specific gravity :

Examples:

In what proportion must glycerin with a specific gravity of 1.25 and water be mixed to give a liquid having a specific gravity of 1.10?

1.25		0.10 parts of glycerin
	1.10	
1.00		0.15 parts of water

Relative amounts: 0.10:0.15, or 2:3, *answer.*

How many milliliters of each of two liquids with specific gravities of 0.950 and 0.875 should be used to prepare 1500 ml. of a liquid having a specific gravity of 0.925?

0.950		0.050, or 50 parts of liquid with specific gravity of 0.950
	0.925	
0.875		0.025, or 25 parts of liquid with specific gravity of 0.875

Relative amounts: 50:25, or 2:1 with a total of 3 parts

$$\frac{3 \text{ (parts)}}{2 \text{ (parts)}} = \frac{1500 \text{ (ml.)}}{x \text{ (ml.)}}$$

x = 1000 ml. of liquid with specific gravity of 0.950, *and*

$$\frac{3 \text{ (parts)}}{1 \text{ (part)}} = \frac{1500 \text{ (ml.)}}{y \text{ (ml.)}}$$

y = 500 ml. of liquid with specific gravity of 0.875, *answers.*

Practice Problems

1. If 250 ml. of a 1:800 (v/v) solution are diluted to 1000 ml., what will be the ratio strength (v/v)?

2. If 1 pint of a 1:500 (w/v) solution is diluted to 24 f℥, what will be the ratio strength (w/v)?

3. If 400 ml. of a 20% (w/v) solution are diluted to 2 liters, what will be the percentage strength (w/v)?

4. If 55 ml. of an 18% (w/v) solution are diluted to 330 ml., what will be the percentage strength (w/v)?

5. If a solution containing 10.5% (w/w) of a chemical is evaporated to 70% of its weight, what per cent (w/w) of the chemical will it then contain?

6. If a solution containing 60% (v/v) of active ingredient is evaporated to 80% of its volume, what will be its percentage strength (v/v)?

7. What is the strength of a sodium chloride solution obtained by evaporating 800 g. of a 10% (w/w) solution to 250 g.?

8. How many grams of 10% (w/w) phosphoric acid can be made from 1 kilogram of 85% (w/w) acid?

9. How many milliliters of 0.45% (w/v) sodium hypochlorite solution can be prepared from 800 ml. of an 11.25% (w/v) solution?

10. How many milliliters of 50% (v/v) solution can be prepared by diluting 800 ml. of 95% (v/v) solution?

11. How many milliliters of 10% (w/v) solution can be made from 50 ml. of 85% (w/v) solution?

12. To what volume must 500 ml. of a 10% (w/v) solution of a chemical be evaporated to produce a 16% (w/v) solution?

13. To what weight must 1360 g. of a 12% (w/w) acid solution be evaporated to produce a 30% (w/w) solution?

14. How many gallons of 70% (v/v) alcohol can be made from 10 gallons of 95% (v/v) alcohol?

15. How many pounds of 10% (w/w) sulfuric acid can be made from 9 lb. of 94% (w/w) sulfuric acid?

16. How many grams of 5% (w/w) zinc chloride solution can be made from 25 ml. of a 50% (w/w) solution having a specific gravity of 1.55?

17. How many milliliters of 0.9% (w/v) sodium chloride solution can be prepared from 250 ml. of 25% (w/v) solution?

18. How many milliliters of a 1:1000 mercury bichloride solution can be prepared from 100 ml. of a 1:50 solution?

19. How many milliliters of a 1:8000 potassium permanganate solution can be prepared from 20 ml. of a 1% solution?

20. If 100 g. of belladonna leaf, assaying 0.35% (w/w) of alkaloids, are required to make 1000 ml. of belladonna tincture, how many milliliters of the tincture can be made from 5 lb. of belladonna leaf containing 0.4% (w/w) of alkaloids?

21. How many fluidounces of 6% (w/v) solution can be made from 2 f℥ of 36% (w/v) solution?

22. How many milliliters of a 1:50 (w/v) stock solution of a chemical should be used to prepare 1 liter of a 1:4000 (w/v) solution?

23. How many milliliters of a 2.5% (w/v) stock solution of potassium permanganate should be used in preparing 5 liters of a 1:5000 (w/v) solution?

24. How many milliliters of water should be added to 5 liters of a 50% solution of dextrose to reduce the concentration to 30% ?

25. A certain product contains benzalkonium chloride in a concentration of 1:5000. How many milliliters of a 17% solution of benzalkonium chloride should be used in preparing 4 liters of the product?

26. How many milliliters of a 10% stock solution of a chemical are needed to prepare 120 ml. of a solution containing 10 mg. of the chemical per ml.?

27. The formula for a buffer solution contains 1.24% (w/v) of boric acid. How many milliliters of a 5% boric acid solution should be used to obtain the boric acid needed in preparing 1 liter of the buffer solution?

28.
Menthol	0.1%
Hexachlorophene	0.1%
Glycerin	10.0%
Alcohol 70%, to make	500 ml.

Label: Menthol and Hexachlorophene Lotion.

How many milliliters of a 5% solution of menthol in alcohol should be used to obtain the amount of menthol needed in preparing the lotion?

29. ℞ Amaranth   1:10000
     Amphogel   ad   180 ml.
     Sig. Tsp. in water.

How many milliliters of a 1% amaranth solution should be used in compounding the prescription?

30. How many milliliters of a 1:50 stock solution of mercuric chloride should be used in preparing 250 ml. of a 0.02% solution?

31. One pint of a stock solution contains 12 gr. of mercuric chloride. How much of this solution should be used to make 8 f℥ of a 1:5000 solution?

32. ℞   Gentian Violet Solution   500 ml.
         1:100,000
        Sig. Mouth wash.

How many milliliters of a ½% solution of gentian violet should be used in compounding the prescription?

33. How many milliliters of a 1:200 stock solution of atropine sulfate are required to prepare 60 ml. of a 0.025% solution?

34. ℞   Potassium Permanganate Solution   500 ml.
         1:8000
        Sig. As directed.

How many milliliters of a 5% stock solution of potassium permanganate should be used in compounding the prescription?

35. How many milliliters of a solution containing 0.275 mg. of histamine phosphate per ml. should be used in preparing 15 ml. of a 1:10000 histamine phosphate solution?

36. ℞   Adrenalin Solution   ℥ss
         1:5000
        Sig. For the nose.

How many minims of a 1:1000 adrenalin solution should be used in compounding the prescription?

37. ℞   Calamine Lotion
        Boric Acid Solution 3%
        White Lotion   aa   ad   240.0
        Sig. Apply.

How many milliliters of 5% boric acid solution and how much water should be used in compounding the prescription?

38. A physician writes for an ophthalmic suspension to contain 100 mg. of cortisone acetate in 8 ml. of normal saline solution. The pharmacist has on hand a 2.5% suspension of cortisone acetate in normal saline solution. How many milliliters of this and how many milliliters of normal saline solution should he use in preparing the prescribed suspension?

39. ℞ Burow's Solution
      1-8
     Isopropyl Alcohol aa ad   120.0
     Sig. Apply locally as directed.

How many milliliters of Burow's Solution should be used in compounding the prescription?

.40. The formula for a mouth wash calls for 0.05% by volume of methyl salicylate. How many milliliters of a 10% (v/v) stock solution of methyl salicylate in alcohol will be needed to prepare 1 gallon of the mouth wash?

41. ℞ Atropine Sulfate Solution   120 ml.
        (Tsp. = gr. $\frac{1}{500}$)
     Sig. Teaspoonful in each feeding.

The atropine sulfate is to be obtained from a stock solution containing $\frac{4}{5}$ grain per fluidounce. How many minims of the stock solution should be used?

42. ℞ Boric Acid Solution 3%
     Burow's Solution
     Aquaphor   aa   ad   60.0
     Sig. For external use.

Only 5% boric acid solution is available. How many milliliters of this and how many milliliters of water should be used in compounding the prescription?

43. ℞ Potassium Permanganate q.s.
     Distilled Water   ad   1000.0
     Sig. 5 ml. diluted to 500 ml. will yield a 1:10000 solution.

(a) How many grams of potassium permanganate should be used?
(b) How many milliliters of a 2.5% stock solution of potassium permanganate should be used to obtain the potassium permanganate needed in (a)?

44. How many grains of mercuric chloride should be used in preparing 6 f℥ of a solution such that f℥i diluted to a pint will give a 1:8000 solution?

45. ℞   Potassium Permanganate q.s.
        Distilled Water   ad   ℥ xvi
        Sig. f℥ii diluted to a pint = 1:5000 solution.

How many grains of potassium permanganate should be used in compounding the prescription?

46. How many grams of silver nitrate are required to make 250 ml. of a solution such that 8 ml. diluted to 1 liter will give a 1:5000 solution?

47. ℞   Benzalkonium Chloride Solution   240 ml.
        Make a solution such that 10 ml. diluted
        to a liter equals a 1:5000 solution.
        Sig. 10 ml. diluted to a liter for external use.

How many milliliters of a 17% solution of benzalkonium chloride should be used in compounding the prescription?

48. How many grains of potassium permanganate should be used in preparing a half pint of a solution such that a half drachm diluted to a pint will equal a 1:2000 solution?

49. How many grams of copper sulfate are required to make 500 ml. of a solution such that 10 ml. diluted to a liter will give a 1:4000 solution?

50. Calculate the quantity of chemicals required to make 16 fluid-ounces of an aqueous solution so that 1 fluidounce added to 3 fluidounces of water will represent 1:500 of ephedrine sulfate and 1:3000 of chloro-butanol.

51. A hospital pharmacist has on hand 500 ml. of a 2% stock solution of mercury bichloride. How many milliliters of water should he add to the stock solution to make a solution such that 10 ml. diluted to 500 ml. will yield a 1:5000 solution?

52. How many milliliters of water should be added to 1500 ml. of a 1:2500 (w/v) solution to make a 1:4000 (w/v) solution?

53. How much water should be added to a liter of 1:3000 (w/v) solution to make a 1:8000 (w/v) solution?

54. How much water should be added to 1 liter of a solution containing 2.5 g. of a chemical to make a 1:2000 solution?

55. How much water should be added to 2500 ml. of 83% (v/v) alcohol to prepare 50% (v/v) alcohol?

56. How many milliliters of water should be mixed with 1200 g. of 65% (w/w) alcohol to make 45% (w/w) alcohol?

57. ℞ Methyl Salicylate 　　　　　　60.0 ml.
　　　Chloroform Liniment 　　　　　60.0 ml.
　　　Alcohol 80%　　　ad　　　　240.0 ml.
　　　Sig. Apply to parts.

How many milliliters of 95% (v/v) alcohol and how much water should be used in compounding the prescription?

58. ℞ Castor Oil 　　　　　　　　　5.0 ml.
　　　Euresol 　　　　　　　　　　15.0 ml.
　　　Alcohol 85%　　　ad　　　　240.0 ml.
　　　Sig. For the scalp.

How many milliliters of 95% (v/v) alcohol and how much water should be used in compounding the prescription?

59. How many milliliters of 95% (w/w) sulfuric acid having a specific gravity of 1.820 should be used in preparing 2 liters of 10% (w/v) acid?

60. How many milliliters of 37% (w/w) hydrochloric acid having a specific gravity of 1.18 should be used in preparing 1000 ml. of 10% (w/v) acid?

61. The formula for Hydriodic Acid Syrup is:
　　　Diluted Hydriodic Acid 　　　140 ml.
　　　Dextrose 　　　　　　　　　450 g.
　　　Water 　　　ad 　　　　　1000 ml.

Diluted hydriodic acid contains 10 g. of HI in each 100 ml. How many milliliters of a 19% (w/w) solution of HI, specific gravity 1.200, should be used in preparing 4000 ml. of hydriodic acid syrup?

62. How many milliliters of a 70% (w/w) sorbitol solution, specific gravity 1.30, should be used in preparing 1 gallon of a 10% (w/v) solution?

63. How many milliliters of 28% (w/w) ammonia water having a specific gravity of 0.89 should be used in preparing 2000 ml. of 10% (w/w) ammonia water with a specific gravity of 0.96?

64. How many milliliters of 92% (w/w) alcohol having a specific gravity of 0.816 should be used in preparing 5 liters of 40% (w/w) alcohol with a specific gravity of 0.939?

65. In compounding a prescription for 500 ml. of diluted phosphoric acid, a pharmacist used 50 ml. of 85% phosphoric acid with a specific gravity of 1.71. What was the percentage strength (w/v) of the finished product?

66. The formula for 1000 ml. of Aromatic Ammonia Spirit calls for 90 ml. of diluted ammonia solution. How many milliliters of a 27% (w/w) solution of ammonia, sp. gr. 0.90, should be used to prepare the diluted ammonia solution required for making 10 liters of the spirit? Diluted ammonia solution contains 9.5% (w/v) of ammonia.

67. Fifty (50) ml. of strong ammonia solution, 27.5% (w/w), sp. gr. 0.90, are diluted with 250 ml. of alcohol, sp. gr. 0.82. What is the concentration of ammonia in the resulting product, calculated on a w/w basis? On a w/v basis?

68. A sample of opium contains 28% of moisture and 10% of morphine. How many grams of morphine could be obtained from 350 g. of the dry opium?

69. How many grams of lactose should be added to 75 g. of belladonna extract assaying 1.50% (w/w) of alkaloids to reduce its strength to 1.40% (w/w)?

70. ℞   Benzocaine Ointment   ℥ii
          2.5%
     Sig. Apply.

How many grains of 20% benzocaine ointment and how many grains of white petrolatum should be used in compounding the prescription?

71. ℞   Hydrocortisone Acetate Ointment   10 g.
          0.25%
     Sig. Apply to the eye.

How many grams of 2.5% ophthalmic hydrocortisone acetate ointment and how many grams of ophthalmic base should be used in compounding the prescription?

72. How many grams of zinc oxide should be added to 3400 g. of a 10% zinc oxide ointment to prepare a product containing 15% of zinc oxide?

73. How many grams of petrolatum should be added to 250 g. of a 25% ichthammol ointment to make a 5% ointment?

74. ℞ Zinc Oxide 1.5
Hydrophilic Petrolatum 2.5
Distilled Water 5.0
Hydrophilic Ointment ad 30.0
Sig. Apply to affected areas.

How much zinc oxide should be added to the product in order to make an ointment containing 10% of zinc oxide?

75. ℞ Coal Tar 5%
Lassar's Paste ad 50.0
Sig. Apply as directed.

In compounding, a pharmacist added 2.5 g. of coal tar to 50 g. of Lassar's Paste. Calculate the concentration of coal tar in the finished product.

76. Liquefied phenol contains 90% of phenol and 10% of water. How many fluidounces of water should be added to 5 lb. of phenol crystals to prepare liquefied phenol?

77. How many grams of coal tar should be added to 925 g. of Zinc Oxide Paste to prepare a 6% ointment?

78. How much lactose and how much atropine sulfate should be used to make ℥iv of a 1:10 trituration of atropine sulfate?

79. A prescription calls for 0.005 g. of atropine sulfate. How much of a 1:10 trituration should be used to obtain the atropine sulfate?

80. If f℥iv of a prescription contain $\frac{1}{160}$ gr. of atropine sulfate per teaspoonful, how many grains of a 10% trituration of atropine sulfate should be used in compounding the prescription?

81. How many milligrams of 1:10 trituration of strychnine sulfate are required to obtain 0.5 mg. of strychnine sulfate?

82. ℞ Atropine Sulfate   0.130 mg.
       Acetylsalicylic Acid   0.3 g.
       Ft. pulv. tal. no. 20
       Sig. One b.i.d.

How many milligrams of a 1:10 trituration of atropine sulfate should be used in compounding the prescription?

83. ℞ Sol. Atropine Sulfate   f℥xvi
       (Each teaspoonful = $\frac{1}{320}$ gr.)
       Sig. Teaspoonful in water as directed.

How many grains of a 10% trituration of atropine sulfate should be used in compounding the prescription?

84. In preparing a 10% trituration of atropine sulfate, a pharmacist used the contents of an original ⅛ oz. bottle and enough lactose to make ℥x. What percentage of error did he incur?

85. Four equal amounts of belladonna extract, containing 1.15%, 1.30%, 1.35%, and 1.20% of alkaloids, respectively, were mixed. What was the percentage strength of the mixture?

86. What is the percentage of alcohol in a lotion containing 1500 ml. of witch hazel (14% alcohol), 2000 ml. of glycerin, and 5000 ml. of 50% alcohol?

87. A pharmacist mixes 200 g. of 10% ichthammol ointment, 450 g. of 5% ichthammol ointment, and 1000 g. of petrolatum (diluent). What is the percentage of ichthammol in the finished product?

88.   Coal Tar Solution   80 ml.   (85% alcohol)
       Glycerin   160 ml.
       Alcohol   500 ml.   (95% alcohol)
       Boric Acid Solution   ad   1000 ml.
       Label: Medicated lotion.

Calculate the percentage of alcohol in the lotion.

89. ℞ Phenobarbital Elixir   30 ml.   (15% alcohol)
       Belladonna Tincture   50 ml.   (65% alcohol)
       Aromatic Elixir   120 ml.   (22% alcohol)
       Distilled Water   ad   250 ml.
       Sig. Teaspoonful t.i.d.

Calculate the percentage of alcohol in the prescription.

90. What is the percentage of zinc oxide in an ointment prepared by mixing 2 lb. of a 20% zinc oxide ointment, 3 lb. of white petrolatum, and 1000 g. of zinc oxide paste (25% of zinc oxide)?

91. ℞ Chloroform Spirit   50.0 ml. (88% alcohol)
       Aromatic Elixir   150.0 ml. (22% alcohol)
       Terpin Hydrate Elixir   300.0 ml. (40% alcohol)
       Sig. 5 ml. for cough.

Calculate the percentage of alcohol in the prescription.

92. Calculate the percentage of alcohol in a lotion containing 2 liters of witch hazel (14% of alcohol), 1 liter of alcohol (95%), and enough boric acid solution to make 5 liters.

93. What is the percentage of alcohol in a liniment containing 1 pint of aconite fluidextract (60% of alcohol), 1 pint of 95% alcohol, 1 pint of chloroform, and 5 pints of soft soap liniment (60% of alcohol)?

94. In what proportion should 95% alcohol be mixed with 30% alcohol to make 70% alcohol?

95. In what proportion should solutions of 1.2% (w/v) and 0.38% (w/v) be mixed to make a 0.5% (w/v) solution?

96. In what proportion should two lots of crude drug containing respectively 2.8% (w/w) and 1.7% (w/w) of active ingredient be mixed to make a mixture containing 2.1% (w/w) of the active ingredient?

97. In what proportion should 10% and 2% coal tar ointments be mixed to prepare a 5% ointment?

98. In what proportion should a 20% zinc oxide ointment be mixed with white petrolatum to produce a 3% zinc oxide ointment?

99. In what proportion should 30% and 1.5% hydrogen peroxide solutions be mixed to prepare a 3% hydrogen peroxide solution?

100. The solvent for the extraction of a vegetable drug is 70% alcohol. In what proportion may 95%, 60%, and 50% alcohol be mixed in order to prepare a solvent of the desired concentration?

101. In what proportion may 15%, 5%, and 3% ointments be mixed to produce a 10% ointment?

102. In what proportion may 15%, 7%, 5%, and 3% zinc oxide ointments be mixed to produce a 10% ointment?

103. How many milliliters of 92.5% (w/v) solution should be mixed with 2175 ml. of 10% (w/v) solution to make a 20% (w/v) solution?

104. How many milliliters of high alcoholic elixir (78% of alcohol) and how many milliliters of low alcoholic elixir (10% of alcohol) should be used in preparing 1 gallon of iso-alcoholic elixir containing 45% of alcohol?

105. How many grams of 25% zinc oxide ointment and how many grams of petrolatum should be used to prepare 2500 g. of a 3% ointment?

106. What is the percentage of iodine in a mixture of 3 liters of 7% (w/v) iodine solution, 10 pints of 2% (w/v) solution, and 2270 ml. of 3.5% (w/v) solution?

107. A manufacturing pharmacist has four lots of ichthammol ointment, containing 50%, 25%, 10%, and 5% of ichthammol. How many grams of each may he use to prepare 4800 g. of a 20% ichthammol ointment?

108. How many grams of 50% ichthammol ointment should be mixed with 250 g. of 15% ointment to make a 20% ichthammol ointment?

109. How many grams of ammoniated mercury should be mixed with 700 g. of 5% ammoniated mercury ointment, 200 g. of 2% ointment, and 100 g. of 1% ointment to make a 10% ointment?

110. How much water must be added to a mixture of 300 g. of 65%, 250 g. of 35%, and 100 g. of 15% acid to produce a 10% acid?

111. How many milliliters of water should be added to 2640 g. of Phenol, U.S.P., containing 98% of phenol, to prepare Liquefied Phenol, U.S.P., containing 88% of phenol?

112. How many milliliters of water should be added to 500 g. of lanolin containing 25% (w/w) of water to prepare a product containing 40% (w/w) of water?

113. How many grams of ichthammol should be added to 1500 g. of 20% ichthammol ointment to make an ointment containing 25% of ichthammol?

114. How many grams of boric acid should be added to 1000 g. of 5% boric acid ointment to make a 20% boric acid ointment?

115. How many grams of coal tar should be added to a mixture of 1000 g. of zinc oxide paste and 500 g. of wool fat to make an ointment containing 10% of coal tar?

116. A sample of lanolin weighing 5 lb. is found to contain 35% of water. How much wool fat must be added to it to reduce the water content to 25%?

117. You have on hand 500 ml. of a 12% and 1 liter of a 6% solution of sodium hypochlorite. How many milliliters of water should be added to a mixture of the two solutions to prepare a solution containing 0.5% of sodium hypochlorite?

118. If wool fat absorbs twice its weight of water, how much additional water will be absorbed by 4000 g. of hydrous wool fat containing 25% of water?

119. You have on hand 800 g. of a 5% coal tar ointment and 1200 g. of a 10% coal tar ointment. (a) If the two ointments are mixed, what is the concentration of coal tar in the finished product? (b) How many grams of coal tar should be added to the product to obtain an ointment containing 15% of coal tar?

120. ℞ Zinc Oxide   20.0
     Wool Fat   60.0
     Water   ad   120.0
     Sig. Apply.

No wool fat is available. How many grams of hydrous wool fat containing 25% of water and how many milliliters of water should be used in compounding the prescription?

121. The formula for Formic Acid Spirit is as follows:
      Formic Acid   40 ml.
      Water   225 ml.
      Alcohol   735 ml.

The specific gravity of formic acid is 1.060 and the specific gravity of the alcohol is 0.800. Calculate the specific gravity of the spirit.

122. What is the specific gravity of a mixture containing 1000 ml. of water, 500 ml. of glycerin having a specific gravity of 1.25, and 1500 ml. of alcohol having a specific gravity of 0.81? (Assume that there is no contraction when the liquids are mixed.)

123. How many milliliters of a liquid with a specific gravity of 1.48 and of a liquid with a specific gravity of 0.71 should be mixed to prepare 100 ml. of a mixture with a specific gravity of 1.05?

124. How many milliliters of each of two liquids with specific gravities respectively of 1.32 and 1.12 should be mixed to make 1000 ml. of a mixture with a specific gravity of 1.20?

125. How many milliliters of a syrup having a specific gravity of 1.350 should be mixed with 3000 ml. of a syrup having a specific gravity of 1.250 to obtain a product having a specific gravity of 1.310?

Chapter 11

Isotonic Solutions

WHEN a solvent passes through a semipermeable membrane from a dilute solution into a more concentrated one with the result that the concentrations tend to become equalized, the phenomenon is known as *osmosis*. The pressure responsible for this phenomenon is called *osmotic pressure*, and it proves to be caused by and to vary with the solute.

If the solute is a non-electrolyte, its solution will contain only molecules, and the osmotic pressure of the solution will vary only with the concentration of the solute. If, on the other hand, the solute is an electrolyte, its solution will contain ions, and the osmotic pressure of the solution will vary not only with the concentration but also with the degree of dissociation of the solute. Obviously then, substances that dissociate have a relatively greater number of particles in solution and should exert a greater osmotic pressure than could undissociated molecules.

Like osmotic pressure, the other colligative properties of solutions, namely, vapor pressure, boiling point, and freezing point, depend upon the number of particles in solution. These properties, therefore, are related, and a change in any one of them will be attended by corresponding changes in the others.

It is generally agreed that many solutions designed to be mixed with body fluids should have the same osmotic pressure—in other words, should be made *isotonic* with those fluids—for greater comfort, efficacy, and safety. Solutions of lower osmotic pressure than that of a body fluid are *hypotonic*, whereas those having a higher osmotic pressure are *hypertonic*. Blood and the fluids of the eye and nose have so far been principally concerned, and of these the pharmacist is most likely to be asked to make ophthalmic solutions, or *collyria*, isotonic with lachrymal fluid.

The calculations involved in preparing isotonic solutions may be made in terms of data relating to the colligative properties of solutions. Theoretically, any one of these properties may be used as a basis for determining tonicity. Practically and most conveniently, a comparison of freezing points may be used for this purpose. At one time, $-0.56\degree$ C. and $-0.80\degree$ C. were generally accepted as the freezing points of blood serum and lachrymal fluid, respectively. However, most investigators now agree that the freezing point of blood serum is $-0.52\degree$ C. and not $-0.56\degree$ C. as previously

(197)

measured, and that the freezing point of lachrymal fluid is the same as that of blood serum.

Now it happens that when one gram molecular weight of any non-electrolyte—that is, a substance with negligible dissociation, such as boric acid—is dissolved in 1000 g. of water, the freezing point of the solution is about 1.86° C. below the freezing point of pure water. By simple proportion, therefore, we may calculate the weight of any non-electrolyte that should be dissolved in each 1000 g. of water if the solution is to be isotonic with the body fluids.

Boric acid, for example, has a molecular weight of 61.8, and hence (in theory) 61.8 g. in 1000 g. of water should produce a freezing point of −1.86° C. Therefore:

$$\frac{1.86 \ (°C.)}{0.52 \ (°C.)} = \frac{61.8 \ (g.)}{x \ (g.)}$$

$$x = 17.3 \ g.$$

In short, 17.3 g. of boric acid in 1000 g. of water, having a weight-in-volume strength of approximately 1.73%, should make a solution isotonic with lachrymal fluid.

With electrolytes, the problem is not quite so simple. Since osmotic pressure depends rather upon the number than upon the kind of particles, substances that dissociate have a tonic effect that increases with the degree of dissociation, and the greater the dissociation, the smaller the quantity required to produce any given osmotic pressure. If we assume that sodium chloride in weak solutions is about 80% dissociated, then each 100 molecules yield 180 particles, or 1.8 times as many particles as are yielded by 100 molecules of a non-electrolyte. This dissociation factor, commonly symbolized by the letter i, must be included in the proportion when we seek to determine the strength of an isotonic solution of sodium chloride (molecular weight, 58.5):

$$\frac{1.86 \ (°C.) \times 1.8}{0.52 \ (°C.)} = \frac{58.5 \ (g.)}{x \ (g.)}$$

$$x = 9.09 \ g.$$

Hence, 9.09 g. of sodium chloride in 1000 g. of water should make a solution isotonic with blood or lachrymal fluid. Actually, a 0.90% (w/v) sodium chloride solution is taken to be isotonic with the body fluids.

Simple isotonic solutions, then, may be calculated by this general formula:

$$\frac{0.52 \times molecular \ weight}{1.86 \times dissociation \ (i)} = g. \ of \ solute \ per \ 1000 \ g. \ of \ water$$

The value of i for many a medicinal salt has not been experimentally determined. Some salts (such as zinc sulfate, with only some 40% dissociation and an i value therefore of 1.4) are exceptional; but most medicinal salts approximate the dissociation of sodium chloride in weak solutions, and if the number of ions is known we may use the following values, lacking better information:

> Non-electrolytes and substances
> of slight dissociation: 1.0
> Substances that dissociate into 2 ions: 1.8
> Substances that dissociate into 3 ions: 2.6
> Substances that dissociate into 4 ions: 3.4
> Substances that dissociate into 5 ions: 4.2

A special problem arises when a prescription directs us to make a solution isotonic by adding the proper amount of some substance other than the active ingredient or ingredients. Given a 0.5% (w/v) solution of sodium chloride, we may easily calculate that 0.9 g. — 0.5 g. = 0.4 g. of additional sodium chloride should be contained in each 100 ml. if the solution is to be made isotonic with a body fluid. But how much sodium chloride should be used in preparing 100 ml. of a 1% (w/v) solution of atropine sulfate, which is to be made isotonic with lachrymal fluid? The answer depends upon *how much sodium chloride is in effect represented by the atropine sulfate.*

The relative tonic effect of two substances—that is, the quantity of one that is the equivalent in tonic effects to a given quantity of the other—may be calculated if the quantity of one having a certain effect in a specified quantity of solvent be divided by the quantity of the other having the same effect in the same quantity of solvent. For example, we have calculated above that 17.3 g. of boric acid per 1000 g. of water and that 9.09 g. of sodium chloride per 1000 g. of water are both instrumental in making an aqueous solution isotonic with lachrymal fluid. But if 17.3 g. of boric acid are the tonicic equivalent of 9.09 g. of sodium chloride, then 1 g. of boric acid must be the equivalent of 9.09 g. ÷ 17.3 g. or 0.52 g. of sodium chloride. And similarly, 1 g. of sodium chloride must be the tonicic equivalent of 17.3 g. ÷ 9.09 g. or 1.90 g. of boric acid.

We have seen that there is one quantity of any substance that should in theory have a constant tonic effect if dissolved in 1000 g. of water: this is one gram molecular weight of the substance divided by its i or dissociation value. Hence, the relative quantity of sodium chloride that is the tonicic equivalent of a quantity of boric acid may be calculated by these ratios:

$$\frac{58.5 \div 1.8}{61.8 \div 1.0} \text{ or } \frac{58.5 \times 1.0}{61.8 \times 1.8}$$

and we may formulate a convenient rule: *quantities of two substances that are tonicic equivalents are proportional to the molecular weights of each multiplied by the i value of the other.*

To return to the problem involving 1 g. of atropine sulfate in 100 ml. of solution:

Molecular weight of sodium chloride = 58.5; i = 1.8
Molecular weight of atropine sulfate = 695; i = 2.6

$$\frac{695 \times 1.8}{58.5 \times 2.6} = \frac{1 \text{ (g.)}}{\text{x (g.)}}$$

x = 0.12 g. of sodium chloride represented by 1 g. of atropine sulfate

Since a solution isotonic with lachrymal fluid should contain the equivalent of 0.90 g. of sodium chloride in each 100 ml. of solution, the difference to be added must be 0.90 g. − 0.12 g. = 0.78 g. of sodium chloride.

The Table on pages 210-213 gives the sodium chloride equivalents of each of the substances listed. These values were calculated according to the rule stated above. If the number of grams (or grains) of a substance included in a prescription be multiplied by its sodium chloride equivalent, the amount of sodium chloride represented by that substance is determined.

The procedure for the *calculation of isotonic solutions with sodium chloride equivalents* may be outlined as follows:

Step 1.   Calculate the amount (in g. or gr.) of sodium chloride represented by the ingredients in the prescription. This may be done by multiplying the amount (in g. or gr.) of each substance by its sodium chloride equivalent.

Step 2.   Calculate the amount (in g. or gr.) of sodium chloride, alone, that would be contained in an isotonic solution of the volume specified in the prescription—namely, *the amount of sodium chloride in a 0.9% solution of the specified volume.* (Such a solution would contain 0.009 g. per ml., or 4.1 gr. per f℥.)

Step 3.   Subtract the amount of sodium chloride represented by the ingredients in the prescription (Step 1) from the amount of sodium chloride, alone, that would be represented in the specified volume of an isotonic solution (Step 2). The answer represents the amount (in g. or gr.) of sodium chloride to be added to make the solution isotonic.

Step 4.   If an agent other than sodium chloride, such as boric acid, dextrose, sodium or potassium nitrate, is to be used to make a solution isotonic, divide the amount of sodium chloride (Step 3) by the sodium chloride equivalent of the other substance.

To calculate the dissociation (i) factor of an electrolyte :

Examples:

> *Zinc sulfate is a 2-ion electrolyte, dissociating 40% in a certain concentration. Calculate its dissociation (i) factor.*

On the basis of 40% dissociation, 100 particles of zinc sulfate will yield:

	40	zinc ions
	40	sulfate ions
	60	undissociated particles
or	140	particles

Since 140 particles represent 1.4 times as many particles as there were before dissociation, the dissociation (*i*) factor is 1.4, *answer.*

> *Zinc chloride is a 3-ion electrolyte, dissociating 80% in a certain concentration. Calculate its dissociation (i) factor.*

On the basis of 80% dissociation, 100 particles of zinc chloride will yield:

	80	zinc ions
	80	chloride ions
	80	chloride ions
	20	undissociated particles
or	260	particles

Since 260 particles represent 2.6 times as many particles as there were before dissociation, the dissociation (*i*) factor is 2.6, *answer.*

To calculate the sodium chloride equivalent of a substance :

Remember that the sodium chloride equivalent of a substance may be calculated as follows:

$$\frac{\text{molecular weight of sodium chloride}}{i \text{ factor of sodium chloride}} \times \frac{i \text{ factor of the substance}}{\text{molecular weight of the substance}} = \text{sodium chloride equivalent}$$

Example:

Papaverine hydrochloride (molecular weight 376) *is a 2-ion electrolyte, dissociating 80% in a given concentration. Calculate its sodium chloride equivalent.*

Since papaverine hydrochloride is a 2-ion electrolyte, dissociating 80%, its *i* factor is 1.8.

$$\frac{58.5}{1.8} \times \frac{1.8}{376} = 0.156, \text{ or } 0.16, \textit{answer.}$$

To calculate the amount of tonicic agent required:

Examples:

How much sodium chloride should be used in compounding the following prescription?

R	Pilocarpine Nitrate	0.3 g.
	Sodium Chloride	q.s.
	Distilled Water ad	30.0 ml.
	Make isoton. sol.	
	Sig. For the eye.	

Step 1.   0.22 × 0.3 g. = 0.066 g. of sodium chloride represented by the pilocarpine nitrate

Step 2.   30 × 0.009 = 0.270 g. of sodium chloride in 30 ml. of an isotonic sodium chloride solution

Step 3.   0.270 g.   (from Step 2)
           −0.066 g.   (from Step 1)
           _____
           0.204 g. of sodium chloride to be used, *answer.*

How many grains of sodium chloride should be used in compounding the following prescription?

R	Atropine Sulfate	gr. v
	Sodium Chloride	q.s.
	Distilled Water ad	℥i
	Make isoton. sol.	
	Sig. One drop in right eye.	

Step 1.   0.12 × 5 gr. = 0.6 gr. of sodium chloride represented by the atropine sulfate

Step 2.   1 × 455 × 0.009 = 4.1 gr. of sodium chloride in ℥i of an isotonic sodium chloride solution

Step 3.   4.1 gr.   (from Step 2)
            −0.6 gr.   (from Step 1)
            _____

            3.5 gr. of sodium chloride to be used, *answer*.

How much boric acid should be used in compounding the following prescription?

> ℞   Holocaine Hydrochloride   1%
>   Chlorobutanol   ½%
>   Boric Acid   q.s.
>   Distilled Water   ad   60.0
>   Make isoton. sol.
>   Sig. One drop in each eye

The prescription calls for 0.6 g. of holocaine hydrochloride and 0.3 g. of chlorobutanol.

Step 1.   0.17 × 0.6 g. = 0.102 g. of sodium chloride represented by holocaine hydrochloride

            0.18 × 0.3 g. = 0.054 g. of sodium chloride represented by
                            _____ chlorobutanol

                   Total: 0.156 g. of sodium chloride represented by both ingredients

Step 2.   60 × 0.009 = 0.540 g. of sodium chloride in 60 ml. of an isotonic sodium chloride solution

Step 3.   0.540 g.   (from Step 2)
            −0.156 g.   (from Step 1)
            _____

            0.384 g. of sodium chloride required to make the solution isotonic

But since the prescription calls for boric acid:

Step 4.   0.384 g. ÷ 0.52 (sodium chloride equivalent of boric acid) = 0.738 g. of boric acid to be used, *answer*.

How much sodium nitrate should be used in compounding the following prescription?

> ℞   Sol. Silver Nitrate   60.0
>   1–500
>   Make isoton. sol.
>   Sig. For eye use.

The prescription contains 0.120 g. of silver nitrate.

Step 1.   0.34 × 0.120 g. = 0.041 g. of sodium chloride represented by silver nitrate

Step 2.   60 × 0.009 = 0.540 g. of sodium chloride in 60 ml. of an isotonic sodium chloride solution

Step 3.   0.540 g.   (from Step 2)
              −0.041 g.   (from Step 1)
              ──────────
              0.499 g. of sodium chloride required to make solution isotonic

But the prescription requires sodium nitrate, since, in this solution, sodium chloride is incompatible with silver nitrate. Therefore,

Step 4.   0.499 g. ÷ 0.69 (sodium chloride equivalent of sodium nitrate) = 0.720 g. of sodium nitrate to be used, *answer.*

How much sodium chloride should be used in compounding the following prescription?

> ℞   Ingredient X   0.5
>   Sodium Chloride   q.s.
>   Distilled Water   ad   50.0
>   Make isoton. sol.
>   Sig. Eye drops.

Let us assume that Ingredient X is a new substance for which no sodium chloride equivalent is to be found in the Table, and that its molecular weight is 295 and its *i* factor is 2.4.

The sodium chloride equivalent of Ingredient X may be calculated as follows:

$$\frac{58.5}{1.8} \times \frac{2.4}{295} = 0.26, \text{ the sodium chloride equivalent for Ingredient X}$$

Then,

Step 1.   0.26 × 0.5 g. = 0.130 g. of sodium chloride represented by Ingredient X

Step 2.   50 × 0.009 = 0.450 g. of sodium chloride in 50 ml. of an isotonic sodium chloride solution

Step 3.   0.450 g.   (from Step 2)
            −0.130 g.   (from Step 1)
            ─────────
            0.320 g. of sodium chloride to be used, *answer*.

Practice Problems

1. Isotonic Sodium Chloride Solution contains 0.9% of sodium chloride. If the sodium chloride equivalent of boric acid is 0.52, what is the percentage strength of an isotonic solution of boric acid?

2. Sodium chloride is a 2-ion electrolyte, dissociating 90% in a certain concentration. Calculate (a) its dissociation factor and (b) the freezing point of a molal solution.

3. A solution of anhydrous dextrose (mol. wt. 180) contains 25 g. in 500 ml. of water. Calculate the freezing point of the solution.

4. Procaine hydrochloride (mol. wt. 273) is a 2-ion electrolyte, dissociating 80% in a certain concentration. (a) Calculate its dissociation factor. (b) Calculate its sodium chloride equivalent. (c) Calculate the freezing point of a molal solution of procaine hydrochloride.

5. The freezing point of a molal solution of a non-electrolyte is −1.86° C. What is the freezing point of an 0.1% solution of zinc chloride (mol. wt. 136), dissociating 80%?[1]

6. The freezing point of a 5% solution of boric acid is −1.55° C. How much boric acid should be used in preparing 1000 ml. of an isotonic solution?

7. ℞   Ephedrine Sulfate   gr. iv
      Sodium Chloride   q.s.
      Distilled Water   ad   ℥i
      Make isoton. sol.
      Sig. Use as directed.

   How many grains of sodium chloride should be used in compounding the prescription?

─────────

[1] For lack of more definite information, the student must assume that the volume of the molal solution is approximately 1 liter.

8. ℞ Dionin $\frac{1}{2}\%$
        Scopolamine Hydrobromide $\frac{1}{3}\%$
        Sodium Chloride   q.s.
        Distilled Water   ad   30.0
        Make isoton. sol.
        Sig. Use in the eye.

How much sodium chloride should be used in compounding the prescription?

9. ℞ Zinc Sulfate   0.06
        Boric Acid   q.s.
        Distilled Water   ad   30.0
        Make isoton. sol.
        Sig. Drop in eyes.

How much boric acid should be used in compounding the prescription?

10. ℞ Atropine Sulfate   1%
        Boric Acid   q.s.
        Distilled Water   ad   30.0
        Make isoton. sol.
        Sig. One drop in each eye.

How much boric acid should be used in compounding the prescription?

11. ℞ Potassium Iodide   gr. v
        Sodium Chloride   q.s.
        Distilled Water   ad   ℥i
        Make isoton. sol.
        Sig. Use in the eye.

How many grains of sodium chloride should be used in compounding the prescription?

12. ℞ Sol. Silver Nitrate   15.0
             0.5%
        Make isoton. sol.
        Sig. For the eyes.

How much sodium nitrate should be used in compounding the prescription?

13. ℞ Cocaine Hydrochloride   0.150
     Sodium Chloride   q.s.
     Distilled Water   ad   15.0
     Make isoton. sol.
     Sig. One drop in left eye.

How much sodium chloride should be used in compounding the prescription?

14. ℞ Cocaine Hydrochloride   0.6
     Eucatropine Hydrochloride   0.6
     Chlorobutanol   0.1
     Sodium Chloride   q.s.
     Distilled Water   ad   30.0
     Make isoton. sol.
     Sig. For the eye.

How much sodium chloride should be used in compounding the prescription?

15. ℞ Tetracaine Hydrochloride   0.1
     Zinc Sulfate   0.05
     Boric Acid   q.s.
     Distilled Water   ad   30.0
     Make isoton. sol.
     Sig. Drop in eye.

How much boric acid should be used in compounding the prescription?

16. ℞ Sol. Homatropine Hydrobromide 15.0
       1%
     Make isoton. sol. with boric acid.
     Sig. For the eyes.

How much boric acid should be used in compounding the prescription?

17. ℞ Procaine Hydrochloride   1%
     Sodium Chloride   q.s.
     Distilled Water   ad   100.0
     Make isoton. sol.
     Sig. For injection.

How much sodium chloride should be used in compounding the prescription?

18. ℞   Phenylephrine Hydrochloride   1.0
        Chlorobutanol   0.5
        Sodium Bisulfite   0.2
        Sodium Chloride   q.s.
        Distilled Water   ad   100.0
        Make isoton. sol.
        Sig. Use as directed.

How many milliliters of an 0.9% solution of sodium chloride should be used in compounding the prescription?

19. ℞   Holocaine Hydrochloride $\frac{1}{2}$%
        Hyoscine Hydrobromide $\frac{1}{3}$%
        Boric Acid Solution   q.s.
        Distilled Water   ad   60.0
        Make isoton. sol.
        Sig. For the eyes.

How many milliliters of a 5% solution of boric acid should be used in compounding the prescription?

20. ℞   Ephedrine Hydrochloride   0.5
        Chlorobutanol   0.25
        Dextrose   q.s.
        Rose Water   ad   50.0
        Make isoton. sol.
        Sig. Nose drops.

How much dextrose should be used in compounding the prescription?

21. ℞   Dionin   5%
        Sodium Chloride   q.s.
        Distilled Water   ad   ℥ i
        Make isoton. sol.
        Sig. Use as directed in the eye.

How many grains of sodium chloride should be used in compounding the prescription?

22. ℞   Oxytetracycline Hydrochloride   0.050
        Chlorobutanol   0.1
        Sodium Chloride   q.s.
        Distilled Water   ad   30.0
        Make isoton. sol.
        Sig. Eye drops.

How many milligrams of sodium chloride should be used in compounding the prescription?

23. ℞ Tetracaine Hydrochloride   0.5%
        Sol. Epinephrine Hydrochloride   10.0
            1:1000
        Boric Acid   q.s.
        Distilled Water   ad   30.0
        Make isoton. sol.
        Sig. Eye drops.

The solution of epinephrine hydrochloride (1:1000) is already isotonic. How much boric acid should be used in compounding the prescription?

24.   Sodium Acid Phosphate, anhydrous   5.6 g.
        Disodium Phosphate, anhydrous   2.84 g.
        Sodium Chloride   q.s.
        Sterile Distilled Water   ad   1000. ml.
        Label: Isotonic Buffer Solution, pH 6.5.

How many grams of sodium chloride should be used in preparing the
solution?

25.   Dextrose, anhydrous   2.5%
        Sodium Chloride   q.s.
        Water for Injection   ad   1000.0 ml.
        Label: Isotonic Dextrose and Saline Solution.

How many grams of sodium chloride should be used in preparing
the solution?

26. ℞ Ephedrine Sulfate   1%
        Chlorobutanol   ½%
        Distilled Water   ad   100.0
        Make isoton. sol. and buffer to pH 6.5.
        Sig. Nose drops.

You have on hand an isotonic buffered solution, pH 6.5. How many
milliliters of distilled water and how many milliliters of the buffered
solution should be used in compounding the prescription?

27. ℞ Oxytetracycline Hydrochloride   0.5%
        Tetracaine Hydrochloride Sol. 2% 15.0 ml.
        Sodium Chloride   q.s.
        Distilled Water   ad   30.0 ml.
        Make isoton. sol.
        Sig. For the eye.

The 2% solution of tetracaine hydrochloride is already isotonic.
How many milliliters of an 0.9% solution of sodium chloride should be used
in compounding the prescription?

TABLE OF SODIUM CHLORIDE EQUIVALENTS

Substance	Molecular weight	Ions	i	Sodium chloride equivalent
Achromycin				
(See Tetracycline hydrochloride)				
Alum (ammonium).12H$_2$O	453	4	3.4	0.24
Alum (potassium).12H$_2$O	474	4	3.4	0.23
Alypin hydrochloride	315	2	1.8	0.19
Ammonium chloride	53.5	2	1.8	1.09
Amphetamine sulfate	368	3	2.6	0.23
Amydricaine				
(See Alypin hydrochloride)				
Amylcaine hydrochloride	287	2	1.8	0.20
Antazoline phosphate	363	2	1.8	0.16
Antipyrine	188	1	1.0	0.17
Antistine				
(See Antazoline phosphate)				
Apothesine hydrochloride	298	2	1.8	0.20
Argyrol				
(See Mild silver protein)				
Atropine sulfate.H$_2$O	695	3	2.6	0.12
Aureomycin				
(See Chlortetracycline hydrochloride)				
Benzalkonium chloride	360	2	1.8	0.16
Benzedrine sulfate				
(See Amphetamine sulfate)				
Benzyl alcohol	108	1	1.0	0.30
Borax				
(See Sodium borate)				
Boric acid	61.8	1	1.0	0.52
Butacaine sulfate	711	3	2.6	0.12
Butyn sulfate				
(See Butacaine sulfate)				
Caffeine	194	1	1.0	0.17
Calcium chloride.2H$_2$O	147	3	2.6	0.57
Calcium gluconate.H$_2$O	448	3	2.6	0.19
Calcium lactate.5H$_2$O	308	3	2.6	0.27
Camphor	152	1	1.0	0.21
Carbachol	183	2	1.8	0.33
Carbamylcholine chloride				
(See Carbachol)				
Chloramphenicol	323	1	1.0	0.10
Chlorobutanol	177	1	1.0	0.18
Chloromycetin				
(See Chloramphenicol)				
Chlortetracycline hydrochloride	515	2	1.8	0.11

TABLE OF SODIUM CHLORIDE EQUIVALENTS (*Continued*)

Substance	Molecular weight	Ions	i	Sodium chloride equivalent
Cocaine hydrochloride	340	2	1.8	0.17
Cupric sulfate.5H$_2$O	250	2	1.4	0.18
Cyclogyl				
(See Cyclopentolate hydrochloride)				
Cyclopentolate hydrochloride	328	2	1.8	0.18
Dextrose (anhydrous)	180	1	1.0	0.18
Dextrose.H$_2$O	198	1	1.0	0.16
Dionin				
(See Ethylmorphine hydrochloride)				
Diothane hydrochloride	434	2	1.8	0.14
Dyclone				
(See Dyclonine hydrochloride)				
Dyclonine hydrochloride	326	2	1.8	0.18
Emetine hydrochloride	554	3	2.6	0.15
Ephedrine hydrochloride	202	2	1.8	0.29
Ephedrine sulfate	429	3	2.6	0.20
Epinephrine hydrochloride	220	2	1.8	0.27
Epinephrine bitartrate	333	2	1.8	0.18
Eserine salicylate				
(See Physostigmine salicylate)				
Eserine sulfate				
(See Physostigmine sulfate)				
Ethylhydrocupreine hydrochloride . . .	377	2	1.8	0.16
Ethylmorphine hydrochloride.2H$_2$O . . .	386	2	1.8	0.15
Eucatropine hydrochloride	328	2	1.8	0.22
Euphthalmine hydrochloride				
(See Eucatropine hydrochloride)				
Fluorescein sodium	376	3	2.6	0.22
Glycerin	92.1	1	1.0	0.36
Holocaine hydrochloride				
(See Phenacaine hydrochloride)				
Homatropine hydrobromide	356	2	1.8	0.16
Hydroxyamphetamine hydrobromide . . .	232	2	1.8	0.25
Hyoscine hydrobromide				
(See Scopolamine hydrobromide)				
Hyoscine hydrochloride				
(See Scopolamine hydrochloride)				
Larocaine hydrochloride	315	2	1.8	0.19
Magnesium sulfate.7H$_2$O	247	2	1.8	0.24
Menthol	156	1	1.0	0.21
Mercuric cyanide	253	3	1.0	0.13
Mercuric oxycyanide	469	3	1.0	0.07
Mercuric succinimide	397	2	1.0	0.08

TABLE OF SODIUM CHLORIDE EQUIVALENTS (*Continued*)

Substance	Molecular weight	Ions	i	Sodium chloride equivalent
Mercury bichloride	272	3	1.0	0.12
Methenamine	140	1	1.0	0.23
Metycaine hydrochloride	298	2	1.8	0.20
Mild protein silver (20% silver)	540 (?)	1	1.0	0.06
Morphine hydrochloride.3H$_2$O	376	2	1.8	0.16
Morphine sulfate.5H$_2$O	759	3	2.6	0.11
Neo-synephrine hydrochloride (See Phenylephrine hydrochloride)				
Novocain (See Procaine hydrochloride)				
Nupercaine hydrochloride	380	2	1.8	0.15
Ophthaine (See Proparacaine hydrochloride)				
Optochin (See Ethylhydrocupreine hydrochloride)				
Oxytetracycline hydrochloride	497	2	1.8	0.12
Paredrine (See Hydroxyamphetamine hydrobromide)				
Phenacaine hydrochloride	353	2	1.8	0.17
Phenobarbital sodium	254	2	1.8	0.23
Phenylephrine hydrochloride	204	2	1.8	0.29
Physostigmine salicylate	413	2	1.8	0.14
Physostigmine sulfate	649	3	2.6	0.13
Pilocarpine hydrochloride	245	2	1.8	0.24
Pilocarpine nitrate	271	2	1.8	0.22
Pontocaine hydrochloride (See Tetracaine hydrochloride)				
Potassium biphosphate	136	2	1.8	0.43
Potassium chloride	74.6	2	1.8	0.78
Potassium iodide	166	2	1.8	0.35
Potassium nitrate	101	2	1.8	0.58
Potassium penicillin G	372	2	1.8	0.16
Procaine hydrochloride	273	2	1.8	0.21
Propadrine	188	2	1.8	0.31
Proparacaine hydrochloride	331	2	1.8	0.18
Protargol (See Strong protein silver)				
Scopolamine hydrobromide.3H$_2$O . . .	438	2	1.8	0.13
Scopolamine hydrochloride.2H$_2$O . . .	376	2	1.8	0.16
Silver nitrate	170	2	1.8	0.34
Sodium bicarbonate	84	2	1.8	0.70
Sodium biphosphate	120	2	1.8	0.49
Sodium biphosphate.H$_2$O	138	2	1 8	0.42

TABLE OF SODIUM CHLORIDE EQUIVALENTS (*Continued*)

Substance	Molecular weight	Ions	i	Sodium chloride equivalent
Sodium bisulfite	104	3	2.6	0.81
Sodium borate.10H$_2$O	381	5	4.2	0.36
Sodium carbonate	106	3	2.6	0.80
Sodium carbonate.H$_2$O	124	3	2.6	0.68
Sodium chloride	58	2	1.8	1.00
Sodium citrate.2H$_2$O	294	4	3.4	0.38
Sodium iodide	150	2	1.8	0.39
Sodium lactate	112	2	1.8	0.52
Sodium nitrate	85	2	1.8	0.69
Sodium phosphate.2H$_2$O	178	3	2.6	0.47
Sodium phosphate.7H$_2$O	268	3	2.6	0.31
Sodium phosphate.12H$_2$O	358	3	2.6	0.24
Sodium sulfite	126	3	2.6	0.64
Strong protein silver (7.5% to 8.5% silver)	1350 (?)	1	1.0	0.024
Sulfadiazine sodium	272	2	1.8	0.21
Sulfanilamide	172	1	1.0	0.19
Sulfapyridine sodium	289	2	1.8	0.20
Sulfathiazole sodium (sesquihydrate)	304	2	1.8	0.19
Tannic acid	324 (?)	1	1.0	0.10
Terramycin (See Oxytetracycline hydrochloride)				
Tetracaine hydrochloride	301	2	1.8	0.19
Tetracycline hydrochloride	481	2	1.8	0.12
Tetrahydrozoline hydrochloride	237	2	1.8	0.25
Tutocaine hydrochloride	287	2	1.8	0.20
Tyzine (See Tetrahydrozoline hydrochloride)				
Urea	60.1	1	1.0	0.54
Zephiran (See Benzalkonium chloride)				
Zinc chloride	136	3	2.6	0.62
Zinc sulfate.7H$_2$O	288	2	1.4	0.16

Chapter 12

Chemical Problems

ATOMIC AND MOLECULAR WEIGHTS

MOST chemical problems involve the use of *atomic* or *combining weights* of the elements, and the validity of their solutions depends upon the *Law of Definite Proportions*.

The *atomic weight* of an element is the ratio of the weight of its atom to the weight of an atom of another element taken as a standard. Long ago, hydrogen, with a weight taken as 1, was used as the standard. For many years, the weight of oxygen, taken as 16, has proved a more convenient standard. In August 1961, however, the International Union of Pure and Applied Chemistry (following similar action by the International Union of Pure and Applied Physics) officially released the most up-to-date table of atomic weights based on carbon, taking 12 as the relative nuclidic mass of the isotope ^{12}C. It should be noted that the rounded-off *approximate* atomic weights in the table given on the inside back cover and those based on the long-familiar oxygen table are identical and continue to be suffiently accurate for most chemical calculations likely to be encountered by pharmacists.

The *combining* or *equivalent weight* of an *element* is that weight of the element which will combine with (or displace) one gram atomic weight of hydrogen (or the equivalent weight of some other element). For example, when hydrogen and chlorine react to form HCl, 1.008 g. of hydrogen react with 35.45 g. of chlorine; therefore the equivalent weight of chlorine is 35.45.

The *equivalent weight* of a *compound* is that weight of a compound which is chemically equivalent to 1.008 g. of hydrogen. Thus, one mole or 36.46 g. of HCl contains 1.008 g. of hydrogen and this is displaceable by one equivalent weight of a metal; hence its equivalent weight is 36.46. Also, one mole or 40.00 g. of NaOH is capable of neutralizing 1.008 g. of hydrogen; therefore its equivalent weight is 40.00. But one mole or 98.08 g. of H_2SO_4 contains 2.016 g. of hydrogen and this is displaceable by *two* equivalent weights of a metal; consequently its equivalent weight is $\frac{98.08}{2}$ or 49.04.

The *Law of Definite Proportions* states that elements invariably combine in the same proportion by weight to form a given compound.

(214)

To calculate molecular weights from atomic weights:

The *molecular weight* of an element or compound is the sum of the weights of the atoms in the molecule.

Example:

Calculate the molecular weight of phosphoric acid, H_3PO_4.

$$\underset{(3 \times 1.008)}{H_3} + \underset{30.97}{P} + \underset{(4 \times 16.00)}{O_4} = 97.99, \; answer.$$

PERCENTAGE COMPOSITION

To calculate the percentage composition of a compound:

Examples:

Calculate the percentage composition of tribasic calcium phosphate, $Ca_3(PO_4)_2$.

$$\underset{(3 \times 40.08)}{Ca_3} + \underset{(2 \times 30.97)}{2P} + \underset{(8 \times 16.00)}{2O_4} =$$

$$120.24 \quad + \quad 61.94 \quad + \quad 128.0 \quad = 310.2$$

$$\frac{310.2}{120.24} = \frac{100 \; (\%)}{x \; (\%)}$$

$x = 38.76\%$ of calcium, *and*

$$\frac{310.2}{61.94} = \frac{100 \; (\%)}{y \; (\%)}$$

$y = 19.97\%$ of phosphorus, *and*

$$\frac{310.2}{128.0} = \frac{100 \; (\%)}{z \; (\%)}$$

$z = 41.27\%$ of oxygen, *answers.*

Check: $38.76\% + 19.97\% + 41.27\% = 100\%$

Calculate the percentage of water in sodium phosphate, $Na_2HPO_4.7H_2O$.

$$\underset{(2 \times 22.99)}{Na_2} + \underset{1.008}{H} + \underset{30.97}{P} + \underset{(4 \times 16.00)}{O_4} + \underset{(7 \times 18.02)}{7H_2O} =$$

$$45.98 \quad + 1.008 + 30.97 + \quad 64.00 \quad + \quad 126.1 \quad =$$

$$268.1, \text{ molecular weight of sodium phosphate}$$

$$\frac{268.1}{126.1} = \frac{100 \; (\%)}{x \; (\%)}$$

$x = 47.03\%$, *answer.*

To calculate the weight of a constituent, given the weight of a compound :

Approximate atomic weights may ordinarily be used in solving problems of this kind.

Example:

> A certain solution contains 500 mg. of sodium fluoride, NaF. How many milligrams of fluoride ion are represented in the solution?

> Na   F
> 23 + 19 = 42

$$\frac{42}{19} = \frac{500 \text{ (mg.)}}{x \text{ (mg.)}}$$

> x = 226 mg., *answer.*

To calculate the weight of a compound, given the weight of a constituent :

Approximate atomic weights may ordinarily be used in solving problems of this kind.

Example:

> A prescription calls for 200 mg. of fluoride ion. How many milligrams of sodium fluoride should be used in order to obtain the prescribed amount of fluoride ion?

> Na   F
> 23 + 19 = 42

$$\frac{19}{42} = \frac{200 \text{ (mg.)}}{x \text{ (mg.)}}$$

> x = 442 mg., *answer.*

CHEMICALS IN REACTIONS

To calculate the weights of pure chemicals involved in reactions :

Approximate atomic weights may ordinarily be used in solving problems of this kind.

Examples:

> *How many grams of absolute hydrochloric acid are required to neutralize 324 g. of anhydrous sodium carbonate?*

$$Na_2CO_3 + 2HCl = 2NaCl + H_2O + CO_2$$
$$\quad 106 \qquad 2(36)$$
$$\qquad\qquad \text{or } 72$$

Molecular weight of $Na_2CO_3 = 106$
Molecular weight of $2HCl = 72$

$$\frac{106}{72} = \frac{324 \text{ (g.)}}{x \text{ (g.)}}$$

x = 223 g., *answer.*

> *How many grams of iron are required to react with 100 g. of iodine?*

$$Fe + \quad I_2 \quad = FeI_2$$
$$56 \quad 2(127)$$
$$\qquad \text{or } 254$$

$$\frac{254}{56} = \frac{100 \text{ (g.)}}{x \text{ (g.)}}$$

x = 22.1 g., *answer.*

> *How many grams of p-aminobenzoic acid and how many grams of sodium bicarbonate should be used to prepare 100 g. of sodium p-aminobenzoate?*

$$NH_2C_6H_4COOH + NaHCO_3 = NH_2C_6H_4COONa + H_2O + CO_2$$
$$\qquad 137 \qquad\qquad 84 \qquad\qquad\quad 159$$

$$\frac{159}{137} = \frac{100 \text{ (g.)}}{x \text{ (g.)}}$$

x = 86.2 g. of p-aminobenzoic acid, *and*

$$\frac{159}{84} = \frac{100 \text{ (g.)}}{y \text{ (g.)}}$$

y = 52.8 g. of sodium bicarbonate, *answers.*

How many grams of anhydrous citric acid are required to react with 25 g. of sodium bicarbonate?

$$3NaHCO_3 + H_3C_6H_5O_7 = Na_3C_6H_5O_7 + 3H_2O + 3CO_2$$
$$\begin{array}{cc} 3(84) & 192 \\ \text{or } 252 & \end{array}$$

$$\frac{252}{192} = \frac{25 \text{ (g.)}}{x \text{ (g.)}}$$

x = 19 g., *answer.*

To calculate the weights of chemicals involved in reactions, with consideration of percentage strengths :

In solving problems of this type, it is important to remember that proportions based upon atomic and molecular weights apply only to *pure* (absolute) or *100%* chemicals. If *volume-in-volume* or *weight-in-volume* strength is specified, *it must be converted to weight-in-weight strength.*

Examples:

How many grams of 85% potassium hydroxide are required to react with 125 g. of mercuric chloride?

$$HgCl_2 + 2KOH = HgO + 2KCl + H_2O$$
$$\begin{array}{cc} 272 & 2(56) \\ & \text{or } 112 \end{array}$$

If

$$\frac{272}{112} = \frac{125 \text{ (g.)}}{x \text{ (g.)}}$$

x = 51.5 g. of 100% KOH,

then

$$\frac{85 \text{ (\%)}}{100 \text{ (\%)}} = \frac{51.5 \text{ (g.)}}{y \text{ (g.)}}$$

y = 60.6 g. of 85% KOH, *answer.*

How many grams of potassium bicarbonate and how many milliliters of 36% acetic acid, sp. gr. 1.045, are required to prepare 200 g. of potassium acetate?

$$KHCO_3 + HC_2H_3O_2 = KC_2H_3O_2 + CO_2 + H_2O$$
$$\quad 100 \qquad\quad 60 \qquad\qquad 98$$

$$\frac{98}{100} = \frac{200 \text{ (g.)}}{x \text{ (g.)}}$$

x = 204 g. of potassium bicarbonate, *and*

If

$$\frac{98}{60} = \frac{200 \text{ (g.)}}{y \text{ (g.)}}$$

y = 122 g. of 100% acetic acid,

then

$$\frac{36 \text{ (\%)}}{100 \text{ (\%)}} = \frac{122 \text{ (g.)}}{z \text{ (g.)}}$$

z = 339 g. of 36% acetic acid

339 g. of water measure 339 ml.

$$\frac{339 \text{ ml.}}{1.045} = 324 \text{ ml. of } 36\% \text{ acetic acid, } answers.$$

To solve problems involving chemically equivalent quantities :

Example:

The formula for a test solution calls for 234 g. of monohydrated sodium carbonate ($Na_2CO_3.H_2O$). Only anhydrous sodium carbonate (Na_2CO_3) is available? How much of it should be used to replace the hydrated salt?

Molecular weights:
$Na_2CO_3.H_2O = 124$ $\qquad\qquad Na_2CO_3 = 106$

$$\frac{124}{106} = \frac{234 \text{ (g.)}}{x \text{ (g.)}}$$

x = 200 g., *answer.*

SAPONIFICATION VALUE

To solve chemical problems based upon saponification value:

Saponification value refers to the number of milligrams of 100% potassium hydroxide required to saponify the free acids and esters in 1 g. of a fat or oil. For example, when we say that olive oil has a saponification value of 190, we mean that 190 mg. of 100% KOH are required to saponify completely 1 g. of olive oil.

Examples:

How many grams of 85% potassium hydroxide are required to saponify completely 100 g. of coconut oil having a saponification value of 260?

$$260 = 260 \text{ mg.} = 0.260 \text{ g.}$$

If

$$\frac{1 \text{ (g.)}}{100 \text{ (g.)}} = \frac{0.260 \text{ (g.)}}{x \text{ (g.)}}$$

$$x = 26 \text{ g. of } 100\% \text{ KOH,}$$

then

$$\frac{85 \text{ (\%)}}{100 \text{ (\%)}} = \frac{26 \text{ (g.)}}{y \text{ (g.)}}$$

$$y = 30.6 \text{ g., } answer.$$

In a formula for soft soap, 100 g. of 88% potassium hydroxide are used to saponify 400 g. of a vegetable oil. Calculate the saponification value of the oil.

If

$$\frac{100 \text{ (\%)}}{88 \text{ (\%)}} = \frac{100 \text{ (g.)}}{x \text{ (g.)}}$$

$$x = 88 \text{ g. of } 100\% \text{ KOH, required to saponify } 400 \text{ g. of the oil,}$$

then

$$\frac{400 \text{ (g.)}}{1 \text{ (g.)}} = \frac{88 \text{ (g.)}}{y \text{ (g.)}}$$

$$y = 0.220 \text{ g.} = 220 \text{ mg.} = 220, answer.$$

ACID VALUE

To solve chemical problems based on acid value :

Acid value refers to the number of milligrams of 100% potassium hydroxide required to neutralize the free fatty acids in 1 g. of a substance. For example, if a wax has an acid value of 22, 1 g. of it will require 22 mg. of 100% KOH (or the equivalent weight of some other alkali) for the neutralization of the free fatty acids.

In the formulation of cold creams and other emulsions containing waxes, the amount of alkali depends upon the acid value of the wax.

Example:

A cold cream formula calls for 1000 g. of white wax having an acid value of 20. (a) How many grams of 85% potassium hydroxide (KOH) should be used in formulating the cream? (b) If sodium borate ($Na_2B_4O_7.10H_2O$) is used in formulating the cream, how many grams are required?

(a)   20 = 20 mg. = 0.020 g.

If

$$\frac{1 \ (g.)}{1000 \ (g.)} = \frac{0.020 \ (g.)}{x \ (g.)}$$

x = 20 g. of 100% KOH,

then

$$\frac{85 \ (\%)}{100 \ (\%)} = \frac{20 \ (g.)}{y \ (g.)}$$

y = 23.5 g. of 85% KOH, *answer.*

(b) Since one molecule of sodium borate (mol. wt. 382) gives two molecules of sodium hydroxide that can react with two atoms of hydrogen, its equivalent weight is ½ of its molecular weight (382 ÷ 2) or 191, and therefore 191 g. are chemically equivalent to 56 g. of KOH (mol. wt. 56).

In (a) it was calculated that 20 g. of 100% KOH are required. Therefore,

$$\frac{56}{191} = \frac{20 \ (g.)}{x \ (g.)}$$

x = 68.2 g. of sodium borate, *answer.*

WEIGHTS AND VOLUMES OF GASES

The methods by which we may calculate the volume of a given weight of any gas—or the weight of a given volume—depend on Avogadro's Law, which states that *under the same conditions of temperature and pressure, equal volumes of all gases contain the same number of molecules.*

When the molecular weight of a gas is taken to indicate a number of grams, the expression is called the *mole* or the *gram-molecular weight* of that gas. By another consequence of Avogadro's Law, the gram-molecular weights of all gases have a common volume, *22.4 liters*, under standard conditions of temperature and pressure (S.T.P.)—that is, at 0° C. and a barometric pressure of 760 mm. Since under normal conditions the molecule of a gas contains two atoms, this volume is shared by 2 × 16 or 32 g. of oxygen, 2 × 1 or 2 g. of hydrogen, 2 × 14 or 28 g. of nitrogen, and so on. Hence, 22.4 liters (S.T.P.) of any gaseous element or compound will weigh a number of grams equal to the number expressing its molecular weight.

To calculate the volume of a gas under standard conditions of temperature and pressure, given its weight:

Example:

> *What is the volume (S.T.P.) of 3.87 g. of hydrogen, H_2?*
>
> > Molecular weight of hydrogen = 2 × 1 = 2
> > 2 g. of hydrogen measure 22.4 liters

$$\frac{2 \text{ (g.)}}{3.87 \text{ (g.)}} = \frac{22.4 \text{ (liters)}}{\text{x (liters)}}$$

> > x = 43 liters, *answer.*

To calculate the volume of a gas formed or used in a reaction under standard conditions of temperature and pressure:

Example:

> *What volume (S.T.P.) of hydrogen sulfide can be produced from 20 g. of iron sulfide?*

$$FeS + 2HCl = FeCl_2 + H_2S\uparrow$$
$$88 \qquad\qquad\qquad\qquad 34$$

88 g. of FeS yield 34 g. of H_2S which measure 22.4 liters

$$\frac{88 \text{ (g.)}}{20 \text{ (g.)}} = \frac{22.4 \text{ (liters)}}{x \text{ (liters)}}$$

x = 5.1 liters, *answer.*

To calculate the weight of a chemical required to make a specified volume of a gas :

Example:

How many grams of zinc are required to make 50 liters (S.T.P.) of hydrogen?

$$Zn + H_2SO_4 = ZnSO_4 + H_2\uparrow$$
$$65 \qquad\qquad\qquad\qquad 2$$

65 g. of Zn will produce 2 g. of hydrogen which measure 22.4 liters

$$\frac{22.4 \text{ (liters)}}{50 \text{ (liters)}} = \frac{65 \text{ (g.)}}{x \text{ (g.)}}$$

x = 145 g., *answer.*

To calculate the volume of a gas when corrections for temperature and pressure must be made :

In the problems above the gases were assumed to be measured at S.T.P. The volume of a gas measured under any conditions of temperature and pressure may be used to calculate the volume of the same gas under different conditions by application of the Laws of Boyle and Charles.

According to Boyle's Law, the *volume of a given mass of gas varies inversely with the pressure, when the temperature is constant.* Thus, an increase in pressure results in a decrease in the volume of a gas and a decrease in pressure results in an increase in its volume.

And according to Charles' Law, the *volume of a gas is proportional to its absolute temperature, when the pressure is constant.* A gas, under constant pressure, will expand, therefore, $\frac{1}{273}$ of its volume when heated through $1° C.$

Examples:

> *The volume of a gas measured at a pressure of 750 mm. is 380 ml. What is its volume at 760 mm., if the temperature remains constant?*

$$\frac{760 \text{ (mm.)}}{750 \text{ (mm.)}} = \frac{380 \text{ (ml.)}}{x \text{ (ml.)}}$$

$$x = 380 \text{ ml.} \times \tfrac{750}{760} = 375 \text{ ml., } \textit{answer.}$$

> *The volume of a gas is 686 ml. at 70° C. What is its volume at 27° C., if the pressure remains constant?*

$$70° \text{ C.} = 343° \text{ Absolute}$$
$$27° \text{ C.} = 300° \text{ Absolute}$$

$$\frac{343 \text{ (°A)}}{300 \text{ (°A)}} = \frac{686 \text{ (ml.)}}{x \text{ (ml.)}}$$

$$x = 686 \text{ ml.} \times \tfrac{300}{343} = 600 \text{ ml., } \textit{answer.}$$

Since the changes in the volume of a gas due to variations in pressure and temperature are *independent* of one another, the corrections may be conveniently made together by combining the proportions used in the preceding examples.

Example:

> *A sample of gas measured 300 ml. at 27° C and 740 mm. Calculate its volume at S.T.P.*

$$27° \text{ C.} = 300° \text{ Absolute}$$
$$0° \text{ C.} = 273° \text{ Absolute}$$

Volume at S.T.P. $= 300 \text{ ml.} \times \tfrac{273}{300} \times \tfrac{740}{760} = 266 \text{ ml., } \textit{answer.}$

Practice Problems

1. Calculate the molecular weight of calcium hydroxide, $Ca(OH)_2$.

2. Calculate the molecular weight of potassium permanganate, $KMnO_4$.

3. Calculate the molecular weight of ethyl alcohol, C_2H_5OH.

4. Calculate the molecular weight of ferrous sulfate, $FeSO_4.7H_2O$.

5. Calculate the molecular weight of acetic acid, CH_3COOH.

6. Calculate the percentage composition of sodium fluoride, NaF.

7. Calculate the percentage composition of ether, $(C_2H_5)_2O$.

8. What is the percentage composition of Sodium Phosphate, N.F., $Na_2HPO_4.7H_2O$?

9. What is the percentage composition of Sodium Biphosphate, N.F., $NaH_2PO_4.H_2O$?

10. Calculate the percentage of water in dextrose, $C_6H_{12}O_6.H_2O$.

11. Calculate the quantity of water in 2000 g. of magnesium sulfate, $MgSO_4.7H_2O$.

12. What is the percentage of iron in ferrous fumarate, $C_4H_2FeO_4$?

13. What is the percentage of copper in cupric sulfate, $CuSO_4.5H_2O$?

14. What is the percentage of iron in ferrous sulfate, $FeSO_4.7H_2O$?

15. What is the percentage of mercury in mercury bichloride, $HgCl_2$?

16. A certain solution contains 110 mg. of sodium fluoride, NaF, in each 1000 ml. How many milligrams of fluoride ion are represented in each 2 ml. of the solution?

17. The usual dose of ferrous sulfate, $FeSO_4.7H_2O$, is 300 mg., three times a day. How many milligrams of elemental iron are represented in the usual daily dose?

18. A prescription calls for 500 ml. of a solution such that each 5 ml. will contain 0.5 mg. of fluoride ion. How many milligrams of sodium fluoride should be used in compounding the prescription?

19. ℞ Sodium Fluoride   q.s.
       Distilled Water   ad   500 ml.
       Sig. 2 ml. diluted to 100 ml. will give a $1:1,000,000$ solution of fluoride ion.

How many milligrams of sodium fluoride, NaF, should be used in compounding the prescription?

20. ℞ Sodium Fluoride   q.s.
       Distilled Water   ad   100 ml.
       Sig. Ten (10) drops diluted to 250 ml. yield a $1:1,000,000$ solution of fluoride ion.

The dispensing dropper calibrates 25 drops per ml. How many milligrams of sodium fluoride should be used in compounding the prescription?

21. ℞　Sol. Sodium Fluoride　　　　　　500 ml.
　　　　(10 ml. = 1500 mcg. of fluoride ion)
　　　　Sig. Dilute and use as directed.

How many grams of sodium fluoride should be used in compounding the prescription?

22. How many milliliters of a solution containing 0.275 mg. of histamine acid phosphate (mol. wt. 307) per ml. should be used in preparing 30 ml. of a solution which is to contain the equivalent of 1:10,000 of histamine (mol. wt. 111)?

23. ℞　Sodium Fluoride　　　　　　　　q.s.
　　　　Multiple Vitamin Drops　　ad　　60.0 ml.
　　　　(Five drops = 1 mg. of fluoride ion)
　　　　Sig. Five drops in orange juice daily.

The dispensing dropper calibrates 20 drops per ml. How many milligrams of sodium fluoride should be used in compounding the prescription?

24. How many grams of potassium iodide are required to react with 250 g. of mercury bichloride?

$$HgCl_2 + 2KI = HgI_2 = 2KCl$$

25. How many grams of potassium bicarbonate (mol. wt. 100) and how many grams of citric acid (mol. wt. 210) should be used in preparing 10 liters of a solution which is to contain 0.3 g. of potassium citrate (mol. wt. 324) per teaspoonful?

26. Starting with the amount of yellow mercuric oxide that can be made from 200 g. of mercury bichloride, how many grams of Yellow Mercuric Oxide Ophthalmic Ointment, containing 1% of yellow mercuric oxide, can be prepared from it?

$$HgCl_2 + 2\,NaOH = HgO + 2NaCl + H_2O$$

27. How many grams of magnesium sulfate and how many grams of 95% sodium hydroxide should be used in preparing 20 liters of milk of magnesia containing 8% (w/v) of magnesium hydroxide?

$$MgSO_4.7H_2O + 2NaOH = Mg(OH)_2 + Na_2SO_4 + 7H_2O$$

28. How many grams of potassium bicarbonate (mol. wt. 100) and how many milliliters of 36% acetic acid (mol. wt. 60), specific gravity 1.050, are required to prepare 1 gallon of a 10% solution of potassium acetate (mol. wt. 98)?

$$KHCO_3 + HC_2H_3O_2 = KC_2H_3O_2 + CO_2 + H_2O$$

29. In preparing Benedict's Solution, you are directed to use 100 g. of anhydrous sodium carbonate (Na_2CO_3) in 1000 ml. of the reagent. Calculate the amount of monohydrated sodium carbonate ($Na_2CO_3.H_2O$) that should be used in preparing 5 liters of the solution.

30. In preparing Sodium Phosphate Solution, N.F., 755 g. of sodium phosphate ($Na_2HPO_4.7H_2O$) are required for 1000 ml. of the product. How many grams of exsiccated sodium phosphate (Na_2HPO_4) may be used in place of the crystallized salt?

31. In preparing Magnesium Citrate Solution, 2.5 g. of potassium bicarbonate ($KHCO_3$) are needed to charge each bottle. If no potassium bicarbonate is available, how much sodium bicarbonate ($NaHCO_3$) should be used?

32. The formula for Albright's Solution "M" calls for 8.84 g. of anhydrous sodium carbonate (Na_2CO_3) per 1000 ml. How many grams of 95% sodium hydroxide (NaOH) should be used to replace the anhydrous sodium carbonate in preparing 5 liters of the solution?

33.   Precipitated Sulfur   50.0 g.
Potassium Hydroxide   10.0 g.
Stearic Acid   200.0 g.
Glycerin   40.0 g.
Water, to make   1000.0 g.
Label: Sulfur cream.

If potassium carbonate ($K_2CO_3.1\frac{1}{2}H_2O$) were to be used in formulating 10 lb. of the cream, how many grams should be used to replace the potassium hydroxide (KOH)?

34. How many grams of p-aminosalicylic acid ($NH_2C_6H_3OHCOOH$) and how many grams of sodium bicarbonate ($NaHCO_3$) should be used in preparing a liter of a solution of sodium p-aminosalicylate ($NH_2C_6H_3OHCOONa$), each 5 ml. of which is to contain the equivalent of 1 g. of p-aminosalicylic acid?

$$NH_2C_6H_3OHCOOH + NaHCO_3 = NH_2C_6H_3OHCOONa$$
$$+ H_2O + CO_2$$

35. Ferrous Sulfate Syrup contains 40 g. of ferrous sulfate ($FeSO_4.7H_2O$) per 1000 ml. How many milligrams of iron (Fe) are represented in the usual dose of 10 ml. of the syrup?

36. How many grams of sodium acid phosphate (NaH_2PO_4) should be used to replace 2500 g. of citric acid $[C_3H_4OH(COOH)_3]$ in a formula for an effervescent salt?

37. How many grams of 42% (MgO equivalent) magnesium carbonate are required to prepare 14 liters of Magnesium Citrate Solution so that each 350 ml. contains the equivalent of 6.0 g. of MgO?

38. Five hundred grams of Effervescent Sodium Phosphate contain 100 g. of dried sodium phosphate (Na_2HPO_4). How much Sodium Phosphate, N.F., ($Na_2HPO_4.7H_2O$) is represented in each 10-g. dose of Effervescent Sodium Phosphate?

39. How many grams of epinephrine bitartrate (mol. wt. 333) should be used in preparing 500 ml. of an ophthalmic solution containing the equivalent of 2% of epinephrine (mol. wt. 183)?

40. One thousand milliliters of Sodium Phosphate Solution, N.F., contain 755 g. of sodium phosphate ($Na_2HPO_4.7H_2O$). How much Dried Sodium Phosphate, N.F., (Na_2HPO_4) is represented in each 10-ml. dose of the solution?

41. Coconut oil has a saponification value of 255. How much 85% potassium hydroxide should be used to saponify completely 750 g. of coconut oil?

42. How much 88% potassium hydroxide should be used to saponify completely 500 ml. of a vegetable oil (sp. gr. 0.850) which has a saponification value of 180?

43. The saponification value of stearic acid is 208. In a vanishing cream formula containing 250 g. of stearic acid, how much 88% potassium hydroxide is required to saponify 20% of the stearic acid?

44. How many grams of 85% potassium hydroxide should be used to saponify completely 2000 ml. of a vegetable oil (sp. gr. 0.90) having a saponification value of 190?

45. In a formula for green soap, 400 g. of 85% potassium hydroxide were used to saponify 1700 g. of a vegetable oil. Calculate the saponification value of the oil.

46.	Stearic Acid	200 g.
	Potassium Hydroxide	q.s.
	Glycerin	100 g.
	Water, to make	1000 g.

If the saponification value of stearic acid is 208, how many grams of 85% potassium hydroxide should be used to saponify 25% of the stearic acid in the formula?

47.	Stearic Acid	120 g.
	Potassium Hydroxide	q.s.
	Propylene Glycol	50 g.
	Water, to make	1000 g.

(a) If the saponification value of stearic acid is 210, how many grams of 88% potassium hydroxide should be used to saponify 30% of the stearic acid?

(b) The equivalent weight of triethanolamine is 143. How many grams of triethanolamine could be used to replace the quantity of potassium hydroxide needed to saponify 30% of the stearic acid in the formula?

48.	Stearic Acid	20.0
	Liquid Petrolatum	5.0
	Triethanolamine	5.0
	Coconut Oil Soap	40.0
	Glycerin	5.0
	Water	25.0

Coconut oil soap contains 40% of coconut oil. How many grams of 85% potassium hydroxide are required to saponify the coconut oil (saponification value 255) needed to prepare the soap for 5 lb. of this formula?

49. A formula for a cold cream calls for 500 g. of white wax. If the sample of white wax used has an acid value of 20, how much 88% potassium hydroxide is required to neutralize the free acids contained in the wax?

50. A cold cream formula contains 1500 g. of white wax. The acid value of the wax is 21.

(a) How many grams of pure KOH should be used?
(b) How many grams of 85% KOH should be used?
(c) The equivalent weight of sodium borate is 191. How many grams of sodium borate should be used?

51. A formula for a cosmetic cream calls for 100 g. of white wax. If the sample of white wax used has an acid value of 22, how much sodium borate (mol. wt. 382) should be used in formulating the cream?

52.

Precipitated Sulfur	7.0
White Wax	10.0
Sodium Borate	q.s.
Mineral Oil	60.0
Rose Water, to make	100.0

The acid value of the white wax is 20, and the equivalent weight of sodium borate is 191. How many grams of sodium borate should be used in preparing 5 lb. of the product?

53.

Stearic Acid	20.0
Potassium Carbonate	q.s.
Propylene Glycol	10.0
Lanolin	5.0
Distilled Water, to make	100.0

How many grams of potassium carbonate ($K_2CO_3.1\frac{1}{2}H_2O$) should be used to saponify 25% of the stearic acid ($C_{17}H_{35}COOH$)? Assume the stearic acid to be 100% pure.

54. What is the volume (S.T.P.) of 75.5 g. of ammonia, NH_3?

55. What is the volume (S.T.P.) of 28.46 g. of oxygen, O_2?

56. How many liters (S.T.P.) of oxygen can be made from 100 g. of potassium chlorate?

$$2KClO_3 = 2KCl + 3O_2 \uparrow$$

57. How many liters (S.T.P.) of sulfur dioxide can be made from 200 g. of sulfur?

$$S + O_2 = SO_2\uparrow$$

58. How many liters (S.T.P.) of ammonia can be made from 684 g. of ammonium sulfate?

$$(NH_4)_2SO_4 + CaO = CaSO_4 + H_2O + 2NH_3\uparrow$$

59. How many grams of potassium chlorate are required to make 60 liters (S.T.P.) of oxygen?

$$2KClO_3 = 2KCl + 3O_2\uparrow$$

60. How many grams of iron are required to make 100 liters (S.T.P.) of hydrogen?

$$Fe + H_2SO_4 = FeSO_4 + H_2\uparrow$$

61. How many grams of sodium sulfite are required to make 65 liters (S.T.P.) of sulfur dioxide?

$$Na_2SO_3 + H_2SO_4 = Na_2SO_4 + H_2O + SO_2\uparrow$$

62. The volume of a gas measured at 780 mm. is 475 ml. What is its volume at 760 mm., if the temperature remains constant?

63. Calculate the volume of 10 g. of hydrogen measured under standard conditions. What would be its volume if the pressure upon the gas were diminished to 750 mm., the temperature remaining constant?

64. The volume of a gas measured at 25° C. is 540 ml. What is its volume at 0° C., if the pressure remains constant?

65. Calculate the volume of 10 g. of oxygen under standard conditions. What would be its volume if the temperature of the gas were increased to 27° C., the pressure remaining constant?

66. A sample of a gas measured 1000 ml. at 27° C. and 770 mm. pressure. Calculate its volume at S.T.P.

67. Calculate the volume (S.T.P.) of a sample of oxygen that occupies 125 ml. at 30° C. and 745 mm. pressure.

Chapter 13

Electrolyte Solutions

As noted in Chapter 11, the molecules of chemical compounds in solution may remain intact, or they may dissociate into particles known as *ions* which carry an electric charge. Substances that are not dissociated in solution are called *non-electrolytes*, and those with varying degrees of dissociation are called *electrolytes*. Urea and dextrose are examples of non-electrolytes in the body water; sodium chloride in body fluids is an example of an electrolyte.

Sodium chloride in solution provides Na^+ and Cl^- ions which carry electric charges. If electrodes carrying a weak current are placed in the solution, the ions move in a direction opposite to their charges. Na^+ ions move to the negative electrode (*cathode*) and are called *cations*. Cl^- ions move to the positive electrode (*anode*) and hence are called *anions*.

Electrolyte ions in the blood plasma include the cations Na^+, K^+, Ca^{++}, and Mg^{++} and the anions Cl^-, HCO_3^-, HPO_4^{--}, SO_4^{--}, organic acids$^-$, and protein$^-$. Electrolytes in body fluids play an important role in maintaining the acid-base balance in the body. They play a part, too, in controlling body water volumes, and they also help to regulate body metabolism.

Electrolyte solutions are liquid preparations used for the treatment of disturbances in the electrolyte and fluid balance of the body. The concentration of these solutions, like the concentration of body electrolytes, used to be commonly expressed in terms of different units, such as g. per 100 ml., volumes %, and mg. %. The term "mg. %" refers to the number of mg. per 100 ml. and represents the older concept of measuring electrolytes in units of weight or *physical units*. However, this concept does not take into consideration chemical equivalence and, consequently, does not indicate the measurement of the chemical combining power of the electrolyte in solution. More significantly, it does not give any direct information as to the number of ions or the charges which they carry. Since the chemical combining power depends not only on the number of particles in solution but also on the total number of ionic charges, the valence of the ions in solution must be taken into consideration in order to make the measurement a meaningful one.

A *chemical unit*, the *milliequivalent*, is now used almost exclusively by clinicians, physicians, and manufacturers to express the concentration of electrolytes in solution. This unit of measure is related to the total number of ionic charges in solution, and it takes note of the valence of the ions. In other words, it is a unit of measurement of the amount of *chemical activity* of an electrolyte.

Under normal conditions blood plasma contains 155 milliequivalents of cations and an equal number of anions. The total concentration of cations always equals the total concentration of anions. Any number of milli-equivalents of Na^+, K^+, or any $cation^+$ always reacts with precisely the same number of milliequivalents of Cl^-, HCO_3^-, or any $anion^-$.

In preparing a solution of K^+ ions, a potassium salt is dissolved in water. In addition to the K^+ ions, the solution will also contain ions of opposite negative charge. These two components will be chemically equal in that the milliequivalents of one are equal to the milliequivalents of the other. The interesting point is that if we dissolve enough potassium chloride in water to give us 40 milliequivalents per liter of K^+, we also have exactly 40 milliequivalents of Cl^-, but the solution will *not* contain the *same weight* of each ion.

A *milliequivalent*, abbreviated mEq, represents the amount, in g. or mg., of a solute equal to $\frac{1}{1000}$ of its gram equivalent weight.

Examples:

> *What is the concentration, in mg. per ml., of a solution containing 2 mEq of potassium chloride (KCl) per ml.?*

Molecular weight of KCl = 74.5

Equivalent weight of KCl = 74.5

1 mEq of KCl = $\frac{1}{1000}$ × 74.5 g. = 0.0745 g. = 74.5 mg.

2 mEq of KCl = 74.5 mg. × 2 = 149 mg. per ml., *answer.*

> *What is the concentration, in g. per ml., of a solution containing 4 mEq of calcium chloride ($CaCl_2.2H_2O$) per ml.?*

It should be recalled that the equivalent weight of a binary compound may be found by dividing the formula weight by the *total valence* of the positive or negative radical.

Formula weight of $CaCl_2.2H_2O$ = 147

Equivalent weight of $CaCl_2.2H_2O$ = $\frac{147}{2}$ = 73.5

1 mEq of $CaCl_2.2H_2O$ = $\frac{1}{1000}$ × 73.5 g. = 0.0735 g.

4 mEq of $CaCl_2.2H_2O$ = 0.0735 g. × 4 = 0.294 g. per ml., *answer.*

A solution contains 10 mg.% of K+ ions. Express this concentration in terms of mEq per liter.

$$\text{Atomic weight of K} = 39$$

$$\text{Equivalent weight of K} = 39$$

$$1 \text{ mEq of K} = \tfrac{1}{1000} \times 39 \text{ g.} = 0.039 \text{ g.} = 39 \text{ mg.}$$

$$10 \text{ mg. \% of K} = \begin{array}{l} 10 \text{ mg. of K per 100 ml. or} \\ 100 \text{ mg. of K per liter} \end{array}$$

$$100 \text{ mg.} \div 39 = 2.56 \text{ mEq per liter, } \textit{answer.}$$

A solution contains 10 mg. % of Ca++ ions. Express this concentration in terms of mEq per liter.

$$\text{Atomic weight of Ca} = 40$$

$$\text{Equivalent weight of Ca} = \tfrac{40}{2} = 20$$

$$1 \text{ mEq of Ca} = \tfrac{1}{1000} \times 20 \text{ g.} = 0.020 \text{ g.} = 20 \text{ mg.}$$

$$10 \text{ mg. \% of Ca} = \begin{array}{l} 10 \text{ mg. of Ca per 100 ml. or} \\ 100 \text{ mg. of Ca per liter} \end{array}$$

$$100 \text{ mg.} \div 20 = 5 \text{ mEq per liter, } \textit{answer.}$$

A person is to receive 2 mEq of sodium chloride per kilogram of body weight. If the person weighs 132 lb., how many milliliters of an 0.9% sterile solution of sodium chloride should be administered?

$$\text{Molecular weight of NaCl} = 58.5$$

$$\text{Equivalent weight of NaCl} = 58.5$$

$$1 \text{ mEq of NaCl} = \tfrac{1}{1000} \times 58.5 = 0.0585 \text{ g.}$$

$$2 \text{ mEq of NaCl} = 0.0585 \text{ g.} \times 2 = 0.117 \text{g.}$$

$$1 \text{ lb.} = 2.2 \text{ lb.} \qquad \text{Weight of person in kg.} = \frac{132 \text{ lb.}}{2.2 \text{ lb.}} = 60 \text{ kg.}$$

Since the person is to receive 2 mEq per kg.,

then   2 mEq or 0.117 g. × 60 = 7.02 g. of NaCl needed

and since 0.9% sterile solution of sodium chloride contains 9.0 g. of NaCl per liter,

then
$$\frac{9.0 \ (g.)}{7.02 \ (g.)} = \frac{1000 \ (ml.)}{x \ (ml.)}$$

$$x = 780 \ ml., \ answer$$

What is the percent (w/v) concentration of a solution containing 100 mEq of ammonium chloride per liter?

Molecular weight of NH_4Cl = 53.5

Equivalent weight of NH_4Cl = 53.5

1 mEq of $NH_4Cl = \frac{1}{1000} \times 53.5 = 0.0535$ g.

100 mEq of NH_4Cl = 0.0535 g. $\times$ 100 = 5.35 g. per liter

or 0.535 g. per 100 ml. or 0.535%, *answer*.

Electrolytes play their part in controlling body water volumes by establishing osmotic pressure. This pressure is proportional to the *total number* of particles in solution. The unit that is used to measure *osmotic activity* is the *milliosmol*, abbreviated mOsm. For dextrose, a non-electrolyte, 1 millimol (1 formula weight in mg.) represents 1 milliosmol. However, this relationship is not the same with electrolytes, since the total number of particles in solution depends upon the degree of dissociation of the substance in question. Assuming complete dissociation, 1 millimol of NaCl represents 2 milliosmols ($Na^+ + Cl^-$) of total particles, and 1 millimol of $CaCl_2$ represents 3 milliosmols ($Ca^+ + 2Cl^-$) of total particles.

The milliosmolar value of *separate* ions of an electrolyte may be obtained by dividing the concentration, in mg. per liter, of the ion by its atomic weight; but the milliosmolar value of the *whole* electrolyte in solution is equal to the sum of the milliosmolar values of the separate ions.

Examples:

A solution contains 5% of anhydrous dextrose in water for injection. How many milliosmols per liter are represented by this concentration?

Formula weight of anhydrous dextrose = 180

1 millimol of anhydrous dextrose (180 mg.) = 1 milliosmol

5% solution contains 50 g. or 50000 mg. per liter

50000 mg. ÷ 180 = 278 mOsm per liter, *answer*.

A solution contains 156 mg. of K+ ions per 100 ml. How many milliosmols are represented in a liter of the solution?

Atomic weight of K = 39

1 millimol of K (39 mg.) = 1 milliosmol

156 mg. of K per 100 ml. = 1560 mg. of K per liter

1560 mg. ÷ 39 = 40 milliosmols, *answer.*

A solution contains 10 mg. % of Ca++ ions. How many milliosmols are represented in 1 liter of the solution?

Atomic weight of Ca = 40

1 millimol of Ca (40 mg.) = 1 milliosmol

10 mg. % of Ca = 10 mg. of Ca per 100 ml. or
100 mg. of Ca per liter

100 mg. ÷ 40 = 2.5 milliosmols, *answer.*

How many milliosmols are represented in a liter of an 0.9% sodium chloride solution?

Osmotic activity (in terms of milliosmols) is a function of the total number of particles present.

Assuming complete dissociation, 1 millimol of sodium chloride (NaCl) represents 2 milliosmols of total particles ($Na^+ + Cl^-$).

Formula weight of NaCl = 58.5

1 millimol of NaCl (58.5 mg.) = 2 milliosmols

$1000 \times 0.009 = 9$ g. or 9000 mg. of NaCl per liter

$$\frac{58.5 \text{ (mg.)}}{9000 \text{ (mg.)}} = \frac{2 \text{ (milliosmols)}}{x \text{ (milliosmols)}}$$

x = 307.7, or 308 milliosmols, *answer.*

Practice Problems

1. What is the concentration, in mg. per ml., of a solution containing 5 mEq of potassium chloride (KCl) per ml.?

2. A solution contains 298 mg. of potassium chloride (KCl) per ml. Express this concentration in terms of milliequivalents of potassium chloride.

3. A 10-ml. ampul of potassium chloride contains 2.98 g. of potassium chloride (KCl). What is the concentration of the solution in terms of mEq per ml.?

4. A person is to receive 36 mg. of ammonium chloride per kilogram of body weight. If the person weighs 154 lb., how many milliliters of a sterile solution of ammonium chloride (NH_4Cl) containing 0.4 mEq per ml. should be administered?

5. A sterile solution of potassium chloride (KCl) contains 2 mEq per ml. If a 20-ml. ampul of the solution is diluted to a liter with sterile distilled water, what is the percentage strength of the resulting solution?

6. A certain electrolyte solution contains, as one of the ingredients, the equivalent of 4.6 mEq of calcium per liter. How many grams of calcium chloride ($CaCl_2.2H_2O$) should be used in preparing 20 liters of the solution?

7. Sterile solutions of ammonium chloride containing 21.4 mg. per ml. are available commercially in 500- and 1000-ml. intravenous infusion containers. Calculate the amount, in terms of milliequivalents, of ammonium chloride (NH_4Cl) in the 500-ml. container.

8. A solution contains, in each 5 ml., 0.5 g. of potassium acetate ($KC_2H_3O_2$), 0.5 g. of potassium bicarbonate ($KHCO_3$), and 0.5 g. of potassium citrate ($K_3C_6H_5O_7$). How many mEq of potassium (K) are represented in each 5 ml. of the solution?

9. How many grams of sodium chloride (NaCl) should be used to prepare a solution containing 154 mEq per liter?

10. Sterile solutions of potassium chloride (KCl) containing 5 mEq per ml. are available in 20-ml. containers. Calculate the amount, in grams, of potassium chloride in the container.

11. How many milliliters of a solution containing 2 mEq of potassium chloride (KCl) per ml. should be used to obtain 2.98 g. of potassium chloride?

12. A patient is to be given 1 g. of sodium methicillin ($C_{17}H_{19}NaO_6S.H_2O$— mol. wt. 420) every six hours for 5 doses. How many mEq of sodium are represented in the prescribed amount of sodium methicillin?

13. A 40-ml. vial of a sodium chloride solution was diluted to a liter with sterile distilled water. The concentration (w/v) of sodium chloride (NaCl) in the finished product was 0.585%. What was the concentration, in mEq per ml., of the original solution?

14. How many grams of sodium bicarbonate (NaHCO$_3$—mol. wt. 84) should be used in preparing a liter of a solution to contain 44.6 mEq per 50 ml.?

15. A solution contains 20 mg. % of Ca^{++} ions. Express this concentration in terms of mEq per liter.

16. Sterile sodium lactate solution is available commercially as a $\frac{1}{6}$-molar solution of sodium lactate in water for injection. How many mEq of sodium lactate (mol. wt. 112) would be provided by a liter of the solution?

17. A solution contains 322 mg. of Na$^+$ ions per liter. How many milliosmols are represented in the solution?

18. A certain electrolyte solution contains 0.9% of sodium chloride in 10% dextrose solution. (a) Express the concentration of sodium chloride (NaCl) in terms of mEq per liter. (b) How many milliosmols of dextrose are represented in 1 liter of the solution?

19. ℞   Potassium Chloride Elixir   240 ml.
             (5 mEq per 5 ml.)
        Sig. One teaspoonful as directed.

    (a) How many grams of potassium chloride (KCl) should be used in compounding the prescription?
    (b) How many milliequivalents of potassium (K) are represented in each prescribed dose?

20. How many mEq of potassium are there in 5 million units of Penicillin V Potassium (C$_{16}$H$_{17}$KN$_2$O$_6$S—mol. wt. 388)? One mg. of Penicillin V Potassium represents 1530 Penicillin Units.

21. The normal potassium level in the blood plasma is 17 mg. %. Express this concentration in terms of mEq per liter.

22. A certain solution contains, among other ingredients, 10% of potassium citrate (K$_3$C$_6$H$_5$O$_7$—mol. wt. 324). How many mEq of potassium (K) are represented in each 5 ml. of the solution?

23. A potassium supplement tablet contains 2.5 g. of potassium bicarbonate (KHCO$_3$—mol. wt. 100). How many mEq of potassium (K) are supplied by the tablet?

24. Ringer's Injection contains 0.86% of sodium chloride, 0.03% of potassium chloride, and 0.033% of calcium chloride. How many mEq of each chloride are contained in 1 liter of the injection?

25. The formula for a potassium ion elixir calls for 5 mEq of potassium chloride per teaspoonful in an elixir base. How many grams of potassium chloride are needed to prepare a liter of the elixir?

26. A 20-ml. vial of a concentrated ammonium chloride solution containing 5 mEq per ml. is diluted to a liter with sterile distilled water. Calculate (a) the total mEq value of the ammonium ion in the dilution and (b) the percentage strength of the dilution.

27. Ringer's Solution contains 0.33 g. of calcium chloride per liter. (a) Express the concentration in terms of mEq of calcium chloride per liter. (b) How many milliosmols of calcium are represented in each liter of the solution?

28. How many milliosmols are represented in a liter of a hypotonic ($\frac{1}{5}$-normal) sodium chloride solution? Isotonic sodium chloride solution (normal) contains 0.9% of sodium chloride. Assume complete dissociation.

29. A solution of sodium chloride contains 77 mEq per liter. Calculate its osmolar strength in terms of milliosmols per liter. Assume complete dissociation.

30. How many mEq of potassium would be supplied daily by the usual dose (0.3 ml. three times a day) of saturated potassium iodide solution? Saturated potassium iodide solution contains 100 g. of potassium iodide per 100 ml.

31. How many milliosmols of dextrose are represented in 50 ml. of a 50% solution?

Chapter 14

Exponential and Logarithmic Notation

EXPONENTIAL NOTATION

MANY physical and chemical measurements deal with either very large or very small numbers. Since it is difficult, in many instances, to handle conveniently numbers of such magnitude in performing even the simplest arithmetic operations in the usual manner, it is best to use exponential notation or *powers of 10* to express them. Thus, we may express *121* as *1.21 × 10^2*, *1210* as *1.21 × 10^3*, and *1,210,000* as *1.21 × 10^6*. Likewise, we may express *0.0121* as *1.21 × 10^{-2}*, *0.00121* as *1.21 × 10^{-3}*, and *0.00000121* as *1.21 × 10^{-6}*.

When numbers are written in this manner, the first part is called the *coefficient*, customarily written with one figure to the left of the decimal point. The second part is the *exponential factor* or *power of ten*.

The exponent represents the number of places that the decimal point has been moved—positive to the left and negative to the right—to form the exponential. Thus, when we convert *19000* to *1.9 × 10^4*, we move the decimal point 4 places to the left; hence the exponent[4]. And when we convert *0.0000019* to *1.9 × 10^{-6}*, we move the decimal point 6 places to the right; hence the *negative* exponent[-6].

FUNDAMENTAL ARITHMETIC OPERATIONS WITH EXPONENTIALS

In the *multiplication* of exponentials, the exponents are *added*. For example, $10^2 × 10^4 = 10^6$. In the multiplication of numbers that are expressed in exponential form, the *coefficients* are multiplied together in the usual manner and this product is then multiplied by the power of *10* found by algebraically *adding* the exponents.

Examples:

$$(2.5 × 10^2) × (2.5 × 10^4) = 6.25 × 10^6, \text{ or } 6.3 × 10^6$$
$$(2.5 × 10^2) × (2.5 × 10^{-4}) = 6.25 × 10^{-2}, \text{ or } 6.3 × 10^{-2}$$
$$(5.4 × 10^2) × (4.5 × 10^3) = 24.3 × 10^5 = 2.4 × 10^6$$

In the *division* of exponentials, the exponents are *subtracted*. For example, $10^2 \div 10^5 = 10^{-3}$. And in the division of numbers that are expressed in exponential form, the *coefficients* are divided in the usual way and the result is multiplied by the power of *10* found by algebraically *subtracting* the exponents.

Examples:

$$(7.5 \times 10^5) \div (2.5 \times 10^3) = 3.0 \times 10^2$$
$$(7.5 \times 10^{-4}) \div (2.5 \times 10^6) = 3.0 \times 10^{-10}$$
$$(2.8 \times 10^{-2}) \div (8.0 \times 10^{-6}) = 0.35 \times 10^4 = 3.5 \times 10^3$$

Note that in each of the examples above the result is rounded off to the number of *significant figures* contained in the *least* accurate factor, and it is expressed with only one figure to the left of the decimal point.

In the *addition* and *subtraction* of exponentials, the expressions must be changed (by moving the decimal points) to forms having any common power of 10 and then the coefficients only are added or subtracted. The result should be rounded off to the number of *decimal places* contained in the *least* precise component, and it should be expressed with only one figure to the left of the decimal point.

Examples:

$$(1.4 \times 10^4) + (5.1 \times 10^3)$$

$$
\begin{array}{r}
1.4 \ \times 10^4 \\
5.1 \times 10^3 = 0.51 \times 10^4 \\
\hline
\end{array}
$$

  Total: 1.91×10^4, or 1.9×10^4, *answer.*

$$(1.4 \times 10^4) - (5.1 \times 10^3)$$

$$
\begin{array}{r}
1.4 \times 10^4 = 14.0 \times 10^3 \\
-5.1 \times 10^3 \\
\hline
\end{array}
$$

Difference: 8.9×10^3, *answer.*

$$(9.83 \times 10^3) + (4.1 \times 10^1) + (2.6 \times 10^3)$$

$$
\begin{array}{r}
9.83 \ \times 10^3 \\
4.1 \times 10^1 = 0.041 \times 10^3 \\
2.6 \ \ \times 10^3 \\
\hline
\end{array}
$$

  Total: 12.471×10^3, or
      $12.5 \ \ \times 10^3 = 1.25 \times 10^4$, *answer.*

Practice Problems

1. Write each of the following in exponential form:

    (a) 12,650
    (b) 0.0000000055
    (c) 451
    (d) 0.065
    (e) 625,000,000

2. Write each of the following in the usual numerical form:

    (a) 4.1×10^6
    (b) 3.65×10^{-2}
    (c) 5.13×10^{-6}
    (d) 2.5×10^5
    (e) 8.6956×10^3

3. Find the product:

    (a) $(3.5 \times 10^3) \times (5.0 \times 10^4)$
    (b) $(8.2 \times 10^2) \times (2.0 \times 10^{-6})$
    (c) $(1.5 \times 10^{-6}) \times (4.0 \times 10^6)$
    (d) $(1.5 \times 10^3) \times (8.0 \times 10^4)$
    (e) $(7.2 \times 10^5) \times (5.0 \times 10^{-3})$

4. Find the quotient:

    (a) $(9.3 \times 10^5) \div (3.1 \times 10^2)$
    (b) $(3.6 \times 10^{-4}) \div (1.2 \times 10^6)$
    (c) $(3.3 \times 10^7) \div (1.1 \times 10^{-2})$

5. Find the sum:

    (a) $(9.2 \times 10^3) + (7.6 \times 10^4)$
    (b) $(1.8 \times 10^{-6}) + (3.4 \times 10^{-5})$
    (c) $(4.9 \times 10^2) + (2.5 \times 10^3)$

6. Find the difference:

    (a) $(6.5 \times 10^6) - (5.9 \times 10^4)$
    (b) $(8.2 \times 10^{-3}) - (1.6 \times 10^{-3})$
    (c) $(7.4 \times 10^3) - (4.6 \times 10^2)$

COMMON LOGARITHMIC NOTATION

We have seen that exponential notation allows us to express any number as a *coefficient times a whole-number power of 10*—as when we interpret *150* to mean *1.5 × 10²*—and that this system of notation offers us a convenient shorthand, as it were, for expressing and manipulating very large or very small numbers.

Still another system, called *common logarithmic notation*, goes the exponential system one better. In common logarithmic notation *every number is expressed simply as a power of 10*—not with absolute precision, but with sufficient accuracy for any given purpose—and we may multiply any two numbers so expressed, or divide one by the other, by the simple process of adding or subtracting their exponents.

The *exponent* that indicates *to what power 10 must be raised to equal approximately a given number* is called the *common logarithm* of that number.

It follows that the logarithm of *10* or of any integral power of *10* is always a positive or negative integer:

$$\log 10 \ (\text{or } 1 \times 10^1) = 1$$
$$\log 100 \ (\text{or } 1 \times 10^2) = 2$$
$$\log 1000 \ (\text{or } 1 \times 10^3) = 3$$

and so on;

$$\log 1 \ (\text{or } 1 \times 10^0) = \quad 0$$
$$\log 0.1 \ (\text{or } 1 \times 10^{-1}) = -1$$
$$\log 0.01 \ (\text{or } 1 \times 10^{-2}) = -2$$

and so on. And if these were the only numbers in existence, no table of logarithms should be needed; for, given a number, say *1,000,000* (or *1 × 10⁶*) if we know the system we can readily supply its logarithm: *6*; or, given the logarithm *6*, we can readily reconstruct the number it represents: *1,000,000*.

But any number *not* in the *10's* series must contain a certain *excess* over some power of *10*—as *150* contains *10²* plus an excess of *50*. Therefore, the logarithm of such a number always consists of a positive or negative whole-number exponent *plus* a positive decimal-fraction exponent (carried to as many decimal places as suit our purpose). As it turns out, the power of *10* that approximates *150* (or *1.5 × 10²*) is *10²·¹⁷⁶¹*, and therefore *log 150 = 2.1761*.

The *whole-number exponent* is called the *characteristic*. It accounts for the integral power of *10* contained in the given number and hence serves to locate the *decimal point* in that number. If a number is given in ordinary notation, you can find the characteristic by converting it to exponential notation, in which the characteristic appears as a power of *10*.

The *decimal-fraction exponent* is called the *mantissa*. You can find the mantissa in a table of logarithms. The mantissa represents the *significant figures* in the given number, regardless of the location of the decimal point. In other words, given the sequence *610*, a four-place table will tell you the mantissa is *7853*, whether the number be *61.0*, or *6.10*, or *0.00610*.

Compare this series of logarithms with the logarithms of the *10's* series given above:

$$\log 6.10 \text{ (or } 6.10 \times 10^0) = 0.7853$$
$$\log 61.0 \text{ (or } 6.10 \times 10^1) = 1.7853$$
$$\log 610 \text{ (or } 6.10 \times 10^2) = 2.7853$$
$$\log 6100 \text{ (or } 6.10 \times 10^3) = 3.7853$$

and so on; and

$$\log 0.610 \text{ (or } 6.10 \times 10^{-1}) = \bar{1}.7853$$
$$\log 0.0610 \text{ (or } 6.10 \times 10^{-2}) = \bar{2}.7853$$
$$\log 0.00610 \text{ (or } 6.10 \times 10^{-3}) = \bar{3}.7853$$

and so on. Note that by putting the minus sign *over* the characteristic we indicate that it alone is negative, and that the mantissa, as always, is positive.

NATURAL LOGARITHMS

The base of the *natural* or *Naperian* system of logarithms is *e* which is the irrational number 2.71828 . . . . When it becomes necessary to change from a natural logarithm to a common logarithm, the computation may be performed by using the following relationship:

$$\log_e n = 2.303 \log_{10} n$$

where 2.303 is the logarithm of 10 to the base 2.71828.

USE OF LOGARITHM TABLES

Logarithm tables give mantissas calculated to four-place, five-place accuracy, and upwards, depending on the table and its purpose. A four-place table insures an accuracy within 0.5% when we work with three figure numbers.

The Table (pp. 250 - 251) has typical features. It contains (1) a column to the left and a row at the top to guide us in locating the mantissas of 3-figure numbers, (2) the 4-place mantissas of all 3-figure numbers, and (3) columns of proportional parts providing us with a quick means of calculating more accurate mantissas when given numbers of 4-figure accuracy—a process called *interpolation*.

To find the logarithm of a number:

First, determine the characteristic, then find the mantissa in the log table.

Examples:

> *Find the log of 262.*
>
>> $262 = 2.62 \times 10^2$
>> By inspection of the ten factor, the characteristic $= 2$.
>> To find the mantissa, focus attention on the digits *262*.
>> In the left-hand column in the log table find *26;* opposite it and in the column numbered *2* is the desired mantissa 0.4183. (The table omits the 0.)
>
> Therefore, log 262 = 2.4183, *answer.*
>
> *Find the log of 2627.*
>
>> $2627 = 2.627 \times 10^3$
>> By inspection of the ten factor, the characteristic $= 3$.
>> In the left-hand column in the table find *26;* opposite it and in the column numbered *2* find the mantissa 0.4183; opposite *26* and in column 7 under proportional parts find 11 (meaning 0.0011 but written without zeros) and add it to 0.4183 to obtain the desired mantissa 0.4194.
>
> Therefore, log 2627 = 3.4194, *answer.*
>
> *Find the log of 0.002627.*
>
>> $0.002627 = 2.627 \times 10^{-3}$
>>
>> By inspection of the ten factor, the characteristic $= \bar{3}$.
>> The mantissa is determined as in the preceding example.
>
> Therefore, log 0.002627 = $\bar{3}$.4194, *answer.*

To find the antilogarithm of a logarithm:

When a problem is solved by logarithms, the result is expressed as the *logarithm* of the answer. This necessitates the finding of the *antilogarithm* or *the number corresponding to the logarithm.* If the mantissa of a logarithm is known, its antilogarithm can be found by a *reverse reading* of the log table.

Examples:

> *Find the antilogarithm of the logarithm 1.7604.*
>
>> The mantissa 0.7604 is found in the column numbered *6* opposite *57*, and the resulting figure is 576.
>> The characteristic is 1 and, the required number is
>>
>> 5.76 × 10¹ or 57.6, *answer.*

> *Find the antilogarithm of the logarithm 3.7607.*
>
>> Since the mantissa 0.7607 is not found in the log table, interpolation must be used. In the log table, 0.7607 falls *between 0.7604 and 0.7612;* therefore, the resulting figure must be between *576 and 577.*
>> The *given* mantissa is 0.0003 (or 3 units) more than the mantissa 0.7604. Therefore opposite 0.7604 find 3 in the column *4* of proportional parts. Then the required figure is *5764.*
>>
>> The characteristic is 3 and the required number is
>>
>> 5.764 × 10³ = 5764, *answer.*

SOME LOGARITHMIC COMPUTATIONS

As shown in the first example below, when a negative number is "added" it is actually *subtracted;* and as shown in the third example, when a negative number is "subtracted" it is actually *added.*

The fourth example shows the curious but consistent fact that, in subtracting one logarithm from another, if you *borrow* from a negative characteristic (as *1* is borrowed from the −*1* of the minuend) you *increase* the value of the negative characteristic (as the −*1* becomes −*2*, which is canceled out when the *2* of the subtrahend is "subtracted" from it).

Examples:

> *Multiply (5.25 × 10³) by (8.92 × 10⁻⁶) by (7.56 × 10⁵).*
>
>> log (5.25 × 10³) = 3.7202
>> log (8.92 × 10⁻⁶) = $\overline{6}$.9504
>> log (7.56 × 10⁵) = 5.8785
>> _____
>> Total: 4.5491

Antilogarithm of $4.5491 = 3.541 \times 10^4 = 35410$, or (retaining only 3 significant figures), 35400, *answer*.

Divide 29600 by 5.544.

$29600 = 2.96 \times 10^4$
$5.544 = 5.544 \times 10^0$
$\log (2.96 \times 10^4) = 4.4713$
$\log (5.544 \times 10^0) = 0.7438$

Difference: 3.7275

Antilogarithm of $3.7275 = 5.34 \times 10^3 = 5340$, *answer*.

Divide 7500 by 0.627.

$7500 = 7.50 \times 10^3$
$0.627 = 6.27 \times 10^{-1}$
$\log (7.50 \times 10^3) = 3.8751$
$\log (6.27 \times 10^{-1}) = \bar{1}.7973$

Difference: 4.0778

Antilogarithm of $4.0778 = 1.196 \times 10^4 = 11960$, or (retaining only 3 significant figures), 12000, *answer*.

Divide 0.191 by 0.0452.

$0.191 = 1.91 \times 10^{-1}$
$0.0452 = 4.52 \times 10^{-2}$
$\log (1.91 \times 10^{-1}) = \bar{1}.2810$
$\log (4.52 \times 10^{-2}) = \bar{2}.6551$

Difference: 0.6259

Antilogarithm of $0.6259 = 4.226 \times 10^0 = 4.226$, or (retaining only 3 significant figures), 4.23, *answer*.

Find the value of $\dfrac{(4.54 \times 10^6) \times (3.25 \times 10^3)}{(1.21 \times 10^8)}$.

$\log (4.54 \times 10^6) = 6.6571$
$\log (3.25 \times 10^3) = 3.5119$

Total: $10.1690 = $ *log of numerator*

$\log (1.21 \times 10^8) = 8.0828 = $ *log of denominator*

Difference: 2.0862

Antilogarithm of $2.0862 = 1.219$ or $1.22 \times 10^2 = 122$, *answer*.

Practice Problems

1. Find the logarithm of each of the following numbers.

(a) 2245   (f) 0.7245
(b) 5.265   (g) 215000
(c) 7000   (h) 0.0001372
(d) 187.9   (i) 68.78
(e) 0.002934   (j) 6.2×10^6

2. Find the antilogarithm corresponding to each of the following logarithms.

(a) 4.4512   (f) 2.1668
(b) 1.1523   (g) 0.0261
(c) 0.3302   (h) $\bar{3}.8902$
(d) $\bar{1}.1105$ (i) 1.9234
(e) 2.7892   (j) $\bar{2}.1234$

3. Compute each of the following by means of logarithms.

(a) 23.87×954.6
(b) 8542×0.8562
(c) 655.7×0.02253
(d) $(8.235 \times 10^2) \times (4.296 \times 10^{-4}) \times (2.325 \times 10^3)$
(e) $26.74 \times 5.987 \times 106.7$

4. Compute each of the following by means of logarithms.

(a) $9525 \div 1.267$
(b) $2500 \div 12.65$
(c) $0.2925 \div 56.85$
(d) $(1.658 \times 10^4) \div (4.689 \times 10^2)$
(e) $0.491 \div 0.0357$

5. Find the value of each of the following by means of logarithms.

(a) $$\frac{(6.29 \times 10^2) \times (1.23 \times 10^4)}{(9.75 \times 10^4)} =$$

(b) $$\frac{1,667,000 \times 0.4101}{(6.31 \times 10^3)} =$$

(c) $$\frac{(7.32 \times 10^2)}{(4.315 \times 10^{-4}) \times (5.795 \times 10^3)} =$$

EXPONENTIAL AND LOGARITHMIC NOTATION

Table of Logarithms

Three-figure numbers	0	1	2	3	4	5	6	7	8	9	Proportional parts (for interpolation)								
											1	2	3	4	5	6	7	8	9
10	0000	0043	0086	0128	0170	0212	0253	0294	0334	0374	4	8	12	17	21	25	29	33	37
11	0414	0453	0492	0531	0569	0607	0645	0682	0719	0755	4	8	11	15	19	23	26	30	34
12	0792	0828	0864	0899	0934	0969	1004	1038	1072	1106	3	7	10	14	17	21	24	28	31
13	1139	1173	1206	1239	1271	1303	1335	1367	1399	1430	3	6	10	13	16	19	23	26	29
14	1461	1492	1523	1553	1584	1614	1644	1673	1703	1732	3	6	9	12	15	18	21	24	27
15	1761	1790	1818	1847	1875	1903	1931	1959	1987	2014	3	6	8	11	14	17	20	22	25
16	2041	2068	2095	2122	2148	2175	2201	2227	2253	2279	3	5	8	11	13	16	18	21	24
17	2304	2330	2355	2380	2405	2430	2455	2480	2504	2529	2	5	7	10	12	15	17	20	22
18	2553	2577	2601	2625	2648	2672	2695	2718	2742	2765	2	5	7	9	12	14	16	19	21
19	2788	2810	2833	2856	2878	2900	2923	2945	2967	2989	2	4	7	9	11	13	16	18	20
20	3010	3032	3054	3075	3096	3118	3139	3160	3181	3201	2	4	6	8	11	13	15	17	19
21	3222	3243	3263	3284	3304	3324	3345	3365	3385	3404	2	4	6	8	10	12	14	16	18
22	3424	3444	3464	3483	3502	3522	3541	3560	3579	3598	2	4	6	8	10	12	14	15	17
23	3617	3636	3655	3674	3692	3711	3729	3747	3766	3784	2	4	6	7	9	11	13	15	17
24	3802	3820	3838	3856	3874	3892	3909	3927	3945	3962	2	4	5	7	9	11	12	14	16
25	3979	3997	4014	4031	4048	4065	4082	4099	4116	4133	2	3	5	7	9	10	12	14	15
26	4150	4166	4183	4200	4216	4232	4249	4265	4281	4298	2	3	5	7	8	10	11	13	15
27	4314	4330	4346	4362	4378	4393	4409	4425	4440	4456	2	3	5	6	8	9	11	13	14
28	4472	4487	4502	4518	4533	4548	4564	4579	4594	4609	2	3	5	6	8	9	11	12	14
29	4624	4639	4654	4669	4683	4698	4713	4728	4742	4757	1	3	4	6	7	9	10	12	13
30	4771	4786	4800	4814	4829	4843	4857	4871	4886	4900	1	3	4	6	7	9	10	11	13
31	4914	4928	4942	4955	4969	4983	4997	5011	5024	5038	1	3	4	6	7	8	10	11	12
32	5051	5065	5079	5092	5105	5119	5132	5145	5159	5172	1	3	4	5	7	8	9	11	12
33	5185	5198	5211	5224	5237	5250	5263	5276	5289	5302	1	3	4	5	6	8	9	10	12
34	5315	5328	5340	5353	5366	5378	5391	5403	5416	5428	1	3	4	5	6	8	9	10	11
35	5441	5453	5465	5478	5490	5502	5514	5527	5539	5551	1	2	4	5	6	7	9	10	11
36	5563	5575	5587	5599	5611	5623	5635	5647	5658	5670	1	2	4	5	6	7	8	10	11
37	5682	5694	5705	5717	5729	5740	5752	5763	5775	5786	1	2	3	5	6	7	8	9	10
38	5798	5809	5821	5832	5843	5855	5866	5877	5888	5899	1	2	3	5	6	7	8	9	10
39	5911	5922	5933	5944	5955	5966	5977	5988	5999	6010	1	2	3	4	5	7	8	9	10
40	6021	6031	6042	6053	6064	6075	6085	6096	6107	6117	1	2	3	4	5	6	8	9	10
41	6128	6138	6149	6160	6170	6180	6191	6201	6212	6222	1	2	3	4	5	6	7	8	9
42	6232	6243	6253	6263	6274	6284	6294	6304	6314	6325	1	2	3	4	5	6	7	8	9
43	6335	6345	6355	6365	6375	6385	6395	6405	6415	6425	1	2	3	4	5	6	7	8	9
44	6435	6444	6454	6464	6474	6484	6493	6503	6513	6522	1	2	3	4	5	6	7	8	9
45	6532	6542	6551	6561	6571	6580	6590	6599	6609	6618	1	2	3	4	5	6	7	8	9
46	6628	6637	6646	6656	6665	6675	6684	6693	6702	6712	1	2	3	4	5	6	7	7	8
47	6721	6730	6739	6749	6758	6767	6776	6785	6794	6803	1	2	3	4	5	5	6	7	8
48	6812	6821	6830	6839	6848	6857	6866	6875	6884	6893	1	2	3	4	4	5	6	7	8
49	6902	6911	6920	6928	6937	6946	6955	6964	6972	6981	1	2	3	4	4	5	6	7	8
50	6990	6998	7007	7016	7024	7033	7042	7050	7059	7067	1	2	3	3	4	5	6	7	8
51	7076	7084	7093	7101	7110	7118	7126	7135	7143	7152	1	2	3	3	4	5	6	7	8
52	7160	7168	7177	7185	7193	7202	7210	7218	7226	7235	1	2	2	3	4	5	6	7	7
53	7243	7251	7259	7267	7275	7284	7292	7300	7308	7316	1	2	2	3	4	5	6	6	7
54	7324	7332	7340	7348	7356	7364	7372	7380	7388	7396	1	2	2	3	4	5	6	6	7

Table of Logarithms—(Continued)

Three-figure numbers	0	1	2	3	4	5	6	7	8	9	Proportional parts (for interpolation)								
											1	2	3	4	5	6	7	8	9
55	7404	7412	7419	7427	7435	7443	7451	7459	7466	7474	1	2	2	3	4	5	5	6	7
56	7482	7490	7497	7505	7513	7520	7528	7536	7543	7551	1	2	2	3	4	5	5	6	7
57	7559	7566	7574	7582	7589	7597	7604	7612	7619	7627	1	2	2	3	4	5	5	6	7
58	7634	7642	7649	7657	7664	7672	7679	7686	7694	7701	1	1	2	3	4	4	5	6	7
59	7709	7716	7723	7731	7738	7745	7752	7760	7767	7774	1	1	2	3	4	4	5	6	7
60	7782	7789	7796	7803	7810	7818	7825	7832	7839	7846	1	1	2	3	4	4	5	6	6
61	7853	7860	7868	7875	7882	7889	7896	7903	7910	7917	1	1	2	3	4	4	5	6	6
62	7924	7931	7938	7945	7952	7959	7966	7973	7980	7987	1	1	2	3	3	4	5	6	6
63	7993	8000	8007	8014	8021	8028	8035	8041	8048	8055	1	1	2	3	3	4	5	5	6
64	8062	8069	8075	8082	8089	8096	8102	8109	8116	8122	1	1	2	3	3	4	5	5	6
65	8129	8136	8142	8149	8156	8162	8169	8176	8182	8189	1	1	2	3	3	4	5	5	6
66	8195	8202	8209	8215	8222	8228	8235	8241	8248	8254	1	1	2	3	3	4	5	5	6
67	8261	8267	8274	8280	8287	8293	8299	8306	8312	8319	1	1	2	3	3	4	5	5	6
68	8325	8331	8338	8344	8351	8357	8363	8370	8376	8382	1	1	2	3	3	4	4	5	6
69	8388	8395	8401	8407	8414	8420	8426	8432	8439	8445	1	1	2	2	3	4	4	5	6
70	8451	8457	8463	8470	8476	8482	8488	8494	8500	8506	1	1	2	2	3	4	4	5	6
71	8513	8519	8525	8531	8537	8543	8549	8555	8561	8567	1	1	2	2	3	4	4	5	5
72	8573	8579	8585	8591	8597	8603	8609	8615	8621	8627	1	1	2	2	3	4	4	5	5
73	8633	8639	8645	8651	8657	8663	8669	8675	8681	8686	1	1	2	2	3	4	4	5	5
74	8692	8698	8704	8710	8716	8722	8727	8733	8739	8745	1	1	2	2	3	4	4	5	5
75	8751	8756	8762	8768	8774	8779	8785	8791	8797	8802	1	1	2	2	3	3	4	5	5
76	8808	8814	8820	8825	8831	8837	8842	8848	8854	8859	1	1	2	2	3	3	4	5	5
77	8865	8871	8876	8882	8887	8893	8899	8904	8910	8915	1	1	2	2	3	3	4	4	5
78	8921	8927	8932	8938	8943	8949	8954	8960	8965	8971	1	1	2	2	3	3	4	4	5
79	8976	8982	8987	8993	8998	9004	9009	9015	9020	9026	1	1	2	2	3	3	4	4	5
80	9031	9036	9042	9047	9053	9058	9063	9069	9074	9079	1	1	2	2	3	3	4	4	5
81	9085	9090	9096	9101	9106	9112	9117	9122	9128	9133	1	1	2	2	3	3	4	4	5
82	9138	9143	9149	9154	9159	9165	9170	9175	9180	9186	1	1	2	2	3	3	4	4	5
83	9191	9196	9201	9206	9212	9217	9222	9227	9232	9238	1	1	2	2	3	3	4	4	5
84	9243	9248	9253	9258	9263	9269	9274	9279	9284	9289	1	1	2	2	3	3	4	4	5
85	9294	9299	9304	9309	9315	9320	9325	9330	9335	9340	1	1	2	2	3	3	4	4	5
86	9345	9350	9355	9360	9365	9370	9375	9380	9385	9390	1	1	2	2	3	3	4	4	5
87	9395	9400	9405	9410	9415	9420	9425	9430	9435	9440	0	1	1	2	2	3	3	4	4
88	9445	9450	9455	9460	9465	9469	9474	9479	9484	9489	0	1	1	2	2	3	3	4	4
89	9494	9499	9504	9509	9513	9518	9523	9528	9533	9538	0	1	1	2	2	3	3	4	4
90	9542	9547	9552	9557	9562	9566	9571	9576	9581	9586	0	1	1	2	2	3	3	4	4
91	9590	9595	9600	9605	9609	9614	9619	9624	9628	9633	0	1	1	2	2	3	3	4	4
92	9638	9643	9647	9652	9657	9661	9666	9671	9675	9680	0	1	1	2	2	3	3	4	4
93	9685	9689	9694	9699	9703	9708	9713	9717	9722	9727	0	1	1	2	2	3	3	4	4
94	9731	9736	9741	9745	9750	9754	9759	9763	9768	9773	0	1	1	2	2	3	3	4	4
95	9777	9782	9786	9791	9795	9800	9805	9809	9814	9818	0	1	1	2	2	3	3	4	4
96	9823	9827	9832	9836	9841	9845	9850	9854	9859	9863	0	1	1	2	2	3	3	4	4
97	9868	9872	9877	9881	9886	9890	9894	9899	9903	9908	0	1	1	2	2	3	3	4	4
98	9912	9917	9921	9926	9930	9934	9939	9943	9948	9952	0	1	1	2	2	3	3	4	4
99	9956	9961	9965	9969	9974	9978	9983	9987	9991	9996	0	1	1	2	2	3	3	3	4

Some Calculations Involving Hydrogen-ion Concentration and pH

WHEN the hydrogen-ion concentration of solutions is expressed quantitatively, it varies from a value of nearly 1 for a normal solution of a strong acid to about 1×10^{-14} for a normal solution of a strong alkali. Consequently, there is a variation of about 100,000,000,000,000 in the numerical values within these two limits. The use of ordinary notation for handling numbers of such magnitude in computations that involve hydrogen-ion concentration is impracticable.

In order to simplify the statement of hydrogen-ion concentration, it is convenient to use logarithmic notation, with the mantissa usually rounded off to one or two places of decimals. It has become customary, therefore, to speak of the hydrogen-ion concentration of a given solution in terms of its pH value which is defined as the *logarithm of the reciprocal of the hydrogen-ion value*. Mathematically, this statement may be expressed as

$$pH = \log \frac{1}{[H^+]}$$

and since the logarithm of a reciprocal equals the negative logarithm of a number, this equation may also be written

$$pH = -\log [H^+]$$

Therefore pH value may also be defined as the *negative logarithm of the hydrogen-ion value*.

Now, the reciprocal, or negative, of a logarithm always contains a *negative mantissa*. *Log* (7×10^{-8}), for example, equals $\bar{8}.8451$ or approximately $\bar{8}.8$, which is interpreted as $-8 + 0.8$. Its reciprocal is $-(-8 + 0.8)$, or $8 - 0.8$. In expressing pH value we eliminate the negative by borrowing *1* from the characteristic and adding it to the mantissa:

$$8 - 0.8 = (8 - 1) + (1 - 0.8) = 7 + 0.2, \text{ or } 7.2$$

If you say this is merely an elaborate way of subtracting 0.8 from 8.0, you are quite right; but the importance of doing it this way becomes clear when you reverse the process.

Given $pH = 7.2$, to convert it to $-\log [H^+]$ as the first step in ascertaining the hydrogen-ion concentration, you must add 1 to the characteristic and subtract it from the mantissa:

$$7.2 \text{ or } 7 + 0.2 = (7 + 1) + (0.2 - 1) = 8 - 0.8$$

Now you can proceed: if $8 - 0.8 = -\log [H^+]$, then
$\log [H^+] = -(8 - 0.8) = -8 + 0.8 \text{ or } \bar{8}.8.$

To calculate the pH value of a solution, given its hydrogen-ion concentration:

Examples:

The hydrogen-ion concentration of a certain solution is 5×10^{-6}. Calculate the pH value of the solution.

$pH = -\log [H^+] = -\log (5 \times 10^{-6})$
$\log (5 \times 10^{-6}) = 6.6990 \text{ or } \bar{6}.7, \text{ or } -6 + 0.7$
$-\log (5 \times 10^{-6}) = -(-6 + 0.7) = 6 - 0.7$
$pH = (6 - 1) + (1 - 0.7) = 5.3, answer.$

The hydrogen-ion concentration of a certain solution is 0.00012 gram-ion per liter. Calculate the pH value of the solution.

$0.00012 = 1.2 \times 10^{-4}$
$pH = -\log [H^+] = -\log (1.2 \times 10^{-4})$
$\log (1.2 \times 10^{-4}) = \bar{4}.08, \text{ or } -4 + 0.08$
$-\log (1.2 \times 10^{-4}) = -(-4 + 0.08) = 4 - 0.08$
$pH = (4 - 1) + (1 - 0.08) = 3.92, answer.$

To calculate the hydrogen-ion concentration of a solution, given its pH value:

Examples:

The pH value of a certain solution is 11.1. Calculate the hydrogen-ion concentration of the solution.

$$pH = 11.1 = -\log [H^+]$$
$$-\log [H^+] = (11 + 1) + (0.1 - 1) = 12 - 0.9$$
$$\log [H^+] = -(12 - 0.9) = -12 + 0.9, \text{ or } \overline{12}.9$$

hydrogen-ion concentration = antilog $\overline{12}.9 = 7.94 \times 10^{-12}$, *answer.*

The pH value of a certain solution is 5.7. Express the hydrogen-ion concentration of the solution as gram-ion per liter.

$$pH = 5.7 = -\log [H^+]$$
$$-\log [H^+] = (5 + 1) + (0.7 - 1) = 6 - 0.3$$
$$\log [H^+] = -(6 - 0.3) = -6 + 0.3 = \overline{6}.3$$

hydrogen-ion concentration = antilog $\overline{6}.3 = 2.0 \times 10^{-6}$, or
0.000002 gram-ion per liter, *answer.*

Practice Problems

1. The hydrogen-ion concentration of a certain solution is 2.5×10^{-11}. Calculate the pH value of the solution.

2. The hydrogen-ion concentration of a certain buffer solution is 2.85×10^{-10}. Calculate the pH value of the solution.

3. The hydrogen-ion concentration of a certain buffer solution is 0.000000603 gram-ion per liter. Calculate the pH of the solution.

4. The hydrogen-ion concentration of a certain solution is 0.0000036 gram-ion per liter. Calculate the pH of the solution.

5. The hydrogen-ion concentration of a buffer solution is 4.4×10^{-8}. Calculate the pH value of the solution.

6. Calculate the pH of a buffer solution which has a hydrogen-ion concentration of 6.5×10^{-7}.

7. A certain elixir has a pH of 2.2. Calculate the hydrogen-ion concentration of the elixir.

8. The pH value of a certain solution is 6.5. Calculate the hydrogen-ion concentration of the solution.

9. The pH value of an 0.1 molar boric acid solution is 5.1. Express the hydrogen-ion concentration of the solution as gram-ion per liter.

10. A prescription for a collyrium calls for a buffer solution having a pH value of 7.2. Calculate the hydrogen-ion concentration of the buffer solution.

11. A 1:200 solution of quinidine sulfate has a pH value of 6.4. Calculate the hydrogen-ion concentration of the solution.

Chapter 16

Some Calculations Involving Buffer Solutions

BUFFERS AND BUFFER SOLUTIONS

WHEN a minute trace of hydrochloric acid is added to pure water, a very significant increase in *hydrogen-ion* concentration occurs immediately. In a similar manner, when a minute trace of sodium hydroxide is added to pure water, it will cause a correspondingly large increase in the *hydroxyl-ion* concentration. These changes take place because water alone cannot neutralize even traces of acid or base. In other words, it has no ability to resist changes in hydrogen-ion concentration or pH. A solution of a neutral salt, such as sodium chloride, also lacks this ability, and therefore it is said to be *unbuffered*.

Now it happens that the presence of certain substances or combinations of substances in aqueous solution imparts to the system the ability to maintain a desired pH at a relatively constant level even upon the addition of materials which may be expected to change the hydrogen-ion concentration. These substances or combinations of substances are called *buffers;* their ability to resist changes in pH is referred to as *buffer action;* their efficiency is measured by the function known as *buffer capacity;* and solutions of them are called *buffer solutions*. By definition, then, a *buffer solution* is a system, usually an aqueous solution, which possesses the property of resisting changes in pH upon the addition of small amounts of a strong acid or base.

Buffers are used to establish and maintain an ion activity within rather narrow limits. In pharmaceutical practice, the most common buffer systems are used (1) in the preparation of dosage forms which approach isotonicity and (2) in the manufacture of formulations in which the pH must be maintained at a relatively constant level in order to insure maximum stability.

Buffer solutions are usually composed of a *weak acid and a salt of the acid,* as for example, acetic acid and sodium acetate, or a *weak base and a salt of the base,* such as ammonium hydroxide and ammonium chloride. Typical buffer systems which may be used in pharmaceutical formulations include the following pairs: acetic acid and sodium acetate, boric acid and sodium borate, and disodium phosphate and sodium acid phosphate. Formulas for several other buffer systems, including those which are suggested for use in ophthalmic solutions, are given in the official compendia.

In the selection of a buffer system, due consideration must be given to the dissociation constant of the weak acid or base so as to insure maximum buffer capacity. This dissociation constant, in the case of an acid, is a measure of the strength of the acid; the more readily the acid dissociates the higher its dissociation constant and the stronger the acid. Selected dissociation constants or K_a values are given in the accompanying table.

Table of Dissociation Constants of Some Weak Acids at 25° C.

Acid	K_a
Acetic	1.75×10^{-5}
Barbituric	1.05×10^{-4}
Benzoic	6.30×10^{-5}
Boric	6.4×10^{-10}
Formic	1.76×10^{-4}
Lactic	1.38×10^{-4}
Mandelic	4.29×10^{-4}
Salicylic	1.06×10^{-3}

The dissociation constant or K_a value of a weak acid is given by the equation:

$$K_a = \frac{(H^+)\ (A^-)}{(HA)} \qquad \text{where } A^- = \text{salt} \\ HA = \text{acid}$$

Since the numerical values of most dissociation constants are very small numbers and may vary over many powers of 10, it is more convenient to express them as negative logarithms, i.e.,

$$pK_a = -\log K_a$$

When equation $K_a = \dfrac{(H^+)\ (A^-)}{(HA)}$ is expressed in logarithmic form, it is written:

$$pK_a = -\log (H^+) - \log \frac{\text{salt}}{\text{acid}}$$

and since $pH = -\log (H^+)$

then $\qquad pK_a = pH - \log \dfrac{salt}{acid}$

and $\qquad pH = pK_a + \log \dfrac{salt}{acid}$

This is the Henderson-Hasselbalch equation for weak acids, commonly known as the *buffer equation*.

Similarly, the dissociation constant or K_b value of a weak base is given by the equation:

$$K_b = \frac{(B^+)\ (OH^-)}{(BOH)} \qquad \begin{array}{l} \text{where } B^+ = salt \\ \text{and } BOH = base \end{array}$$

and the buffer equation for weak bases which is derived from this relationship may be expressed as:

$$pH = pK_w - pK_b + \log \frac{base}{salt}$$

The buffer equation is useful (1) for calculating the pH of a buffer system if its composition is known and (2) for calculating the molar ratio of the components of a buffer system required to give a solution of a desired pH. The equation may also be used to calculate the change in pH of a buffered solution upon the addition of a given amount of acid or base.

To calculate the pK_a value of a weak acid, given its dissociation constant, K_a:

Example:

The dissociation constant of acetic acid is 1.75×10^{-5} at $25°$ C. Calculate its pK_a value.

$\qquad\qquad K_a = 1.75 \times 10^{-5}$

and $\qquad \log K_a = \log 1.75 + \log 10^{-5}$

$\qquad\qquad\qquad = 0.2430 - 5 = -4.757 \text{ or } -4.76$

Since $\qquad pK_a = -\log K_a$

$\qquad\qquad pK_a = -(-4.76) = 4.76, \text{ } answer.$

To calculate the pH value of a salt/acid buffer system :

Example:

What is the pH of a buffer solution prepared with 0.05 M sodium borate and 0.005 M boric acid? The pK_a value of boric acid is 9.24 at 25° C.

It should be noted that the ratio of the components of the buffer solution is given in molar concentrations.

Using the buffer equation for weak acids,

$$pH = pK_a + \log \frac{\text{salt}}{\text{acid}}$$

$$= 9.24 + \log \frac{0.05}{0.005}$$

$$= 9.24 + \log 10$$

$$= 9.24 + 1$$

$$= 10.24, \text{ } answer.$$

To calculate the pH value of a base/salt buffer system :

Example:

What is the pH of a buffer solution prepared with 0.05 M ammonia and 0.05 M ammonium chloride? The K_b value of ammonia is 1.80 × 10^{-5} at 25° C.

Using the buffer equation for weak bases,

$$pH = pK_w - pK_b + \log \frac{\text{base}}{\text{salt}}$$

Since the K_w value for water is 10^{-14} at 25° C., $pK_w = 14$.

$$K_b = 1.80 \times 10^{-5}$$

and $\log K_b = \log 1.8 + \log 10^{-5}$

$$= 0.2553 - 5 = -4.7447 \text{ or } -4.74$$

$$pK_b = -\log K_b$$

$$= -(-4.74) = 4.74$$

and $\qquad$ $pH = 14 - 4.74 + \log \dfrac{0.05}{0.05}$

$$= 9.26 + \log 1$$

$$= 9.26, \ answer.$$

To calculate the molar ratio of salt/acid required to prepare a buffer system having a desired pH value :

Example:

    What molar ratio of salt/acid is required to prepare a sodium acetate-acetic acid buffer solution having a pH of 5.76? The pK_a value of acetic acid is 4.76 at 25° C.

    Using the buffer equation,

$$pH = pK_a + \log \dfrac{salt}{acid}$$

$$\log \dfrac{salt}{acid} = pH - pK_a$$

$$= 5.76 - 4.76 = 1$$

antilog of $1 = 10$

    ratio $= 10/1$ or 10:1, *answer.*

To calculate the amounts of the components of a buffer solution required to prepare a desired volume, given the molar ratio of the components and the total buffer concentration :

Example:

    The molar ratio of sodium acetate to acetic acid in a buffer solution having a pH of 5.76 is 10:1. Assuming that the total buffer concentration is 2.2×10^{-2} mole/liter, how many grams of sodium acetate (mol. wt. — 82) and how many grams of acetic acid (mol. wt. — 60) should be used in preparing a liter of the solution?

    Since the molar ratio of sodium acetate to acetic acid is 10:1

the mole fraction of sodium acetate $= \dfrac{10}{1 + 10}$ or $\dfrac{10}{11}$

and the mole fraction of acetic acid $= \dfrac{1}{1 + 10}$ or $\dfrac{1}{11}$

If the total buffer concentration $= 2.2 \times 10^{-2}$ mole/liter,

the concentration of sodium acetate $= \dfrac{10}{11} \times (2.2 \times 10^{-2})$

$= 2.0 \times 10^{-2}$ mole/liter

and the concentration of acetic acid $= \dfrac{1}{11} \times (2.2 \times 10^{-2})$

$= 0.2 \times 10^{-2}$ mole/liter

then 2.0×10^{-2} or $0.02 \times 82 = 1.64$ g. of sodium acetate per liter of solution, *and*

0.2×10^{-2} or $0.002 \times 60 = 0.120$ g. of acetic acid per liter of solution, *answers.*

The efficiency of buffer solutions, that is their specific ability to resist changes in pH, is measured in terms of *buffer capacity*; and the *smaller* the pH change upon the addition of a given amount of acid or base, the *greater* the buffer capacity of the system. Among other factors, the buffer capacity of a system depends upon (1) the relative concentration of the buffer components and (2) the ratio of the components. For example, a 0.5 M acetate buffer at a pH of 4.76 would have a higher buffer capacity than a 0.05 M buffer.

Now, if a strong base such as sodium hydroxide is added to a buffer system consisting of equimolar concentrations of sodium acetate and acetic acid, the base is neutralized by the acetic acid forming more sodium acetate, and the resulting *increase* in pH is slight. Actually, the addition of the base increases the concentration of sodium acetate and decreases *by an equal amount* the concentration of acetic acid.

In a similar manner, the addition of a strong acid to a buffer system consisting of a weak base and its salt would produce only a small *decrease* in pH.

To calculate the change in pH of a buffer solution upon the addition of a given amount of acid or base:

Example:

Calculate the change in pH upon adding 0.04 mole of sodium hydroxide to a liter of a buffer solution containing 0.2 M concentrations of sodium acetate and acetic acid. The pK$_a$ value of acetic acid is 4.76 at 25° C.

The pH of the buffer solution is calculated by using the buffer equation as follows:

$$pH = pK_a + \log \frac{salt}{acid}$$

$$= 4.76 + \log \frac{0.2}{0.2}$$

$$= 4.76 + \log 1$$

$$= 4.76$$

The addition of 0.04 mole of sodium hydroxide converts 0.04 mole of acetic acid to 0.04 mole of sodium acetate. Consequently, the concentration of acetic acid is *decreased* and the concentration of sodium acetate is *increased* by equal amounts according to the following equation:

$$pH = pK_a + \log \frac{salt + base}{acid - base}$$

$$\text{and} \quad pH = pK_a + \log \frac{0.2 + 0.04}{0.2 - 0.04}$$

$$= pK_a + \log \frac{0.24}{0.16}$$

$$= 4.76 + 0.1761 = 4.9361 \text{ or } 4.94$$

Since the pH before the addition of the sodium hydroxide was 4.76, the change in pH $= 4.94 - 4.76 = 0.18$ unit, *answer*.

Practice Problems

1. The dissociation constant of lactic acid is 1.38×10^{-4} at 25° C. Calculate its pK_a value.

2. Calculate the pK_a value of an acid having a dissociation constant of 1.75×10^{-10} at 25° C.

3. The dissociation constant of ethanolamine is 2.77×10^{-5} at 25° C. Calculate its pK_b value.

4. Calculate the pK_b value of urea which has a dissociation constant of 1.5×10^{-14} at $25°$ C.

5. What is the pH of a buffer solution prepared with 0.055 M sodium acetate and 0.01 M acetic acid? The pK_a value of acetic acid is 4.76 at $25°$ C.

6. Calculate the pH of a buffer solution containing 0.1 mole of acetic acid and 0.2 mole of sodium acetate per liter. The pK_a value of acetic acid is 4.76 at $25°$ C.

7. What is the pH of a buffer solution prepared with 0.5 M disodium phosphate and 1 M sodium acid phosphate? The pK_a value of sodium acid phosphate is 7.21 at $25°$ C.

8. What molar ratio of salt/acid is required to prepare a sodium borate-boric acid buffer solution having a pH of 9.44? The pK_a value of boric acid is 9.24 at $25°$ C.

9. What molar ratio of salt to acid would be required to prepare a buffer solution having a pH of 4.5? The pK_a value of the acid is 4.05 at $25°$ C.

10. What molar ratio of base to salt would be required to prepare a buffer solution having a pH of 6.8? The dissociation constant of the base is 4.47×10^{-5} at $25°$ C.

11. What is the change in pH upon adding 0.02 mole of sodium hydroxide to a liter of a buffer solution containing 0.5 M of sodium acetate and 0.5 M acetic acid? The pK_a value of acetic acid is 4.76 at $25°$ C.

12. What is the change in pH upon the addition of 0.01 hydrochloric acid to a liter of a buffer solution containing 0.05 M of ammonia and 0.05 M of ammonium chloride? The K_b value of ammonia is 1.80×10^{-5} at $25°$ C.

13. The molar ratio of salt to acid needed to prepare a sodium acetate-acetic acid buffer solution is 1:1. Assuming that the total buffer concentration is 0.1 mole/liter, how many grams of sodium acetate (mol. wt. — 82) and how many grams of acetic acid (mol. wt. — 60) should be used in preparing 2 liters of the solution?

Chapter 17

Some Calculations Involving Radioisotopes

RADIOISOTOPES

THE atoms of a given element are not necessarily alike. In fact, certain elements actually consist of several different components, called *isotopes*, which are chemically identical but which physically may differ slightly in mass. Isotopes, then, may be defined as atoms having the same nuclear charge, and hence the same atomic number, but having masses differing from each other. The mass number physically characterizes a particular isotope.

Isotopes may be classified as stable and unstable. Those which are stable never change unless affected by some outside force; but those which are unstable are distinguishable by radioactive transformations and hence are said to be radioactive. The radioactive isotopes of the elements are called *radioisotopes* or *radionuclides*. They may be divided into two different types: the naturally occurring and the artificially produced radionuclides.

The use of naturally occurring radioisotopes in medicine dates back some 60 years when radium was first introduced in radiological practice. However, it was not until after 1946 that artificially produced radioisotopes became readily available to hospitals and to the medical profession. Since that time radionuclides have become important tools in medical research, and selected radioisotopes have been recognized as extremely valuable diagnostic and therapeutic agents. Monographs on sixteen radiopharmaceuticals are now included in the official compendia. The official radioactive products are listed in the table which follows:

Table of Official Radiopharmaceuticals

Iodinated I 125 Serum Albumin, U.S.P.
Iodinated I 131 Serum Albumin, U.S.P.
Chlormerodrin Hg 197 Injection, U.S.P.
Chlormerodrin Hg 203 Injection, U.S.P.
Cyanocobalamin Co 57 Capsules, U.S.P.
Cyanocobalamin Co 57 Solution, U.S.P.
Cyanocobalamin Co 60 Capsules, N.F.
Cyanocobalamin Co 60 Solution, N.F.
Gold Au 198 Injection, U.S.P.
Sodium Chromate Cr 51 Injection, U.S.P.
Sodium Iodide I 125 Solution, U.S.P.
Sodium Iodide I 131 Capsules, U.S.P.
Sodium Iodide I 131 Solution, U.S.P.
Sodium Iodohippurate I 131 Injection, U.S.P.
Sodium Phosphate P 32 Solution, U.S.P.
Sodium Rose Bengal I 131 Injection, U.S.P.

These and many other radiopharmaceutical products are commercially available to properly trained and licensed personnel. Pharmacists, especially those engaged in hospital practice, who have a knowledgeable background of radioisotopes may be required to make certain modifications and dilutions of the products which are usually available from pharmaceutical manufacturers. They may also be required to make certain corrections for radioactive decay in making dosage calculations.

RADIOACTIVITY

The breakdown of an unstable isotope is characterized by radioactivity. In the process of radioactivity an unstable isotope undergoes changes until a stable state is reached and in the transformation emits energy in the form of radiation. This radiation may consist of *alpha particles*, *beta particles*, and *gamma rays*. The stable state is reached as a result of *radioactive decay* which is characteristic of all types of radioactivity. Individual radioisotopes differ in the rate of radioactive decay, but in each case a definite time is required for half of the original atoms to decay. This time is called the *half-life* of the radioisotope. Each radioisotope, then, has a distinct half-life. The half-lives of some commonly used radioisotopes are given in the accompanying Table:

Table of Half-lives of Some Radioisotopes

Radioisotope	Half-life
^{198}Au	2.70 days
^{14}C	5,700 years
^{45}Ca	180 days
^{57}Co	270 days
^{60}Co	5.27 years
^{51}Cr	27.8 days
^{59}Fe	45.1 days
^{197}Hg	64.8 hours
^{203}Hg	46.6 days
^{125}I	60 days
^{131}I	8.08 days
^{42}K	12.4 hours
^{99}Mo	2.6 years
^{22}Na	2.6 years
^{24}Na	15.0 hours
^{32}P	14.3 days
^{35}S	87.2 days
^{75}Se	120 days
^{85}Sr	64 days

The rate of decay is always a constant fraction of the total number of undecomposed atoms present. Mathematically, the rate of disintegration may be expressed as follows:

$$-\frac{dN}{dt} = \lambda N \tag{1}$$

where N is the number of undecomposed atoms at time t, and λ is the decay constant or the fraction disintegrating per unit of time.

The constant may be expressed in any unit of time, *i.e.*, reciprocal seconds, minutes, hours, etc. The numerical value of the decay constant will be 24 times as great when expressed in days, for example, as when expressed in hours. This equation may be integrated to give the expression of the *exponential decay law* which may be written,

$$N = N_o e^{-\lambda t} \tag{2}$$

where N is the number of atoms remaining at elapsed time t, N_o is the number of atoms originally present (when $t = 0$), λ is the decay constant for the unit of time in terms of which the interval t is expressed, and e is the base of the natural logarithm 2.71828.[1]

Since the rate of decay may also be characterized by the half-life $(T_{\frac{1}{2}})$, the value of N in equation (2) at the end of a half period is $\frac{1}{2}N_o$. The equation then becomes,

$$\tfrac{1}{2}N_o = N_o e^{-\lambda T_{\frac{1}{2}}} \tag{3}$$

Solving equation (3) by natural logarithms results in the following expression:

$$\ln \tfrac{1}{2} = -\lambda T_{\frac{1}{2}}$$

$$\text{or} \quad \lambda T_{\frac{1}{2}} = \ln 2$$

$$\text{then} \quad \lambda T_{\frac{1}{2}} = 2.303 \log 2$$

$$\text{and} \quad T_{\frac{1}{2}} = \frac{0.693}{\lambda} \tag{4}$$

The half-life $(T_{\frac{1}{2}})$, then, is related to the disintegration constant (λ) by equation (4). Hence, if one value is known, the other can be readily calculated.

[1]See p. 245

UNITS OF RADIOACTIVITY

The quantity of activity of a radioisotope is expressed in absolute units (total number of atoms disintegrating per unit time). The basic unit is the *curie* (Ci) which is defined as that quantity of a radioisotope in which 3.7×10^{10} (37 billion) atoms disintegrate per second. The *millicurie* (mCi) is one-thousandth of a curie and the *microcurie* (μCi) is one-millionth of a curie. The doses of the official radiopharmaceuticals are expressed in terms of millicuries and microcuries.

Other units which may be encountered in practice—but which will not be used in the calculations which follow—include the roentgen and the rad. The *roentgen* is the international unit of X rays or gamma radiation. It is the quantity of X rays or gamma radiation that will produce under standard conditions of temperature and pressure ions carrying 1 electrostatic unit of electrical charge of either sign. The *rad* (acronym for radiation absorbed dose) is a unit of measurement of the absorbed dose of ionizing radiation. It corresponds to an energy transfer of 100 ergs per gram of any absorbing material (including tissues).

To calculate the half-life of a radioisotope when its disintegration constant is given:

Example:

> *The disintegration constant of a radioisotope is 0.02496 day⁻¹. Calculate the half-life of the radioisotope.*

$$T_{\frac{1}{2}} = \frac{0.693}{\lambda}$$

Substituting, $\quad T_{\frac{1}{2}} = \dfrac{0.693}{0.02496 \ \text{day}^{-1}}$

$$T_{\frac{1}{2}} = 27.76 \text{ or } 27.8 \text{ days, } \textit{answer.}$$

To calculate the disintegration constant of a radioisotope when its half-life is given:

Example:

> *The half-life of ¹⁹⁸Au is 2.70 days. Calculate its disintegration constant.*

$$T_{\frac{1}{2}} = \frac{0.693}{\lambda}$$

Substituting, $2.70 \text{ days} = \dfrac{0.693}{\lambda}$

$$\lambda = \frac{0.693}{2.70 \text{ days}} = 0.2567 \text{ day}^{-1}, \textit{ answer.}$$

To calculate the disintegration constant and the half-life of a radioisotope when its initial activity and its activity at time t are given:

Example:

   The original quantity of a radioisotope is given as 500 microcuries per ml. If the quantity remaining after 16 days is 125 microcuries per ml., calculate (a) the disintegration constant and (b) the half-life of the radio-isotope.

(a) Equation (2), written in logarithmic form, becomes

$$\ln \frac{N}{N_o} = -\lambda t$$

or $\lambda = \dfrac{2.303}{t} \log \dfrac{N_o}{N}$

Substituting, $\lambda = \dfrac{2.303}{16} \log \dfrac{500}{125}$

$$\lambda = \frac{2.303}{16} \left(0.6021 \right)$$

$$\lambda = 0.08666 \text{ day}^{-1}, \textit{ answer.}$$

(b) Equation (4) may now be used to calculate the half-life.

$$T_{\frac{1}{2}} = \frac{0.693}{\lambda}$$

Substituting, $T_{\frac{1}{2}} = \dfrac{0.693}{0.08666 \text{ day}^{-1}} = 8.0 \text{ days}, \textit{ answer.}$

To calculate the activity of a radioisotope remaining at any time t after the original assay :

Examples:

A sample of ^{131}I has an initial activity of 30 microcuries. Its half-life is 8.08 days. Calculate its activity, in microcuries, at the end of exactly 20 days.

By substituting $\lambda = \dfrac{0.693}{T_{\frac{1}{2}}}$ and $e^{-0.693} = 2$

in equation (2), the activity of a radioactive sample decreases with time according to the following expression:

$$N = N_o \left(2^{-t/T_{\frac{1}{2}}} \right) = N_o \left(\frac{1}{2^{t/T_{\frac{1}{2}}}} \right)$$

Since $\quad t/T_{\frac{1}{2}} = \dfrac{20}{8.08} = 2.475$

then $\quad N = 30 \left(\dfrac{1}{2^{2.475}} \right)$

Solving by logarithms
$$\log N = \log 30 - \log 2\ (2.475)$$
$$= 1.4771 - 0.7450$$
$$\log N = 0.7321$$
$$N = 5.39 \text{ or } 5.4 \text{ microcuries, } answer.$$

A vial of Sodium Phosphate ^{32}P Solution has a labeled activity of 500 microcuries per ml. How many milliliters of this solution should be administered exactly 10 days after the original assay to provide an activity of 250 microcuries? The half-life of ^{32}P is 14.3 days.

The activity exactly 10 days after the original assay is given by

$$N = N_o \left(\frac{1}{2^{t/T_{\frac{1}{2}}}} \right)$$

Since $\quad t/T_{\frac{1}{2}} = \dfrac{10}{14.3} = 0.6993$

then $\qquad N = 500 \left(\dfrac{1}{2^{0.6993}}\right)$

$$\log N = \log 500 - \log 2 \ (0.6993)$$

$$= 2.6990 - 0.2105$$

$$\log N = 2.4885$$

$N = 308$ microcuries per ml., activity after
radioactive decay

$$\frac{308 \ (\mu Ci)}{250 \ (\mu Ci)} = \frac{1 \ (ml.)}{x \ (ml.)}$$

$$x = 0.81 \ ml., \ answer.$$

Practice Problems

1. Calculate the half-life of a radioisotope which has a disintegration constant of 0.00456 day^{-1}.

2. Calculate the half-life of ^{203}Hg which has a disintegration constant of 0.0149 day^{-1}.

3. Calculate the disintegration constant of ^{64}Cu which has a half-life of 12.8 hours.

4. Calculate the disintegration constant of ^{35}S which has a half-life of 87.2 days.

5. The original quantity of a radioisotope is given as 100 millicuries. If the quantity remaining after 6 days is 75 millicuries, calculate the disintegration constant and the half-life of the radioisotope.

6. A series of measurements on a sample of a radioisotope gave the following data:

Days	Counts per minute
0	5600
4	2000

Calculate the disintegration constant and the half-life of the radioisotope.

7. The original activity of a radioisotope is given as 10 millicuries per 10 ml. If the quantity remaining after exactly 15 days is 850 microcuries per ml., calculate the disintegration constant and the half-life of the radioisotope.

8. If the half-life of a radioisotope is 12 hours, what will be the activity after 4 days of a sample which has an original activity of 1 curie? Express the activity in terms of microcuries.

9. A Sodium Iodide ^{131}I Capsule has a labeled potency of 100 microcuries. What will be its activity exactly 3 days after the stated assay date? The half-life of ^{131}I is 8.08 days.

10. A Sodium Chromate ^{51}Cr Injection has a labeled activity of 50 millicuries at 5:00 p.m. on April 19. Calculate its activity at 5:00 p.m. on May 1. The half-life of ^{51}Cr is 27.8 days.

11. Iodinated I 125 Serum Albumin contains 0.5 millicurie of radioactivity per ml. How many milliliters of the solution should be administered exactly 30 days after the original assay to provide an activity of 60 microcuries? The half-life of ^{125}I is 60 days.

12. A Chlormerodrin Hg 203 Injection has a labeled radioactivity of 50 microcuries per ml. How many milliliters of the injection should be administered 10 days after the original assay to provide an activity of 2 microcuries per kilogram of body weight for a person weighing 110 lb.? The half-life of ^{203}Hg is 46.6 days.

Chapter 18

Basic Statistical Concepts

STATISTICS may be defined as the science of the collection, classification, and interpretation of facts on the basis of relative number or occurrence as a ground for induction. Accordingly, all statistical studies begin with the gathering of reliable data. This information, or "raw data," whether it deals with measurements in business or science, is subsequently tabulated and analyzed for significance and validity by means of a number of mathematical and graphical procedures.

In this brief presentation some of the elementary concepts which form the basis for these procedures will be discussed in order to acquaint the student with the fundamentals of the "statistical approach."

THE ARRAY

When numerical facts are collected, they are initially recorded in haphazard fashion. But before the data can be effectively analyzed, a logical arrangement of it must be made. In other words, the "raw data" must be tabulated. One such simple arrangement is called the *array*. It consists of listing the items in a set of values in order of their magnitude from smallest to largest or from largest to smallest. Thus, the array rearranges the values but does not summarize them. The data are organized but not reduced.

Example:

Prepare an array of the following set of body temperatures (° F.) of 20 individuals.

98.3	98.6	98.6	98.8	98.5
98.6	98.7	98.4	98.5	98.6
98.7	98.4	98.6	98.7	98.6
98.5	99.0	98.9	98.6	98.9

The array is made by listing the body temperature (° F.) from the lowest to the highest.

Temperatures (°F.)

98.3	98.5	98.6	98.6	98.8
98.4	98.5	98.6	98.7	98.8
98.4	98.6	98.6	98.7	98.9
98.5	98.6	98.6	98.7	99.0

answer.

THE FREQUENCY DISTRIBUTION

A more precise tabulation consists of arranging the given data in classes and listing their frequencies. Such an arrangement is called the *frequency distribution*. In this arrangement the data are both organized and reduced.

Example:

Prepare a frequency distribution of the body temperatures given in the preceding example.

The frequency distribution of the body temperatures is made by separating the values into classes and listing the number of times a value appears in each class. If 5 classes of 0.2 beginning with 98.15 are chosen, the tabulation is made in the following manner.

Class	Tally	Frequency
98.15 — 98.35	I	1
98.35 — 98.55	++++	5
98.55 — 98.75	++++ ++++	10
98.75 — 98.95	III	3
98.95 — 99.15	I	1
	Total:	20

This tabulation shows that there is a concentration of values in the 98.55 — 98.75 class.

In general, frequency distributions should have not less than 5 classes and not more than 15. Unequal class intervals should be avoided for ease of understanding.

AVERAGES

Mean, Median, and Mode

One of the commonly used summary measures, or measures of central tendency, is the *arithmetic mean* or *average*. This is computed by adding the values of all the items in a set of data and dividing by the number of items. The formula for the arithmetic mean or average is:

$$\overline{X} = \frac{\text{Sum of values (X)}}{\text{Number of values}} = \frac{\Sigma X}{n}$$

The notation $\overline{X}$ (read X-bar) is the symbol for the average. The symbol Σ (the Greek capital letter sigma) means the summation of all the items of the variable X, and n refers to the number of values in the given set of data.

Example:

Referring to the array of the set of body temperatures, find the arithmetic mean of the recorded values.

$$\overline{X} = \frac{\Sigma X}{n}$$

$$\frac{1(98.3)+2(98.4)+3(98.5)+7(98.6)+3(98.7)+2(98.8)+1(98.9)+1(99.0)}{20}$$

$$= \frac{1972.4}{20} = 98.6, \text{ answer.}$$

Another type of average is called the *median*, sometimes referred to as the *middle* item in a series. It *is* the middle item if there is an odd number of items in the tabulation. However, in a tabulation with an even number of items, the median may be considered as the average of the two middle items or, if greater precision is desired, it is the *weighted average* of the two middle items.

Example:

Referring to the array of the set of body temperatures, find the median of the recorded values.

Average of the two middle temperatures =

$$\frac{98.6 + 98.7}{2} = \frac{197.3}{2} = 98.65, \text{ or } 98.7, \text{ answer.}$$

or, Weighted average of the two middle temperatures =

$$\frac{7(98.6) + 3(98.7)}{10} = \frac{986.3}{10} = 98.63, \text{ or } 98.6, \text{ } answer.$$

A third type of summary measure is the *mode*. It is the item that appears most *frequently* in a set of values. The mode in the array of the set of body temperatures is 98.6 because that temperature appears the greatest number of times in the tabulation. The mode and the median are considered as "positional averages" since they are determined by location. The arithmetic mean is a "computed average."

MEASURES OF VARIATION

Range, Average Deviation, and Standard Deviation

The measures of central tendency which have been discussed offer one characteristic of a distribution. Another characteristic is the measure of variation within the distribution. The simplest measure of variation is the *range* or the difference between the largest and smallest item in a distribution. The range is symbolized by the capital letter R. For the body temperature distribution previously cited, $R = 0.7$.

The amount by which a given single item in a set of values differs from the mean of those values is the *deviation*. A deviation is considered positive if the item is larger than the mean, and negative if it is smaller. One of the measures used to describe how much, on an average, an item deviates from the mean is called the *average deviation*. It is obtained by summing all the deviations from the mean without regard to algebraic sign and dividing by the number of deviations. The formula for average deviations, abbreviated *A.D.*, is:

$$\text{A.D.} = \frac{\text{Sum of absolute deviations}}{\text{Number of deviations}} = \frac{\Sigma|X - \overline{X}|}{n} = \frac{\Sigma d}{n}$$

Example:

> *Using a micrometer caliper, the diameter of a sample of a nylon suture material at different points on the strand was found to be: 0.230 mm., 0.265 mm., 0.225 mm., 0.240 mm., 0.250 mm., 0.240 mm., 0.260 mm., 0.235 mm., 0.225 mm., and 0.270 mm. Calculate the mean and the average deviation.*

Diameter mm.	Absolute Deviation mm.
0.230	0.014
0.265	0.021
0.225	0.019
0.240	0.004
0.250	0.006
0.240	0.004
0.260	0.016
0.235	0.009
0.225	0.019
0.270	0.026
2.440	0.138

$$\text{Mean} = \frac{2.440}{10} = 0.244 \text{ mm., } and$$

$$\text{A.D.} = \frac{0.138}{10} = 0.0138 \text{ or } 0.014 \text{ mm., } answers.$$

The more commonly used measure of variation is the *standard deviation* of the items in a given set of values. It is a measure of the precision of the mean and is obtained by (1) squaring the deviations, (2) summing the squared deviations and dividing by the number of deviations *minus one*, and (3) finding the square root of the quotient of the division. The formula for standard deviation, abbreviated S.D., is:

$$\text{S.D.} = \sqrt{\frac{\text{Sum of (deviations)}^2}{\text{Number of deviations minus one}}} = \sqrt{\frac{\Sigma d^2}{n-1}}$$

(The minus one in this formula is referred to as a "degree of freedom.")

Example:

In checking the weights of a set of divided powders, the following values were obtained: 304 mg., 295 mg., 310 mg., 305 mg., 290 mg., 306 mg., 298 mg., 293 mg., 302 mg., and 297 mg. Calculate the mean and the standard deviation.

Weight mg.	Deviation mg.	(Deviation)²
304	+ 4	16
295	− 5	25
310	+10	100
305	+ 5	25
290	−10	100
306	+ 6	36
298	− 2	4
293	− 7	49
302	+ 2	4
297	− 3	9
3000		368

$$\text{Mean} = \frac{3000}{10} = 300 \text{ mg.,} \textit{ and}$$

$$\text{S.D.} = \sqrt{\frac{\Sigma d^2}{n\text{-}1}} = \sqrt{\frac{368}{9}} = \sqrt{40.9} = 6.4 \text{ mg.,} \textit{ answers.}$$

In general, the following approximate relationships may be used to compare the accuracy of measures of variation:

(1) The average deviation is approximately $\frac{4}{5}$ of the standard deviation.

(2) The range is never less than the standard deviation nor more than 7 times the standard deviation.

SOME ASPECTS OF PROBABILITY

When you speak of "probability" you should make sure that both you and your listener know the sense in which you are using the word.

In our everyday speech, "probably" often expresses merely a hunch about some likelihood or possibility, and we may indicate the strength of our hunch in phrases ranging from "extremely probable" to "very unlikely." Sometimes the hunch can be supported—like the predictions of a competent weather prophet—by very good evidence. But sometimes we have no other evidence except a vague "feeling"—and this lacks the degree of reliability sought in the world of mathematics and science.

To the mathematician, "probability"—in a usage that has nicely been termed "classical"—is a kind of *certainty*. Not certainty that an event E

will take place. Certainty, rather, about the *chance* that E will take place in competition with a number N of alternate events that might happen to take place instead. The mathematician envisions an ideal or abstract world in which the chances of every competing event are *absolutely equal*. This basic premise is called the *Principle of Indifference*. It can claim 100% accuracy in some formulas only when referring imaginatively to an infinite number of cases.

As soon as "classical" probability formulas were devised they were predictably seized by gamblers and financial speculators, and the literature abounds with references to coin tossing, dice rolling, and card dealing, as well as to expectations of births, deaths, and shipwrecks. But, warn the mathematicians, the rules apply only if we respect the Principle of Indifference: our coins must not be bent, nor our dice loaded, nor our cards marked or stacked.

The statistician, whose research now carries him into every field of human interest and activity, has been forced to recognize and overcome a two-fold handicap. For one thing, actual events rarely and perhaps never are patterned by the Principle of Indifference. For another thing, equally significant, the statistician deals with a total number of cases (which he likes to call his "population") that lies a long way this side of infinity.

True, when the "population" is enormous—such as the number of molecules of gas in a chamber, or even the far lesser number of fine particles in a trituration—you can regard the great postulate of science that *like causes always produce like effects* as if it were a certainty. As a chemist, for example, you may feel certain that your gas laws will not be broken by random molecules all at once heading toward one end of the chamber; and as a pharmacist you may feel certain that with proper trituration a small amount of a potent substance like atropine sulfate will be uniformly distributed throughout a larger amount of a diluent such as powdered lactose.

Even when dealing with much smaller "populations" the statistician has found a very satisfactory substitute for "classical" probability. His "applied" probability, as indicated in the definition of statistics in the opening paragraph of this chapter, is revealed by the *relative frequency* of an event shown by an *actual survey* of cases.

An extended treatment of the subject is beyond the scope of this book. The odds are that you will find delight and profit if you explore this increasingly important area of study. Meantime, you may be interested in the following elementary observations. You may find ways to apply them in your own practice.

(1) When an event E is one of a total N of equally likely alternatives, the chance, or probability p, of its occurrence is one in that total number:

$$p = \frac{1}{N} \text{ or 1 chance in N}$$

The fraction $\frac{1}{N}$ may be expressed as a percentage.

The so-called "odds" are 1 to $N - 1$.

Example:

> *If a question on a multiple-choice examination directs you to underscore one of five alternative answers, what is your chance of guessing the correct answer?*

$$\frac{1}{N} = \frac{1}{5} \text{ or 1 chance in 5, or 20\%, } answer.$$

> *What are the odds in favor of a correct guess?*

> 1 to $N - 1$ = 1 to 4, *answer.*

(2) The probability q of the non-occurrence of E in the preceding example is

$$q = \frac{N - 1}{N} = N - 1 \text{ in } N = 4 \text{ in 5, or } 80\%$$

The *odds* in favor of q are $N - 1$ to 1 = 4 to 1.

(3) If E has several (or n) chances of occurring among a given total N of alternatives, its chances are

$$p = \frac{n}{N} \text{ or n chances in N}$$

A "classic" example is the drawing of a playing card from a pack. The chance of drawing the Queen of Spades is 1 in 52, but the chances of drawing any *one* of the *four* queens are

$$\frac{n}{N} = \frac{4}{52} = \frac{1}{13} \text{ or 1 chance in 13}$$

Example:

> *If you are asked to underscore the two correct answers among six alternatives in a multiple-choice examination, what are your chances of guessing one correct answer?*

$$\frac{n}{N} = \frac{2}{6} = \frac{1}{3} \text{ or 1 chance in 3, } answer.$$

(4) A succession of events may or may not one by one exhaust the total of possible alternatives. If you draw a queen from a pack and then restore it before a second drawing, you have restored the $\frac{4}{52}$ or $\frac{1}{13}$ ratio. But if you withdraw a queen and then draw again, hoping for another queen, you have a new ratio: three remaining queens among 51 remaining cards gives 3 in 51 or 1 in 17. A third drawing after two queens have been removed faces a ratio of two queens in 50 cards, or 1 in 25, and if this succeeds, a fourth attempt will face 1 in 49. You combine odds by multiplying, and your chances of drawing four queens in succession are only 1 in 270,725. Perhaps you can figure out why your chances of drawing them in the order of spades, hearts, diamonds, clubs are only 1 in 6,497,400.

You must be alert to such shifting odds if you are to avoid one of the most treacherous pitfalls in the game of probability.

Example:

> *Referring to the multiple-choice question cited in (3) above, what are your chances of guessing both correct answers among the six alternatives?*

By analysis of the chances you face in each step of your two-part answer, you may reckon chances of 2 in 6 or 1 in 3 for a correct first step; but then you face a chance of 1 in 5 for a correct second step. Combining the two ratios, you have the following chance of being twice correct:

$$\frac{1}{3} \times \frac{1}{5} = \frac{1}{15} \text{ or 1 chance in 15, } answer.$$

A clear proof of this analytical calculation may be charted. Presented with six alternatives—a, b, c, d, e, f—you may pair them in fifteen possible ways, and only one pair will contain the two correct answers:

a	a	a	a	a
b	c	d	e	f
b	b	b	b	c
c	d	e	f	d
c	c	d	d	e
e	f	e	f	f

Therefore you have only a 1 in 15 chance of guessing the correct pair.

(5) Often the probability of the occurrence of an event or the percentage of occurrences in a total number of cases cannot be calculated in advance of research. Recall that the *relative frequency* of the event is the number of times it actually occurs in a total number of *observations*. *Statistical probability* (in contrast to "classical" probability) may be defined as *the limit of the relative frequency as the number of observations increases*. To illustrate, you may be curious about the extent of your vocabulary. The mean average percentage of words you know on a few representative pages of your dictionary will enable you to calculate very roughly—perhaps within a limit of five percentage points more or less—how many words you know in the entire dictionary. Test yourself on several dozen more pages, and your score will approach a limit of one percentage point.

(6) When a limited number of samplings is supposed to represent an unattainable whole "population" the selection of samples should be as *random* as possible, so that every member of the whole (in theory at least) has an equal chance of being selected. A survey of public opinion should not be limited to the dwellers on one or two streets in a city, or to people whose names begin with *A*, or to members of a particular club.

Example:

Criticize the procedure of a tablet maker who selected for assay every fiftieth tablet during the first part of a run.

Since a machine might conceivably have regular cycles of varying dependability, the selection of samples should be at random intervals scattered throughout the entire run, *answer*.

(7) In any survey-by-sampling, the greater the number of measurements, the greater the probability that their mean average will approach the true one being sought. Therefore, in appraising the value of a statistical report of apparent general reliability, be ready to question any "break-downs" into components that may be individually unreliable. For example, a survey of the hair-grooming habits of 5000 American males may appear to be representative of American males in general; but if it is "broken down" into special groups (460 lawyers, 57 clergymen, 275 teachers, 13 convicts, etc.) can we fairly generalize about American lawyers, clergymen, teachers, convicts, etc.?

For comparing two surveys of a similar kind it has been found that *the probability of a truer mean average varies as the square root of the number of measurements.*

Example:

Two groups of researchers made a series of freezing point determinations on an 0.9% solution of sodium chloride which, theoretically, freezes at −0.52° C. Group A made 36 measurements, Group B 16. Assuming equal skill, which group probably found a truer average?

$$\frac{A}{B} = \frac{\sqrt{36}}{\sqrt{16}} = \frac{6}{4} = \frac{3}{2} \text{ or a 3 to 2 probability in favor of Group A, } \textit{answer.}$$

(8) Another means of comparing the reliability of two sets of measurements involves the average deviations from the mean averages. *The reliability varies inversely as the deviations.*

Example:

In the preceding example, if given the average deviation of report A as 0.006° C. and of report B as 0.012° C., you could compare their reliability as follows:

$$\frac{A}{B} = \frac{\dfrac{1}{0.006}}{\dfrac{1}{0.012}} = \frac{0.012}{0.006} = \frac{2}{1} \text{ or a 2 to 1 probability in favor of group A, } \textit{answer.}$$

(9) If the results of two investigations differ both in number of measurements and in average deviation from the mean average, you can use both factors together in comparing relative trustworthiness, keeping in mind that this varies *directly with the square root of the number of measurements and inversely as the average deviation from the mean average.*

Example:

Combine the data in the two preceding examples.

$$\frac{A}{B} = \frac{\sqrt{36}}{\sqrt{16}} \times \frac{\dfrac{1}{0.006}}{\dfrac{1}{0.012}} = \frac{0.072}{0.024} = \frac{3}{1} \text{ or 3 to 1 in favor of A,} \quad answer.$$

Or, combining the separate answers in (7) and (8):

$$\frac{A}{B} = \frac{3}{2} \times \frac{2}{1} = \frac{6}{2} = \frac{3}{1} \text{ or 3 to 1 in favor of A, } answer.$$

(10) In many a survey, particularly if of a social nature, the reliability of some of the measurements may be open to question, or a reported measurement may be irrelevant to the purpose of the survey. Any measurement that is widely out of line with others of its kind may be rejected, since its inclusion would have a disproportionate and misleading influence on the mean average and other calculations.

For example, a pharmacist in a small isolated town that had lost its only resident physician headed a committee to investigate the possibility of arranging a subsidy to attract some young general practitioner. The inhabitants consisted of several score householders, most of whom worked in a mill that was the only local industry. There were also an eccentric, uncooperative recluse, rumored to be rich, and the mill owner, a man of known considerable means. The committee decided that its survey to ascertain the average family income need not include the recluse and should not include the mill owner. The latter's income would have raised the mean average from about $4700 to over $7000.

Practice Problems

1. The blood pressures of a group of 15 individuals were recorded as follows:

125	130	127	136	132
126	134	125	120	125
138	119	130	126	124

Prepare an array of the data, calculate the mean, and find the median and the mode from the array.

2. A sample of catgut was measured for diameter by use of a micrometer caliper. The values obtained at 10 different points on the strand were:

0.230 mm.	0.225 mm.	0.240 mm.	0.250 mm.
0.225 mm.	0.260 mm.	0.270 mm.	0.265 mm.
0.235 mm.	0.255 mm.		

Calculate the mean, the range, and the average deviation.

3. In checking the weights of a set of 15 tablets, the following values were obtained:

95 mg.	100 mg.	98 mg.	103 mg.	100 mg.
102 mg.	105 mg.	104 mg.	97 mg.	99 mg.
104 mg.	101 mg.	105 mg.	96 mg.	101 mg.

Calculate the mean, the average deviation, and the standard deviation for the set of values.

4. In determining the viscosity of a liquid in terms of centipoises, 10 observations were made and the following values were recorded:

10.5 cps.	9.6 cps.	10.0 cps.	9.5 cps.
10.0 cps.	10.3 cps.	9.9 cps.	11.0 cps.
9.8 cps.	10.0 cps.		

Calculate the mean, the average deviation, and the standard deviation for the recorded values.

5. A series of 15 samples of a solution were assayed. The results, in terms of percent of active ingredient, were as follows:

5.05%	4.92%	4.85%	5.23%	5.05%
4.89%	5.05%	5.20%	5.15%	4.96%
4.95%	5.00%	5.02%	5.10%	4.87%

Calculate the mean, and find the median and the mode for the recorded data.

6. During a year-long community centennial celebration, the local pharmacist collaborated by keeping 300 tags identifying his regular customers in a drum. Each week for 50 weeks a tag was drawn from the drum, a souvenir prize awarded, and the tag returned to the drum.

(a) In any drawing, what was any customer's chance of winning the prize?

(b) During the series of drawings, what was a customer's chance of winning two prizes?

(c) What was a customer's chance of winning two prizes in a row?

(d) If the tags, once drawn, had not been returned to the drum, what would have been a previously unawarded customer's chance of winning in the last drawing?

7. In choosing a sample of 25 subjects for a certain experiment, a researcher has a group of 50 individuals available to him from which he is to select the sample. He assigns a number to each of the 50 subjects corresponding to an identical number on each of 50 buttons. He shakes the buttons in a container, draws one button, shakes the remaining buttons, then draws another button, shakes the buttons again, draws a third one, and so on until he has 25 buttons. The subjects whose numbers correspond to the numbers on the buttons which were drawn are chosen for the experiment. Is this a random selection? Justify your answer.

8. Report A on a reduction in absenteeism in an industrial institution attributed to vaccination during an outbreak of influenza: among the 1,952 employees there were 183 cases (9.4%) of clinical influenza; in the vaccinated group of 847, only 15 cases (1.77%) appeared.

Report B on a similar study: in a total of 3,497 employees, of which 1,148 received vaccination, the influenza attack rate was 10.8% as compared with 15.02% in the controls.

Comparing only the total "population" in these reports, calculate the odds that Report B may have produced more reliable percentages.

9. An old-time check of the body temperature of 25 people "in normal health" found an average of 98.4° F. with an average deviation of 0.18° F. A later check of 100 people found an average temperature of 98.6° F. with an average deviation of 0.12° F. By comparing both "population" and average deviation, calculate the ratio of the reliability of the two checks.

10. An aptitude test being devised for undergraduate applicants to graduate school was experimentally tested on fifteen subjects. With a possible score of 200, the results were as follows:

141	115	153
119	109	132
108	127	138
69	126	114
157	132	120

Compare the mean averages and average deviations calculated with and without the inclusion of the low 69. Which figures would probably be more reliable?

Appendix A
Thermometry

A *thermometer* is an instrument for measuring temperature, or intensity of heat. For practical purposes, a liquid such as alcohol or mercury undergoes a constant and measurable expansion or contraction with a rising or lowering of temperature. If contained in a small rigid bulb attached to a hermetically sealed extension tube, the liquid forces a column upwards in the tube upon expanding and draws the column down again upon contracting. If the tube has a uniform bore and we mark it with evenly spaced lines, we have a thermometer.

Obviously, any number of degrees of temperature may be marked off between any two fixed points on the tube, and similar degrees can then be uniformly extended above and below them. Late seventeenth-century physicists suggested the constant temperatures of melting ice and of pure water boiling under normal atmospheric pressure as offering the most convenient fixed points.

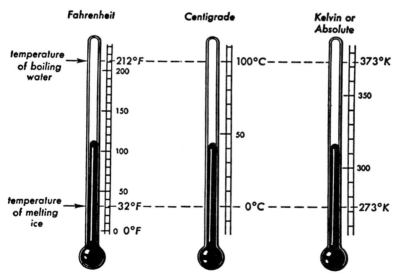

Mercury thermometers showing the Fahrenheit, Centigrade, and Kelvin scales (White's *Modern College Physics*, Copyright 1962, D. Van Nostrand Company, Inc., Princeton, N. J.).

In 1709, the German scientist Gabriel Fahrenheit (who improved the construction of thermometers and was the first to use mercury instead of alcohol) took for 0° the temperature of a mixture of snow and sal ammoniac (equal parts by weight). He discovered that by the scale he had marked on his thermometer ice melted at 32° and water boiled at 212°—with a difference of 180 degrees between these two points. The *Fahrenheit thermometer* is still commonly used in the United States.

In 1742, Anders Celsius, a Swedish astronomer, suggested the convenience of a thermometer with a scale having a difference of 100° between two fixed points, and the *centigrade thermometer* was devised, with 0° for the freezing and 100° for the boiling points of water.

On each thermometer, negative numbers are used to designate degrees "below" the arbitrarily selected zero.

Since 100 centigrade degrees (100° – 0°) measure the same difference in temperature that is measured by 180 Fahrenheit degrees (212° – 32°), each centigrade degree is the equivalent of 1.8 or $\frac{9}{5}$ the size of each Fahrenheit degree, and therefore any given rise or fall in temperature is measured by $\frac{9}{5}$ as many Fahrenheit degrees as centigrade degrees. So, we may construct a general formula for converting from one system to the other:

$$\frac{\text{Number of centigrade degrees above or below any degree centigrade}}{\text{Number of Fahrenheit degrees above or below an equivalent degree Fahrenheit}} = \frac{5}{9}$$

In other words, every 5° change in temperature as measured by the centigrade thermometer is a 9° change as measured by the Fahrenheit.

To derive a specific working proportion, it remains for us only to select points on the two thermometers that are known to be equivalent, are easy to remember, and are convenient to use in calculations.

Here are some equivalent readings above and below the melting point of ice:

0° C.	=	32° F.	0° C.	=	32° F.
5° C.	=	41° F.	−5° C.	=	23° F.
10° C.	=	50° F.	−10° C.	=	14° F.
15° C.	=	59° F.	−15° C.	=	5° F.
20° C.	=	68° F.	−20° C.	=	−4° F.
30° C.	=	86° F.	−30° C.	=	−22° F.
40° C.	=	104° F.	−40° C.	=	−40° F.
50° C.	=	122° F.	−50° C.	=	−58° F.
75° C.	=	167° F.	−75° C.	=	−103° F.
100° C.	=	212° F.	−100° C.	=	−148° F.
and so on.			and so on.		

First or fundamental method :

Modern physicists not only have verified the hypothesis that "cold" is lower "heat" activity but have found the point at which no such activity would be present, called *absolute zero*. Temperatures which are measured from this point are called *absolute temperatures* or temperatures on the *Kelvin scale*. Absolute zero has been computed as approximately $-273°$ centigrade or $-459.4°$ Fahrenheit. Consequently, this temperature may be considered the basic point of equivalence in the two systems:

$$-273°\ \text{C.} = -459.4°\ \text{F.}$$

By subtracting -273 from any given number of degrees centigrade we get the number of centigrade degrees above absolute zero. But subtracting a negative number is the same as adding its positive counterpart, so we may express this operation as $C + 273$. Similarly, any number of Fahrenheit degrees above absolute zero may be expressed as $F + 459.4$.

Our general proportion can now be specifically revised:

$$\frac{C + 273}{F + 459.4} = \frac{5}{9}$$

Using this proportion, if given the value of C we could compute the corresponding value of F, and *vice versa*.

But this can scarcely be called a working formula, since the numbers involved would not permit swift calculation. There are at least two other points of equivalence that are both easy to remember and easy to use: (1) the temperature at which both thermometers happen to register the same number of degrees and (2) the temperature of melting ice.

Second method :

The temperature registered as $-40°$ centigrade happens also to be $-40°$ Fahrenheit. The difference between any number of degrees centigrade and $-40°$ C. may be expressed as $C + 40$, and the difference between any number of degrees Fahrenheit and $-40°$ F. may be expressed as $F + 40$. By our general proportion, then,

$$\frac{C + 40}{F + 40} = \frac{5}{9}$$

Since this proportion is easy to remember, it is favored by many students, who usually sum up a working procedure as follows:

(1) To convert centigrade to Fahrenheit, *add 40 to the given number of centigrade degrees, multiply by $\frac{9}{5}$, and subtract 40.*

(2) To convert Fahrenheit to centigrade, *add 40 to the given number of Fahrenheit degrees, multiply by $\frac{5}{9}$, and subtract 40.*

These rules interpret the following derived equations:

$$(1) \quad F = \tfrac{9}{5}(C + 40) - 40$$

$$(2) \quad C = \tfrac{5}{9}(F + 40) - 40$$

Third or standard method:

The method of conversion most commonly employed, since its calculations are simplest, is based on the fact that $0°$ centigrade is equivalent to $32°$ Fahrenheit. Any number of centigrade degrees above or below $0°$ C. may be expressed as $C - 0$, or simply C. Any number of Fahrenheit degrees above or below $32°$ Fahrenheit may be expressed as $F - 32$. Hence:

$$(1) \qquad \frac{C}{F - 32} = \frac{5}{9}$$

$$(2) \qquad C = \tfrac{5}{9}(F - 32)$$

$$(3) \qquad F = 32 + \tfrac{9}{5} C$$

Perhaps a majority of scientists use equations (2) and (3), depending upon the direction of conversion, and resolve them by simple arithmetic.

Fourth and easiest method:

Here is a noteworthy fact: *no matter what specific proportion we select, if we multiply means and extremes and simplify the result we get the same working equation.*

$$(1) \qquad \frac{C + 273}{F + 459.4} = \frac{5}{9}$$

$$9\,C + 2457 = 5\,F + 2297$$
$$9\,C = 5\,F - 160$$

$$(2) \qquad \frac{C + 40}{F + 40} = \frac{5}{9}$$

$$9\,C + 360 = 5\,F + 200$$
$$9\,C = 5\,F - 160$$

$$(3) \qquad \frac{C}{F - 32} = \frac{5}{9}$$

$$9\,C = 5\,F - 160$$

Once the principle is understood, therefore, it would seem advisable to use this equation (by the rules of elementary algebra) for conversion in either direction. It is easy to remember; it is convenient to use; it prevents the errors that frequently arise from careless interchange of $\frac{5}{9}$ and $\frac{9}{5}$ or confusion of the minus and plus signs in the other equations.

Examples:

Convert 26° C. to Fahrenheit.

$$9\ C = 5\ F - 160$$
$$9 \times 26 = 5\ F - 160$$
$$234 + 160 = 5\ F$$
$$5\ F = 394$$
$$F = 78.8°,\ answer.^{1}$$

Convert −12° C. to Fahrenheit.

$$9\ C = 5\ F - 160$$
$$9 \times -12 = 5\ F - 160$$
$$-108 + 160 = 5\ F$$
$$5\ F = 52$$
$$F = 10.4°,\ answer.$$

Convert 162° F. to centigrade.

$$9\ C = 5\ F - 160$$
$$9\ C = (5 \times 162) - 160$$
$$9\ C = 650$$
$$C = 72\tfrac{2}{9}°,\ answer.$$

Convert −62° F. to centigrade.

$$9\ C = 5\ F - 160$$
$$9\ C = (5 \times -62) - 160$$
$$9\ C = -470$$
$$C = -52\tfrac{2}{9}°,\ answer.$$

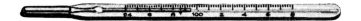

Clinical thermometer showing the average normal oral body temperature (98.6° F.)

[1] When centigrade degrees are converted to Fahrenheit, fractions are fifths and are customarily expressed as decimals; but when Fahrenheit degrees are converted to centigrade, fractions are ninths.

Practice Problems

1. Convert 10° C. to Fahrenheit.

2. Convert −30° C. to Fahrenheit.

3. Convert 4° C. to Fahrenheit.

4. Convert −173° C. to Fahrenheit.

5. Convert 77° F. to centigrade.

6. Convert 240° F. to centigrade.

7. The normal temperature of the human body is 98.6° F. Express this temperature on the centigrade scale.

8. A saturated solution of sodium chloride boils at 227.1° F. What is its boiling point on the centigrade scale?

9. The range of a centigrade thermometer is −5° to 300°. What is this range on the Fahrenheit scale?

10. Liquid Petrolatum has a kinematic viscosity of 38.1 centistokes at 37.8° C. Express this temperature on the Fahrenheit scale.

11. If a chemical reaction takes place at 71° C., at what temperature on the Fahrenheit scale will it take place?

12. If a person shows a temperature of 102.5° F. on a clinical thermometer, what temperature would he show on the centigrade scale?

13. If mercury freezes at −40° F., what is its freezing point on the centigrade scale?

14. The N.F. directs that in the preparation of Starch Glycerite the temperature must be kept between 140° and 144° C. What would be the range if a Fahrenheit thermometer were used?

15. Theobroma Oil melts between 30° and 35° C. What is the range of its melting point on the Fahrenheit scale?

16. If the maximum density of water is reached at 4° C., what would this point be on the Fahrenheit scale?

17. A specific gravity determination was made at 20° C. What was the temperature on the Fahrenheit scale?

18. Oxygen can be liquefied at −119° C. Express this temperature on (a) the Fahrenheit scale and (b) the absolute scale.

19. Rabies Vaccine must be stored at a temperature between 2° and 5° C. What are these limits on the Fahrenheit scale?

20. Petrolatum melts between 38° and 50° C. What is this range on the Fahrenheit scale?

21. In preparing a vanishing cream, you are directed to heat the oil phase to 80° C. and the aqueous phase to 82° C. Express these temperatures on the Fahrenheit scale.

22. The directions for the preparation of a certain formulation specified that the ingredients were to be heated for fifteen minutes at 70° F. This was a typographical error; it should have read 70° C. What is the difference in centigrade degrees between these two readings?

23. The critical temperature of a certain aerosol propellent is 388.4° F. and its freezing point is −168° F. Express these temperatures on the centigrade scale.

24. Dry ice vaporizes at −112° F. What is the corresponding temperature on (a) the centigrade scale and (b) the Kelvin scale?

25. A pharmacist purchased a biological refrigerator which is equipped with a centigrade thermometer. At what temperature should the refrigerator be set for storing insulin which is directed to be kept at 40° F.?

26. Rubber closures for containers for injections are sterilized preferably with moist heat in an autoclave at 121° C. for 15 to 20 minutes. Express this temperature on the Fahrenheit scale.

Proof Strength

IT IS customary to express the percentage strength of an aqueous solution of alcohol in volume-in-volume percentage, reckoned from the number of milliliters or minims or fluidounces of pure or *absolute* alcohol contained in 100 of the same unit. Consequently, if weight-in-weight percentage is specified, it should be clearly identified.

The legal and official temperature for the specific gravity of alcohol of all strengths is 60° F., or 15.56° C., at which temperature the specific gravity of absolute alcohol is 0.794.

Proof spirit is an aqueous solution containing 50% (v/v) of absolute alcohol. Alcohols of other percentage strengths are said to be *above proof* or *below proof*, depending upon whether they contain more or less than 50% (v/v) of absolute alcohol.

Proof strength of alcohol is expressed by taking 50% alcohol, or proof spirit, as *100 proof*. Then 100% or *absolute* alcohol is twice as strong, or 200 proof; 25% alcohol is half as strong, or 50 proof; and, inevitably, proof strength is always numerically twice as great as percentage strength (v/v). Hence, if percentage strength (v/v) is multiplied by 2, we have the corresponding proof strength—so 35% alcohol is 70 proof, 95% alcohol is 190 proof, and so on. Conversely, if proof strength is divided by 2, we have percentage strength (v/v)—so 160 proof alcohol is 80% (v/v) strength, 90 proof alcohol is of 45% (v/v) strength, and so on.

Alcoholic and alcoholic beverages are generally measured in gallons, for purposes of taxation, whatever their percentage strengths; and for this and other reasons, a unit called the *proof gallon* is frequently used to measure, or evaluate, alcohols of given quantities and strengths. The tax on alcohol or alcoholic liquors is quoted at a definite figure per proof gallon. A *drawback* or refund of the tax paid on distilled spirits which are used in the manufacture of medicines and medicinal preparations is allowed by the government and may be obtained by eligible claimants. Like the tax on distilled spirits, the drawback is quoted at a definite rate per proof gallon.

A *proof gallon* is 1 wine gallon (a gallon by measure) of proof spirit. In other words, 1 proof gallon = 1 wine gallon of an alcohol solution containing $\frac{1}{2}$ wine gallon of absolute alcohol and having therefore a strength of 100 proof or 50% (v/v). Any quantity of alcohol containing $\frac{1}{2}$ wine gallon of absolute alcohol is said "to be the equivalent of" or "to contain" 1 proof gallon. So, 2 wine gallons of 50 proof or 25% (v/v) alcohol would contain $\frac{1}{2}$ wine gallon of absolute alcohol, and would therefore be the equivalent of 1 proof gallon; but 3 wine gallons of such a solution would contain $1\frac{1}{2}$ proof gallons.

To calculate the number of proof gallons contained in a given quantity of alcohol of specified strength:

Since a proof gallon has a percentage strength of 50 per cent (v/v), the equivalent number of proof gallons may be calculated by the formula:

$$\text{Proof gallons} = \frac{\text{Wine gallons} \times \text{Percentage strength of solution}}{50\ (\%)}$$

And since proof strength is twice percentage strength, the formula may validly be revised as follows:

$$\text{Proof gallons} = \frac{\text{Wine gallons} \times \text{Proof strength of solution}}{100\ (\text{proof})}$$

Example:

How many proof gallons are contained in 5 wine gallons of 75% (v/v) alcohol?

First method:

1 proof gallon = 1 wine gallon of 50% (v/v) strength

$$\frac{5\ (\text{wine gallons}) \times 75\ (\%)}{50\ (\%)} = 7.5 \text{ proof gallons, } \textit{answer.}$$

Second method:

75% (v/v) = 150 proof

$$\frac{5\ (\text{wine gallons}) \times 150\ (\text{proof})}{100\ (\text{proof})} = 7.5 \text{ proof gallons, } \textit{answer.}$$

To calculate the number of wine gallons of alcohol of specified strength equivalent to a given number of proof gallons:

$$\text{Wine gallons} = \frac{\text{Proof gallons} \times 50\ (\%)}{\text{Percentage strength of solution}}$$

or,

$$\text{Wine gallons} = \frac{\text{Proof gallons} \times 100\ (\text{proof})}{\text{Proof strength of solution}}$$

Example:

> *How many wine gallons of 20% (v/v) alcohol would be the equivalent of 20 proof gallons?*

First method:

1 proof gallon = 1 wine gallon of 50% (v/v) strength

$$\frac{20 \text{ (proof gallons)} \times 50 \text{ (\%)}}{20 \text{ (\%)}} = 50 \text{ wine gallons, } answer.$$

Second method:

20% (v/v) = 40 proof

$$\frac{20 \text{ (proof gallons)} \times 100 \text{ (proof)}}{40 \text{ (proof)}} = 50 \text{ wine gallons, } answer.$$

To calculate the tax on a given quantity of alcohol of a specified strength :

Example:

> *If the tax on alcohol is quoted at $10.50 per proof gallon, how much tax would be collected upon 10 wine gallons of alcohol marked "190 proof"?*

$$\frac{10 \text{ (wine gallons)} \times 190 \text{ (proof)}}{100 \text{ (proof)}} = 19 \text{ proof gallons}$$

$10.50 × 19 (proof gallons) = $199.50, *answer.*

Practice Problems

1. How many proof gallons are represented by 54 wine gallons of 95% (v/v) alcohol?

2. How many gallons of proof spirit are there in 25 wine gallons of a sample that contains 70% (v/v) of pure alcohol?

3. How many proof gallons are contained in 500 wine gallons of Diluted Alcohol, U.S.P., that contains 49% (v/v) of pure alcohol?

4. During a certain month, a hospital pharmacist used 54 gallons of 95% alcohol and 5 gallons of absolute (100%) alcohol. How many proof gallons did he use?

5. How many wine gallons of 60% (v/v) alcohol are the equivalent of 100 proof gallons?

6. How many wine gallons of 95% (v/v) alcohol would contain 91.2 proof gallons?

7. Calculate the volume, in wine gallons, represented by 175 proof gallons of 70% (v/v) alcohol.

8. If a drum contains 54 wine gallons of 95% (v/v) alcohol, how much tax must be paid on it at the rate of $10.50 per proof gallon?

9. If the tax on alcohol is $10.50 per proof gallon, how much tax must be paid on 5 wine gallons of Alcohol, U.S.P., that contains 94.9% (v/v) of pure alcohol?

10. If alcohol is taxed at the rate of $10.50 per proof gallon, compute the tax on 6 wine gallons of 65% (v/v) alcohol.

11. The drawback on alcohol is $9.50 per proof gallon. If an eligible claimant has used 18 gallons of 95% alcohol, to how much drawback is he entitled?

12. A manufacturing pharmacist received a drawback of $790 on the alcohol that he used during a certain period. If the drawback on alcohol is $9.50 per proof gallon, how many wine gallons of 95% alcohol did he use?

13. The formula for an elixir calls for 4 gallons of 95% alcohol. Alcohol (95%) costs $25.00 per gallon and the drawback is $9.50 per proof gallon. Calculate the net cost of the alcohol in the formula.

14. The drawback on a quantity of 95% alcohol used in the manufacture of a certain medicinal preparation was $180.50, and the net cost of the alcohol was $67.00. If the rate of drawback is $9.50 per proof gallon, what was the original purchase price per gallon of the alcohol?

15. On the first of the month, a hospital pharmacist had on hand a drum containing 54 gallons of 95% alcohol. During the month he used the following amounts:

    (a) 10 gallons in the manufacture of bathing lotion.
    (b) 20 gallons in the manufacture of medicated alcohol.
    (c) 5 gallons in the manufacture of soap solution.

How many proof gallons of alcohol did he have on hand at the end of the month?

16. A hospital pharmacist had two drums (108 gallons) of 95% alcohol and 10 pints of absolute (100%) alcohol on hand on the first of the month. During the month he prepared 20 gallons of 70% (v/v) alcohol and 30 gallons of 50% (v/v) alcohol. He also dispensed 2 pints of absolute alcohol. How many proof gallons did his alcohol inventory show at the end of the month?

Appendix C

Alcoholometric Tables

THE percentage strengths of mixtures of alcohol and water can be calculated from their specific gravities by reference to alcoholometric tables; and conversely, their specific gravities can be calculated from the tables when their percentage strengths are known.

It happens that alcoholometric tables, like other tables of data and of numerical figures (such as acid and alkali tables and logarithmic tables), give values of variables at certain intervals only. Consequently, when it becomes necessary to determine values between those actually given in a table, *interpolation*—a method of estimating intermediate values by proportional parts—must be used.

The alcoholometric table of the *United States Pharmacopeia* gives, under its several headings, *percentage strengths by volume* and *by weight* of mixtures of alcohol and water, together with the *corresponding specific gravities* at 15.56° C. and 25° C. Only two of these headings, each with its column of values, will be used here to illustrate the method of interpolation in finding values of variables not given in the table. It should be noted that, in alcoholometric tables, as the percentage strength increases, the specific gravity decreases.

To find the percentage strength of alcohol when its known specific gravity is not included in the table:

Example:

A *sample of alcohol has a specific gravity of 0.8601 at 15.56° C. By reference to the alcoholometric table, find the percentage of alcohol, by volume, in the sample.*

The known specific gravity lies between the figures 0.8608 and 0.8580 included in the table, and the difference between these figures is 0.0028. The table tells us that the percent by volume will lie between 81 and 82, and the difference between these is 1%.

If we interpolate the known 0.8601 and the unknown $x\%$ in the table, we can calculate the value of x by proportion, and the percentage of alcohol, by volume, in the sample will be *81 + x.*

(298)

$$\frac{0.0028}{0.0007} = \frac{1\ (\%)}{x\ (\%)}$$

or,

$$\frac{28}{7} = \frac{1\ (\%)}{x\ (\%)}$$

$$x = \tfrac{7}{28} \times 1\ (\%) = 0.25\%$$

$$81\% + 0.25\% = 81.25\%,\ answer.$$

To find the specific gravity of alcohol when its known percentage strength is not given in the table:

Example:

By reference to the alcoholometric table, find the specific gravity of a sample of alcohol whose percentage strength by volume is 86.4% at 15.56° C.

Since the percentage strength lies between 86% and 87%, the table tells us that the specific gravity lies between 0.8462 and 0.8432, and using the same procedure as in solving the preceding problem, we can find its value by proportion. But note that this value will be 0.8462 − x.

$$\frac{1\ (\%)}{0.4\ (\%)} = \frac{0.0030}{x}$$

$$x = 0.0012$$

$$0.8462 - 0.0012 = 0.8450,\ answer.$$

ALCOHOLOMETRIC TABLE

Percent of C_2H_5OH by volume at 15.56° C.	Specific gravity in air at 15.56° C. / 15.56° C.	Percent of C_2H_5OH by volume at 15.56° C.	Specific gravity in air at 15.56° C. / 15.56° C.	Percent of C_2H_5OH by volume at 15.56° C.	Specific gravity in air at 15.56° C. / 15.56° C.
		31	0.9641	66	0.8995
		32	0.9629	67	0.8972
		33	0.9617	68	0.8948
		34	0.9604	69	0.8923
0	1.0000	35	0.9590	70	0.8899
1	0.9985	36	0.9576	71	0.8874
2	0.9970	37	0.9562	72	0.8848
3	0.9956	38	0.9548	73	0.8823
4	0.9942	39	0.9533	74	0.8797
5	0.9928	40	0.9517	75	0.8771
6	0.9915	41	0.9501	76	0.8745
7	0.9902	42	0.9485	77	0.8718
8	0.9890	43	0.9469	78	0.8691
9	0.9878	44	0.9452	79	0.8664
10	0.9866	45	0.9434	80	0.8636
11	0.9854	46	0.9417	81	0.8608
12	0.9843	47	0.9399	82	0.8580
13	0.9832	48	0.9380	83	0.8551
14	0.9821	49	0.9361	84	0.8522
15	0.9810	50	0.9342	85	0.8493
16	0.9800	51	0.9322	86	0.8462
17	0.9789	52	0.9302	87	0.8432
18	0.9779	53	0.9282	88	0.8401
19	0.9769	54	0.9262	89	0.8369
20	0.9759	55	0.9241	90	0.8336
21	0.9749	56	0.9220	91	0.8303
22	0.9739	57	0.9199	92	0.8268
23	0.9729	58	0.9177	93	0.8233
24	0.9719	59	0.9155	94	0.8196
25	0.9708	60	0.9133	95	0.8158
26	0.9697	61	0.9111	96	0.8118
27	0.9687	62	0.9088	97	0.8077
28	0.9676	63	0.9065	98	0.8033
29	0.9664	64	0.9042	99	0.7986
30	0.9653	65	0.9019	100	0.7936

Practice Problems

1. An alcohol sample has a specific gravity of 0.9280 at 15.56° C. By referring to the alcoholometric table determine the percentage of alcohol, by volume, in the sample.

2. The specific gravity of a sample of alcohol is 0.9784 at 15.56° C. Calculate the percentage of alcohol, by volume, in the sample.

3. The specific gravity of an alcoholic distillate observed at 15.56° C. is 0.9692. By referring to the alcoholometric table determine the percentage of alcohol, by volume, in the distillate.

4. If the specific gravity of an alcoholic distillate observed at 15.56° C. is 0.9666, what is the percentage of alcohol, by volume, in the distillate?

5. A sample of alcohol has a specific gravity of 0.8425 at 15.56° C. By referring to the alcoholometric table determine its percentage strength by volume.

6. The specific gravity of an alcoholic liquid taken at 15.56° C. is 0.9813. Calculate the percentage strength by volume of the liquid.

7. By referring to the alcoholometric table determine the specific gravity of a sample of alcohol whose percentage strength is 92.3%, by volume, at 15.56° C.

8. A sample contains 12.35% of alcohol, by volume, at 15.56° C. By referring to the alcoholometric table determine the specific gravity of the sample.

9. What is the specific gravity of an alcoholic distillate that contains 25.75%, by volume, of alcohol?

10. By referring to the alcoholometric table determine the specific gravity of an alcoholic liquid whose percentage strength is 45.7%, by volume, at 15.56° C.

Appendix D

Solubility Ratios

THE *solubility* of a substance is the ratio between the amount of it contained in a given amount of saturated solution (at a given temperature) and the amount of solvent therein. For instance, if 400 g. of saturated solution contain 100 g. of solute and 300 g. of solvent, the solubility of the active ingredient (at that temperature) is 100:300 and may be expressed as 1:3. The relative amounts of solute and solvent may be calculated from various data, such as the ratio or percentage strength of the saturated solution.

The official compendia express solubilities as 1 g. of solute in so many ml. of solvent (for example, *1 g. of sodium chloride is soluble in 2.8 ml. of water*). Solubilities may also be expressed as so many grams of solute in 100 ml. of a saturated solution.

To calculate the solubility of a substance :

This procedure will work for any kind of solution: (1) use the data to set up a proportion including the ratio *1:x*, *x* being the number of parts by weight containing *1* part by weight of active ingredient, and (2) if required, calculate the *volume* of *x* weight parts of solvent.

Examples:

What is the solubility of an anhydrous chemical if 100 g. of a saturated aqueous solution leave a residue of 25 g. after evaporation?

100 g. — 25 g. = 75 g. of water

$$\frac{25 \text{ (g.)}}{75 \text{ (g.)}} = \frac{1 \text{ (part)}}{x \text{ (parts)}}$$

x = 3 parts of water, indicating a solubility of 1:3, or 1 g. in 3 g. or ml. of water, *answer*.

What is the solubility of an anhydrous chemical if 100 g. of a saturated alcoholic solution leave a residue of 20 g. after evaporation? (The sp. gr. of the alcohol is 0.80.)

100 g. $-$ 20 g. $=$ 80 g. of alcohol

$$\frac{20 \ (g.)}{80 \ (g.)} = \frac{1 \ (part)}{x \ (parts)}$$

x $=$ 4 parts of alcohol, indicating a solubility of 1:4, or 1 g. in 4 g. of alcohol

4 g. of water measure 4 ml.

$$\frac{4 \ ml.}{0.80} = 5 \ ml.,$$ indicating a solubility of 1 g. in 5 ml. of alcohol, *answer.*

A saturated aqueous solution contains, in each 100 ml., 25 g. of a substance. The specific gravity of the solution is 1.15. Calculate the solubility of the substance.

100 ml. of water weigh 100 g.

100 g. $\times$ 1.15 $=$ 115 g. (weight of 100 ml. of saturated solution)

115 g. $-$ 25 g. $=$ 90 g. of water

$$\frac{25 \ (g.)}{90 \ (g.)} = \frac{1 \ (part)}{x \ (parts)}$$

x $=$ 3.6 parts of water, indicating a solubility of 1:3.6, or 1 g. in in 3.6 g. or ml. of water, *answer.*

What is the solubility of the active ingredient if a saturated aqueous solution has a strength of 20% (w/w)?

100 parts $-$ 20 parts $=$ 80 parts of solvent in every 100 parts of solution

$$\frac{20 \ (parts)}{80 \ (parts)} = \frac{1 \ (part)}{x \ (parts)}$$

x $=$ 4 parts of solvent, indicating a solubility of 1:4, or 1 g. in 4 g. or ml. of water, *answer.*

To determine the percentage strength (w/w) of a saturated solution when the solubility is given:

Examples:

> *One gram of boric acid is soluble in 18 ml. of water. What is the percentage strength (w/w) of a saturated aqueous solution?*

1 g. + 18 g. (18 ml. of water) = 19 g.

$$\frac{19 \text{ (g.)}}{1 \text{ (g.)}} = \frac{100 \text{ (\%)}}{x \text{ (\%)}}$$

x = 5.26%, *answer.*

> *One gram of boric acid is soluble in 18 ml. of alcohol. What is the percentage strength (w/w) of a saturated alcoholic solution? (The specific gravity of the alcohol is 0.80.)*

18 ml. of water weigh 18 g.

18 g. × 0.80 = 14.4 g., weight of 18 ml. of alcohol

1 g. + 14.4 g. = 15.4 g. of solution

$$\frac{15.4 \text{ (g.)}}{1 \text{ (g.)}} = \frac{100 \text{ (\%)}}{x \text{ (\%)}}$$

x = 6.49%, *answer.*

Practice Problems

1. What is the solubility of a substance in water if 125 g. of a saturated aqueous solution yield a 20-g. residue upon evaporation?

2. What is the solubility of a chemical if a saturated aqueous solution has a strength of 15% (w/w)?

3. A saturated aqueous solution contains 30 g. of a substance in each 100 ml. The specific gravity of the solution is 1.10. Calculate the solubility of the substance.

4. One gram of calcium hydroxide is soluble in 630 ml. of water at 25° C. Calculate the percentage strength (w/w) of a saturated solution.

5. The solubility of potassium chlorate is 1 g. in 16.5 ml. of water at 25° C. What is the percentage strength (w/w) of a saturated solution?

6. A saturated aqueous solution contains, in each 500 ml., 400 g. of a substance. The specific gravity of the solution is 1.30. What is the solubility of the substance?

7. The solubility of a substance is 1 g. in 3 ml. of water. When 5 g. of it are dissolved in 15 ml. of water, the volume of the resulting solution is 16.8 ml. How many grams of the substance and how many milliliters of water should be used to make 200 ml. of a saturated solution?

8. One gram of a substance is soluble in 0.55 ml. of water. When 20 g. of it are dissolved in 11 ml. of water, the volume of the resulting solution is 23.5 ml.

(a) How many grams of the substance and how many milliliters of water should be used in preparing 1000 ml. of a saturated solution?

(b) Calculate the percentage strength (w/w) of the solution.

(c) Calculate the percentage strength (w/v) of the solution.

(d) What is the specific gravity of the saturated solution?

9. A saturated solution of potassium iodide contains, in each 100 ml., 100 g. of potassium iodide. The specific gravity of the solution is 1.7. Calculate the solubility of potassium iodide.

10. The solubility of magnesium sulfate is 1 g. in 0.8 ml. of water at 25° C. How many grams of magnesium sulfate should be used in preparing a liter of a saturated solution? Assume a specific gravity of 1.30 of the saturated solution at 25° C.

11. If the percentage strength (w/v) of a saturated aqueous solution of sucrose is 85% and the specific gravity of the solution is 1.313, what is the solubility of sucrose in water?

Appendix E

Emulsion Nucleus

In the preparation of emulsions by the *Continental Method* ("4-2-1 Method"), the proportions for the *nucleus* or *primary emulsion* are "fixed oil 4 parts by volume, water 2 parts by volume, and acacia 1 part by corresponding weight." The weight is measured in grams when volumes are measured in milliliters, and in apothecaries' ounces when volumes are measured in fluidounces. The mixture therefore contains one half as much water by volume as oil and one quarter as much acacia by "corresponding" weight.

When emulsions of volatile oils are prepared by this method, the proportions are "volatile oil 2 parts by volume, water 2 parts by volume, and acacia 1 part by corresponding weight."

To calculate the quantities of ingredients required for a nucleus or primary emulsion :

Examples:

> *A castor oil emulsion contains 30% of castor oil. How much castor oil, water, and acacia are required to prepare the primary emulsion in the formulation of a liter of the emulsion?*

$$1 \text{ liter} = 1000 \text{ ml.}$$

$$1000 \text{ ml.} \times 30\% = 300 \text{ ml. of castor oil required}$$

Since castor oil is a *fixed* oil, the ratio *4–2–1* is used.

4	—	*2*	—	*1*	
300 ml.		150 ml.		75 g.	
oil		water		acacia	*answers.*

In preparing the emulsion, the castor oil and acacia are mixed, the water is added, and the mixture is emulsified forming the primary emulsion which is then diluted to the required volume.

A mineral oil emulsion contains 25% of mineral oil. How much mineral oil, water, and acacia are required to prepare the primary emulsion in the formulation of a pint of the emulsion?

$$1 \text{ pint } = 16 \text{ f℥}$$

$$16 \text{ f℥} \times 25\% = 4 \text{ f℥ of mineral oil required}$$

Since mineral oil is a *fixed* oil, the ratio *4–2–1* is used.

4	—	*2*	—	*1*
4 f℥		2 f℥		1℥ (480 grains)
oil		water		acacia

answers.

A turpentine emulsion contains 15% of turpentine oil. How much turpentine oil, water, and acacia are required to prepare the primary emulsion in the formulation of 4 liters of the emulsion?

$$4 \text{ liters } = 4000 \text{ ml.}$$

$$4000 \text{ ml.} \times 15\% = 600 \text{ ml. of turpentine oil required}$$

Since turpentine oil is a *volatile* oil, the ratio *2–2–1* is used.

2	—	*2*	—	*1*
600 ml.		600 ml.		300 g.
oil		water		acacia

answers.

Practice Problems

In each of the following formulas or prescriptions, calculate (a) the amount of acacia and (b) the amount of water to be used in preparing the nucleus or primary emulsion.

1. Mineral Oil   500 ml. (A *fixed* oil.)
    Acacia   q.s.
    Syrup   100 ml.
    Vanillin   40 mg.
    Alcohol   60 ml.
    Purified Water, to make 1000 ml.
    Label: Mineral Oil Emulsion.

2. Castor Oil   (A *fixed* oil.)
    Chocolate Syrup   aa   25%
    Acacia   q.s.
    Purified Water, to make 2000 ml.
    Label: Castor Oil Emulsion.

3. Cod Liver Oil   50%   (A *fixed* oil.)
   Acacia   q.s.
   Syrup   10%
   Peppermint Water, to make   5000 ml.
   Label: Cod Liver Oil Emulsion.

4. Turpentine Oil   150 ml. (A *volatile* oil.)
   Syrup   100 ml.
   Acacia   q.s.
   Purified Water, to make   1000 ml.
   Label: Turpentine Oil Emulsion.

5. ℞ Aspidium Oleoresin   4.0   (Treat as a *volatile* oil.)
   Syrup   5.0
   Vanilla Tincture   2.0
   Acacia   q.s.
   Water   ad   60.0
   Sig. Take at one dose.

6. ℞ Castor Oil   ℥iv   (A *fixed* oil.)
   Chocolate Syrup   ℥iv
   Acacia   q.s.
   Water   ad   ℥xvi
   Sig. Emulsion of Castor Oil 25%.

7. ℞ Copaiba Balsam   20.0   (Treat as a *volatile* oil.)
   Olive Oil   30.0   (A *fixed* oil.)
   Glycyrrhiza Syrup   30.0
   Acacia   q.s.
   Purified Water   ad   240.0
   Sig. 5 ml. t.i.d.

HLB System: Problems Involving HLB Values

THE systematic choice of emulsifying agents in the formulation of many emulsion systems depends upon their HLB (Hydrophile-Lipophile-Balance) values. These values form the basis of the so-called HLB System which was developed by Griffin.[1] The system presupposes a scale of HLB numbers and is based upon the facts (1) that every surfactant or emulsifier molecule is partly hydrophilic and partly lipophilic in character, and (2) that a certain balance between these two parts is necessary for various types of surfactant functions. In this scheme, each surfactant or emulsifying agent is assigned a number which varies from 1 to 20. The lower values are assigned to substances which are predominantly lipophilic (oil-loving) and which have a tendency to form water-in-oil (w/o) emulsions. The higher values are given to those materials which show hydrophilic (water-loving) characteristics and which favor the formation of oil-in-water (o/w) emulsions. Consequently, the HLB number of an emulsifying agent is an index of the type of emulsion which it has the greatest tendency to form. The HLB values of a few selected surfactants are given in the table which follows:

Table of HLB Values of Some Surfactants

Surfactant	*HLB*
Sorbitan trioleate (Span 85)*	1.8
Sorbitan sesquioleate (Arlacel 83)*	3.7
Glyceryl monostearate	3.8
Sorbitan monooleate (Span 80)*	4.3
Sorbitan monostearate (Span 60)*.	4.7
Sorbitan monopalmitate (Span 40)*	6.7
Sorbitan monolaurate (Span 20)*	8.6
Polyoxyethylene sorbitan trioleate (Tween 85)*.	11.0
Polyethylene glycol 400 monostearate	11.6
Polyoxyethylene sorbitan monostearate (Tween 60)*	14.9
Polyoxyethylene sorbitan monooleate (Tween 80)*.	15.0
(Polysorbate 80, U.S.P.)	
Polyoxyethylene sorbitan monopalmitate (Tween 40)*.	15.6
Polyoxyethylene sorbitan monolaurate (Tween 20)*	16.7

* Atlas Powder Company, Wilmington, Delaware.

[1] Griffin, W. C., *J. Soc. Cos. Chem.*, *1*, 311 (1949).

Just as surfactants and emulsifiers are assigned HLB numbers, so, too, the ingredients to be emulsified have been given certain "required HLB" numbers. These have been determined experimentally and are necessary for the proper emulsification of the dispersed phase. The "required HLB" values for some of the more commonly used ingredients in emulsion formulation are given in the accompanying table:

Table of "Required HLB" Values of Some Ingredients

| | "Required HLB" for | |
| | w/o | o/w |
Ingredient	emulsion	
Acid, Stearic	6	15
Alcohol, Cetyl	–	15
Alcohol, Stearyl	–	14
Lanolin, Anhydrous	8	10
Oil, Mineral	5	12
Petrolatum	5	12
Wax, Beeswax	4	12

To calculate the HLB of a blend of emulsifying agents :

When two or more emulsifiers are combined, the HLB of the combination is determined arithmetically by adding the contribution that each makes to the HLB total of the mixture.

Example:

What is the HLB of a mixture of 40% of Span 60 and 60% of Tween 60?

$$\text{HLB of Span 60} = 4.7$$
$$\text{HLB of Tween 60} = 14.9$$

	HLB		% of mixture		
Span 60	4.7	×	40%	=	1.9
Tween 60	14.9	×	60%	=	8.9
			HLB of mixture	=	10.8, *answer.*

To calculate the "required HLB" of a combination of ingredients which are to be emulsified :

The "required HLB" of each ingredient is multiplied by the percentage or the fraction of the oil phase that the ingredient represents; the products are then added to give the "required HLB" for emulsification of the oil phase.

Example:

> *Calculate the "required HLB" for the oil phase of the following o/w emulsion.*

Cetyl Alcohol	15.0 g.
White Wax	1.0 g.
Lanolin, Anhydrous	2.0 g.
Emulsifier	q.s.
Glycerin	5.0 g.
Distilled Water ad	100.0 g.

The oil phase represents *18 parts* of the entire formula.

Cetyl Alcohol	$= \frac{15}{18}$ of the oil phase
White Wax	$= \frac{1}{18}$ of the oil phase
Lanolin, Anhydrous	$= \frac{2}{18}$ of the oil phase

	"Required HLB"		Fraction of oil phase		
Cetyl Alcohol	15	$\times$	$\frac{15}{18}$	=	12.5
White Wax	12	$\times$	$\frac{1}{18}$	=	0.7
Lanolin, Anhydrous	10	$\times$	$\frac{2}{18}$	=	1.1

"Required HLB" of the oil phase = 14.3, *answer.*

To calculate the relative amounts of emulsifiers that should be used to obtain a "required HLB":

Problems of this type are conveniently solved by alligation alternate (p. 175).

Examples:

> *In what proportion should Tween 80 and Span 80 be blended to obtain a "required HLB" of 12.0?*

HLB of Tween 80 = 15.0

HLB of Span 80   =   4.3

By alligation,

15.0		7.7 parts of Tween 80
	12.0	
4.3		3.0 parts of Span 80

Relative amounts: 7.7:3.0 or 72%:28%, *answer.*

A formula for a cosmetic cream calls for 35 g. of an emulsifier blend consisting of Tween 40 and Span 20. If the "required HLB" is 12.6, how many grams of each emulsifier should be used in preparing the cream?

$$\text{HLB of Tween 40} = 15.6$$
$$\text{HLB of Span 20} \ \ = \ \ 8.6$$

By alligation,

15.6		4.0 parts of Tween 40
	12.6	
8.6		3.0 parts of Span 20

Relative amounts: 4:3 with a total of 7 parts

$$\frac{4 \ (\text{parts})}{7 \ (\text{parts})} = \frac{\text{x (g.)}}{35 \ (\text{g.})}$$

$$\text{x} = 20 \text{ g. of Tween 40, } and$$

$$\frac{3 \ (\text{parts})}{7 \ (\text{parts})} = \frac{\text{y (g.)}}{35 \ (\text{g.})}$$

$$\text{y} = 15 \text{ g. of Span 20, } answers.$$

Practice Problems

1. What is the HLB of an emulsifier blend consisting of 25% of Span 20 and 75% of Tween 20?

2. Calculate the HLB of a mixture of 45 g. of Span 80 and 55 g. of Polysorbate 80.

3. What is the HLB of an emulsifier blend consisting of 20% of Span 60, 20% of Span 80, and 60% of Tween 60?

4. Calculate the "required HLB" for the oil phase of the following ointment.

Stearyl Alcohol	250 g.
White Petrolatum	250 g.
Propylene Glycol	120 g.
Emulsifier	q.s.
Preserved Water ad	1000 g.

5. Calculate the "required HLB" for the oil phase of the following oil-in-water type lotion.

Mineral Oil	30%
Lanolin, Anhydrous	2%
Cetyl Alcohol	3%
Emulsifier	q.s.
Preserved Water ad	100%

6. In what proportion should Tween 60 and Arlacel 83 be blended to obtain a "required HLB" of 11.5?

7. The "required HLB" of an oil phase is 13.2. What percentage of Tween 40 and of Span 40 should be used to give the "required HLB"?

8. The formula for a greaseless ointment calls for 100 g. of an emulsifier blend consisting of Polysorbate 80 and Span 80. If the "required HLB" of the oil phase is 11.5, how many grams of each emulsifier should be used in preparing the ointment?

9. The formula for a cosmetic cream calls for 5% of an emulsifier blend consisting of Span 60 and Tween 20. If the "required HLB" of the oil phase is 14.0, how many grams of each emulsifier should be used in preparing 500 g. of the cream?

10.

Stearic Acid	8.0%
Cetyl Alcohol	1.0%
Lanolin, Anhydrous	1.0%
Emulsifier	4.0%
Glycerin	10.0%
Preserved Water ad	100.0%

(a) Calculate the "required HLB" of the oil phase.

(b) How many grams of Span 80 and how many grams of Tween 60 should be used in formulating 1000 g. of the product?

Appendix G

Miscellaneous Problems in Dispensing Pharmacy

PROBLEMS INVOLVING THE RELATIONSHIP BETWEEN PREPARATIONS OF VEGETABLE DRUGS

THE unavailability of a preparation of a vegetable drug may necessitate a replacement by an equivalent amount of some other preparation of the drug. If, for example, a prescription or a formula calls for an extract which is not available, an equivalent amount of the corresponding fluidextract or tincture may be used provided the replacement will present no compounding or formulating difficulties.

To calculate the amount of a tincture equivalent to its corresponding extract:

Example:

Belladonna tincture (*10%*) is the only preparation of belladonna available. If 1 g. of the extract represents 4 g. of the drug, how many ml. of the tincture should be used in compounding the following prescription?

    R   Ephedrine Sulfate   150 mg.
         Belladonna Extract   15 mg.
         Carbowax Base   q.s.
         Make 10 such suppositories
         Sig. Insert one at night.

15 mg. or 0.015 g. × 10 = 0.150 g. of extract needed

Belladonna extract		Belladonna		Belladonna tincture
1 g.	represents	4 g.	represented by	40 ml.

Therefore, the extract is 40 times as strong as the tincture.

$$\frac{1 \text{ (g.)}}{0.15 \text{ (g.)}} = \frac{40 \text{ (ml.)}}{x \text{ (ml.)}}$$

(314)

x = 6 ml., *answer.*

Dispensing note: The volume of the tincture must be reduced by evaporation at a controlled temperature before incorporation with the carbowax base.

To calculate the amount of an extract equivalent to its corresponding tincture :

One gram of belladonna extract represents 4 g. of the drug. How many milligrams of belladonna extract should be used to replace the tincture (10%) in the following prescription?

R   Belladonna Tincture   0.6 ml.
     Aspirin   0.3 g.
     Make 20 such capsules
     Sig.   One capsule as directed.

0.6 ml. $\times$ 20 = 12 ml. of tincture needed

Belladonna tincture is $\frac{1}{40}$ as strong as the extract.

$$\frac{40 \text{ (ml.)}}{12 \text{ (ml.)}} = \frac{1 \text{ (g.)}}{\text{x (g.)}}$$

x = 0.3 g. or 300 mg., *answer.*

PROBLEMS INVOLVING THE USE OF TABLETS TO OBTAIN DESIRED QUANTITIES OF MEDICINAL SUBSTANCES

There can be little justification for the use of tablets or dispensing tablets as a standard procedure for obtaining small quantities of medicinal substances, since greater accuracy may be achieved by the use of the aliquot method (see Chapter 1). The availability of materials, however, may restrict the choice of the method that can be employed for this purpose to the use of tablets.

To obtain a desired quantity of a medicinal substance by the use of tablets :

Examples:

The only source of sodium chloride is in the form of dispensing tablets each containing 1 g. Explain how you would obtain the amount of sodium chloride needed for the following prescription.

R̶   Ephedrine Sulfate   0.5
    Isotonic Sodium Chloride Solution (0.9%)   50.0
    Sig. For the nose.

50 (g.) × 0.009 = 0.450 g. of sodium chloride needed

Since one dispensing tablet contains 1 g. of sodium chloride or $\frac{20}{9}$ *times* the amount desired, $\frac{9}{20}$ of the tablet will contain the required quantity or 0.450 g. The required amount of sodium chloride may be obtained as follows:

Step 1. Dissolve *one* dispensing tablet in enough distilled water to make 20 ml. of dilution.

Step 2. Take 9 ml. of the dilution, *answer.*

The only source of potassium permanganate is in the form of dispensing tablets each containing 0.2 g. Explain how you would obtain the amount of potassium permanganate needed for the following prescription.

R̶   Potassium Permanganate Solution   250 ml.
         1:5000
    Sig. Use as directed.

         1:5000 = 0.02%

250 (g.) × 0.0002 = 0.050 g. or 50 mg. of potassium permanganate needed

Since one dispensing tablet contains 200 mg. of potassium permanganate or 4 *times* the amount needed, $\frac{1}{4}$ of the tablet will contain the required amount or 50 mg. The required quantity of potassium permanganate may be obtained as follows:

Step 1. Dissolve *one* dispensing tablet in enough distilled water to make 40 ml. of dilution.

Step 2. Take 10 ml. of the dilution, *answer.*

Only tablets, each containing $\frac{1}{150}$ gr. of scopolamine hydrobromide, are available. How many tablets should be used to obtain the amount of scopolamine hydrobromide needed in preparing the following solution?

Scopolamine Hydrobromide   0.0065 g.
Morphine Hydrochloride   0.5   g.
Ethylmorphine Hydrochloride   1.0   g.
Distilled Water   ad   25.0 ml.
Label: Schlesinger's Solution.

0.0065 g. = $\frac{1}{10}$ gr. of scopolamine hydrobromide needed

Changing $\frac{1}{10}$ gr. to a fraction having 150 as the denominator,
$\frac{1}{10}$ gr. = $\frac{15}{150}$ gr. of scopolamine hydrobromide needed

Since the available tablets contain $\frac{1}{150}$ gr. of scopolamine hydrobromide, $\frac{15}{150} \div \frac{1}{150}$ = 15 tablets, *answer*.

PROBLEMS INVOLVING UNITS OF POTENCY

The potency of many antibiotics and endocrine preparations as well as most of the enzymes, serums, toxins, vaccines and related products is expressed in terms of *units*. Officially, these units refer to U.S.P. or N.F. units of activity, and they are equivalent to the corresponding international units, where such exist, and to the units of activity established by the Food and Drug Administration in the case of antibiotics, and by the National Institutes of Health in the case of biological products. There is no relationship between the unit of potency of one drug and the unit of potency of another drug.

A comparison of units of potency of some official drugs and their respective weight equivalents is given in the table which follows:

TABLE OF DRUG UNITAGE EQUIVALENTS

Drug	Units of Potency	Weight Equivalents
Bacitracin	40 to 50 Units	1 mg. of bacitracin
Ergocalciferol	400 U.S.P. Vitamin D Units	10 mcg. of vitamin D
Hyaluronidase	1 N.F. Hyaluronidase Unit	0.25 mcg. of tyrosine
Insulin	22 (approx.) U.S.P. Insulin Units	1 mg. of crystallized insulin
Potassium Penicillin G	1595 Penicillin Units	1 mg. of potassium penicillin G
Sodium Heparin	120 U.S.P. Heparin Units	1 mg. of sodium heparin
Sodium Penicillin G	1667 Penicillin Units	1 mg. of F.D.A. sodium penicillin G master standard

Just as potencies of certain drugs are designated in units, so too, the doses of these drugs and of their preparations are measured in units; and problems involving the computation of the amount of a drug or its preparation corresponding to a prescribed dose are usually solved by simple proportion.

Of the drugs whose potency is expressed in units, insulin and the antibiotics are perhaps the most commonly used. In the case of insulin, several types which may vary according to the time of onset of action and the duration of action are commercially available in different strengths. These strengths are designated as U-40, U-80 and U-100, and their potencies refer to 40, 80 and 100 U.S.P. Insulin Units per ml. of solution or suspension. Special syringes are available for measuring units of insulin, but frequently a 1 ml. tuberculin syringe or a regular syringe of 1 or 2 ml. capacity is used, and the required dosage is then measured in milliliters or minims depending upon the calibration of the syringe.

To calculate the amount of a drug or preparation equivalent to a dose expressed in units :

Examples:

How many milliliters of U-80 insulin should be used to obtain 32 units of insulin?

U-80 insulin contains 80 units per ml.

$$\frac{80 \ (units)}{32 \ (units)} = \frac{1 \ (ml.)}{x \ (ml.)}$$

$$x \ = \ 0.4 \ ml., \ answer.$$

How many minims of U-40 insulin zinc suspension should be used to obtain 17 units of insulin?

U-40 insulin zinc suspension contains 40 units per ml.

Using 16 minims as the equivalent for 1 ml.,

$$\frac{40 \ (units)}{17 \ (units)} = \frac{16 \ (minims)}{x \ (minims)}$$

$$x \ = \ 6.8 \ or \ 7 \ minims, \ answer.$$

How many milliliters of a sodium heparin injection containing 200,000 units in 10 ml. should be used to obtain 5,000 sodium heparin units which are to be added to an intravenous dextrose solution?

$$\frac{200,000 \ (units)}{5,000 \ (units)} = \frac{10 \ (ml.)}{x \ (ml.)}$$

$$x \ = \ 0.25 \ ml, \ answer.$$

PROBLEMS INVOLVING THE USE OF DRUGS PACKAGED AS DRY POWDERS AND INTENDED FOR RECONSTITUTION

Many drugs which are unstable in solution, notably the penicillins and other antibiotics, are usually packaged and marketed in the dry form. The dry powder is dissolved in water or other aqueous diluent when the dosage form is dispensed or when it is to be used by the pharmacist as the source of a prescribed quantity of the drug. In the case of most antibiotics the reconstituted product retains practically full activity for a limited period of time, especially if it is refrigerated.

If the prescribed amount of the drug does not significantly increase the final volume of the reconstituted solution, the quantity of diluent which is added to the dry powder corresponds to the desired volume of the prepared solution. For example, if 1000 units of a certain antibiotic in dry form are to be dissolved and if the powder does not account for any significant portion of the final volume, the addition of 5 ml. of diluent will produce a solution containing 200 units per ml.

But if the dry powder, because of its bulk, contributes to the final volume of the reconstituted solution, the increase in volume produced by the drug must be taken into consideration, and this factor must then be used in calculating the amount of diluent to be used in preparing a solution of a desired concentration. For example, the package directions for making solutions of streptomycin sulfate specify that 9.2 ml. of sterile diluent be added to 1 g. of the dry powder to produce 10 ml. of a solution which is to contain 100 mg. per ml. The drug, in this case, accounts for 0.8 ml. of the final volume. And again, in dissolving 20,000,000 units of potassium penicillin G, the addition of 42 ml. of sterile diluent provides a total volume of 50 ml. of a solution which contains 400,000 units per ml. The dry powder now accounts for 8 ml. of the final volume.

Information concerning this increase in volume is particularly useful to the pharmacist when he prepares solutions of these drugs in concentrations other than those which are specifically mentioned in the package literature. The reconstituted solutions of the dry powders are most frequently prescribed alone, but they may also be used by the pharmacist to obtain desired quantities of the powders when they are prescribed in combination with other medicaments.

To calculate the amount of diluent to be used for a given vial content of a dry powder to produce a desired concentration when the solid material does not significantly account for any portion of the reconstituted solution:

Examples:

Using a vial containing 200,000 units of potassium penicillin G, how many milliliters of diluent should be added to the dry powder in preparing a solution having a concentration of 25,000 units per ml.?

$$\frac{25,000 \ (\text{units})}{200,000 \ (\text{units})} = \frac{1 \ (\text{ml.})}{x \ (\text{ml.})}$$

$$x = 8 \text{ ml.}, \textit{answer.}$$

Using a vial containing 200,000 units of penicillin sodium and isotonic sodium chloride solution as the diluent, explain how you would obtain the penicillin sodium needed in compounding the following prescription.

℞ Penicillin Sodium	15,000 units per ml.	
Streptomycin Sulfate	100 mg.	
Isotonic Sodium Chloride Solution ad	10 ml.	
Sig. Nose drops.		

15,000 units × 10 = 150,000 units of penicillin sodium needed

Since the dry powder represents 200,000 units of penicillin sodium or $\frac{4}{3}$ *times* the number of units desired, $\frac{3}{4}$ of the powder will contain the required number of units.

Step 1. Dissolve the dry powder in 4 ml. of isotonic sodium chloride solution.

Step 2. Use 3 ml. of the reconstituted solution, *answer.*

To calculate the amount of diluent to be used for a given vial content of a dry powder to produce a desired concentration when the solid material accounts for a definite volume of the reconstituted solution:

Examples:

The package information enclosed with a vial containing 5,000,000 units of potassium penicillin G (buffered) specifies that when 23 ml. of a sterile diluent are added to the dry powder the resulting concentration is 200,000 units per ml. On the basis of this information, how many milliliters of water for injection should be used in preparing the following solution?

℞   Potassium Penicillin G (buffered)   5,000,000 units
Water for Injection   q.s.
Make solution containing 500,000 units per ml.
Sig. One ml. = 500,000 units of Potassium
                    Penicillin G.

It should be noted from the package information that the reconstituted solution prepared by dissolving 5,000,000 units of the dry powder in 23 ml. of sterile diluent has a final volume of 25 ml. The dry powder, then, accounts for 2 ml. of this volume.

Step 1. The final volume of the prescription is determined as follows:

$$\frac{500,000 \text{ (units)}}{5,000,000 \text{ (units)}} = \frac{1 \text{ (ml.)}}{x \text{ (ml.)}}$$

$$x = 10 \text{ ml.}$$

Step 2. 10 ml. − 2 ml. (dry powder accounts for this volume) = 8 ml., *answer.*

Streptomycin sulfate is available in 1-g. vials, and the dry powder accounts for 0.8 ml. of the volume of the reconstituted solution. Using a 1-g. vial of streptomycin sulfate and isotonic sodium chloride solution as the diluent, explain how you would obtain the streptomycin sulfate needed for the following prescription.

R̸ Penicillin Sodium   15,000 units per ml.
   Streptomycin Sulfate   250 mg.
   Isotonic Sodium Chloride Solution   ad   15 ml.
   Sig. For the nose.

Step 1. Dissolve the dry powder in 9.2 ml. of isotonic sodium chloride solution. The reconstituted solution will measure 10 ml. and will contain 100 mg. of streptomycin sulfate per ml.

Step 2. Use 2.5 ml. of the reconstituted solution, *answer.*

SOME PROBLEMS INVOLVING PARENTERAL ADMIXTURES

The preparation of parenteral admixtures usually involves the addition of one or more drugs to large volume solutions such as intravenous and nutrient fluids. Although a wide variety of drugs and drug combinations have been used in preparing dilute infusions for intravenous therapy and in formulating hyperalimentation solutions, some of the more commonly used additives include electrolytes, antibiotics, vitamins and trace minerals.

In any properly administered parenteral additives program, all basic fluids (large volume solutions), additives (already in solution or extemporaneously reconstituted), and *calculations* must be very carefully checked against the medication orders. The discussion which follows concerns itself *solely* with some calculations that may be encountered in the extemporaneous compounding and dispensing of typical parenteral admixtures.

To calculate the amount of additive(s) to be admixed with a large volume intravenous or nutrient fluid to produce an infusion containing a required quantity of a drug or combination of drugs :

Examples:

A medication order for a patient weighing 154 lb. calls for 0.25 mg. of amphotericin B per kg. of body weight to be added to 500 ml. of 5% dextrose injection. If the amphotericin B is to be obtained from a reconstituted injection which contains 50 mg. per 10 ml., how many milliliters should be added to the dextrose injection?

$$1 \text{ kg.} = 2.2 \text{ lb.}$$

$$\frac{154 \text{ (lb.)}}{2.2 \text{ (lb.)}} = 70 \text{ kg.}$$

$$0.25 \text{ mg.} \times 70 = 17.5 \text{ mg.}$$

Reconstituted solution contains 50 mg. per 10 ml.

$$\frac{50 \text{ (mg.)}}{17.5 \text{ (mg.)}} = \frac{10 \text{ (ml.)}}{x \text{ (ml.)}}$$

$$x = 3.5 \text{ ml., } answer.$$

An intravenous infusion is to contain 15 mEq of potassium ion and 20 mEq of sodium ion in 500 ml. of 5% dextrose injection. Using an injection of potassium chloride containing 6 g. per 30 ml. and 0.9% injection of sodium chloride, how many milliliters of each should be used to supply the required ions?

15 mEq of K+ ion will be supplied by 15 mEq of KCl

and   20 mEq of Na+ ion will be supplied by 20 mEq of NaCl
$$1 \text{ mEq of KCl} = 74.5 \text{ mg.}$$

$$15 \text{ mEq of KCl} = 1117.5 \text{ mg. or } 1.118 \text{ g.}$$

$$\frac{6 \text{ (g.)}}{1.118 \text{ (g.)}} = \frac{30 \text{ (ml.)}}{x \text{ (ml.)}}$$

$$x = 5.59 \text{ or } 5.6 \text{ ml., } and$$

$$1 \text{ mEq of NaCl} = 58.5 \text{ mg.}$$

$$20 \text{ mEq of NaCl} = 1170 \text{ mg. or } 1.170 \text{ g.}$$

$$\frac{0.9 \ (g.)}{1.17 \ (g.)} = \frac{100 \ (ml.)}{x \ (ml.)}$$

$$x \ = \ 130 \ ml., \ answers.$$

A medication order for a child weighing 44 lb. calls for polymyxin B sulfate to be administered by the intravenous drip method in a dosage of 7500 units per kg. of body weight in 500 ml. of 5% dextrose injection. Using a vial containing 500,000 units of polymyxin B sulfate and sodium chloride injection as the solvent, explain how you would obtain the polymyxin B sulfate needed in preparing the infusion.

$$1 \ kg. \ = \ 2.2 \ lb.$$

$$\frac{44}{2.2} \ = \ 20 \ kg.$$

$$7500 \ units \times 20 \ = \ 150,000 \ units$$

Step 1. Dissolve *contents* of vial (500,000 units) in 10 ml. of sodium chloride injection.

Step 2. Add 3 ml. of reconstituted solution to 500 ml. of 5% dextrose injection, *answer.*

It should be clearly understood that the physician specifies the rate of flow of intravenous fluids in ml. per minute, drops per minute, or more frequently, as the approximate time of administration of the total volume of the infusion. In the latter instance, the pharmacist may be requested to make or to check the calculations involved in converting the desired total time interval into a flow rate of drops per minute.

To calculate the rate of flow needed to administer a large volume intravenous fluid during a desired time interval:

Examples:

Ten (10) ml. of 10% calcium gluconate injection and 10 ml. of multivitamin infusion are mixed with 500 ml. of 5% dextrose injection. The infusion is to be administered over a period of five hours. If the dropper in the venoclysis set calibrates 15 drops per ml., at what rate, in drops per minute, should the flow be adjusted in order to administer the infusion over the desired time interval?

Total volume of infusion =

10 ml. + 10 ml. + 500 ml. = 520 ml.

Dropper calibrates 15 drops per ml.

520 + 15 drops = 7800 drops

$$\frac{7800 \text{ (drops)}}{300 \text{ (minutes)}} = 26 \text{ drops per minute, } answer.$$

An intravenous infusion contains 10 ml. of a 1:5000 solution of isoproterenol hydrochloride and 500 ml. of a 5% dextrose injection. At what flow rate should the infusion be administered to provide 5 mcg. of isoproterenol hydrochloride per minute and what time interval will be necessary for the administration of the entire infusion?

10 ml. of a 1:5000 solution contain 2 mg.

2 mg. or 2000 mcg. are contained in a volume of 510 ml.

$$\frac{2000 \text{ (mcg.)}}{5 \text{ (mcg)}} = \frac{510 \text{ (ml.)}}{x \text{ (ml.)}}$$

x = 1.275 or 1.28 ml. per minute, *and*

$$\frac{1.28 \text{ (ml.)}}{510 \text{ (ml.)}} = \frac{1 \text{ (minute)}}{x \text{ (minutes)}}$$

x = 398 minutes or approx. $5\frac{1}{2}$ hours, *answers.*

Practice Problems

1. ℞   Belladonna Extract   0.005 g.
     Phenobarbital   0.03 g.
     Salicylamide   0.3   g.
     Make 24 such capsules
     Sig. One capsule as directed.

Only belladonna tincture (10%) is available. If 1 g. of belladonna extract represents 4 g. of the drug, how many milliliters of belladonna tincture should be used in compounding the prescription?

2. ℞ Hydrastis Extract   0.2 g.
    Tannic Acid   0.2 g.
    Carbowax Base   q.s.
    Make 12 such suppositories
    Sig. Insert one at night.

Only hydrastis tincture (20%) is available. If 1 g. of the extract represents 4 g. of the drug, how many milliliters of hydrastis tincture should be used in compounding the prescription?

3. ℞ Belladonna Tincture   0.3 ml.
    Aspirin   0.3 g.
    Make 24 such capsules
    Sig. One capsule b.i.d.

One gram of belladonna extract represents 4 g. of the drug. How many milligrams of belladonna extract could be used to replace the tincture (10%) in this prescription?

4. A hospital pharmacist is requested to prepare 200 suppositories each containing $\frac{1}{4}$ gr. of belladonna extract and $\frac{1}{2}$ gr. of opium extract. His narcotic stock includes only powdered opium. If 1 g. of opium extract represents 2 g. of powdered opium, how many grams of powdered opium should he use in preparing the suppositories?

5. ℞ Powdered Opium   0.06 g.
    Belladonna Extract   0.02 g.
    Pentobarbital Sodium   0.05 g.
    Carbowax Base   q.s
    Make 25 such suppositories
    Sig. Insert one at night.

The only preparation of belladonna available is the fluidextract. If 1 g. of the extract represents 4 g. of the drug and 1 g. of the drug yields 1 ml. of the fluidextract, how many milliliters of the fluidextract should be used in compounding the prescription?

6.   Belladonna Extract   0.5 g
    Phenobarbital   0.4 g.
    Bismuth Subnitrate   24.0 g.
    Kaolin   45.0 g.
    Peppermint Oil   0.1 g.
    Label: Diarrhea Powder.

If the only preparation of belladonna available is the tincture (10%), how many milliliters should be used in preparing 5 lb. of the powder? One (1) g. of the extract represents 4 g. of the drug.

7. ℞ Potassium Permanganate Solution   500 ml.
        1:10,000
      Sig. Use as directed.

Using tablets, each containing 0.3 g. of potassium permanganate, explain how you would obtain the amount of potassium permanganate needed for the prescription.

8. A pediatric prescription calls for 250 ml. of a solution, each teaspoonful to contain $\frac{1}{1000}$ gr. of atropine sulfate. How many tablets, each containing $\frac{1}{150}$ gr. of atropine sulfate, should be used in preparing the solution?

9. How many milliliters of a 0.9% solution of sodium chloride can be made from 10 dispensing tablets each containing 2.25 g. of sodium chloride?

10. ℞ Holocaine Hydrochloride Solution 1%   7.5 ml.
       Scopolamine Hydrobromide Solution 0.2%   7.5 ml.
       Sig. For the eye.

How many tablets, each containing 600 mcg. of scopolamine hydrobromide, should be used in compounding the prescription?

11. ℞ Hexachlorophene
       Hydrocortisone   aa   0.25%
       Coal Tar Solution   30.0 ml.
       Hydrophilic Ointment ad   120.0 g.
       Sig. Apply.

How many tablets, each containing 20 mg. of hydrocortisone, should be used in compounding the prescription?

12. ℞ Atropine Sulfate   gr. $\frac{1}{200}$ per teaspoonful
       B Complex Elixir   ad   240 ml.
       Sig. Teaspoonful in water.

Only $\frac{1}{150}$ gr. tablets of atropine sulfate are available. How many tablets should be used to obtain the required amount of atropine sulfate?

13. ℞ Vitamin B$_{12}$ 0.6 mg.
       Lactated Pepsin Elixir
       Phenobarbital Elixir aa 120 ml.
       Sig. 5 ml. t.i.d.

How many soluble tablets of vitamin B_{12}, each containing 25 mcg., should be used in compounding the prescription?

14. A prescription for 240 ml. of a cough mixture calls for 2 mg. of hydrocodone bitartrate per teaspoonful. How many tablets, each containing 5 mg. of hydrocodone bitartrate, should be used in preparing the cough mixture?

15. ℞ Atropine Sulfate   0.3 mg.
    Aspirin   300   mg.
    Make 20 such capsules
    Sig. One capsule as directed.

How many tablets, each containing 400 mcg. of atropine sulfate, should be used to obtain the atropine sulfate needed for the prescription?

16. ℞ Cocaine Hydrochloride   1 g.
    Isotonic Sodium Chloride Solution   100 ml.
    Sig. For the nose.

The only source of sodium chloride is in the form of dispensing tablets each containing 2.25 g. Explain how you would obtain the amount of sodium chloride needed for the prescription. Isotonic sodium chloride solution contains 0.9% of sodium chloride.

17. ℞ Colchicine   gr. $\frac{1}{150}$
    Sodium Salicylate   gr. v
    Make 20 such capsules
    Sig. One for pain.

How many granules, each containing $\frac{1}{120}$ gr. of colchicine, should be used to obtain the amount of colchicine required for the prescription?

18. ℞ Solution of
        Codeine Phosphate   gr. $\frac{1}{50}$ per drop
        Atropine Sulfate   gr. $\frac{1}{1500}$ per drop
    Dispense 5 ml. of solution.
    Sig. One drop every 4 hours.

The only source of codeine phosphate is in the form of tablets, each containing $\frac{1}{8}$ grain, and the only source of atropine sulfate is in the form of tablets, each containing $\frac{1}{120}$ grain. Assuming that the dispensing dropper calibrates 20 drops per ml., how many tablets of codeine phosphate and of atropine sulfate should be used in compounding the prescription?

19. How many milliliters of U-80 insulin zinc suspension should be used to obtain 36 units of insulin?

20. A patient is required to take 9 units of U-40 crystalline insulin and 16 units of U-80 protamine zinc insulin. What volume, in minims, of each type will provide the desired dosage?

21. How many minims of U-100 insulin should be used to obtain 60 units?

22. How many milliliters of U-80 isophane insulin suspension should be used to provide 28 units of insulin?

23. A physician prescribes 60 ml. of phenoxymethyl penicillin for oral suspension containing 4,800,000 units. How many penicillin units will be represented in each teaspoonful dose of the prepared suspension?

24. The contents of a vial of potassium penicillin G weigh 600 mg. and represent one million units. How many milligrams are needed to prepare 15 g. of an ointment which is to contain 15,000 units of potassium penicillin G per g.?

25. If 10 mcg. of ergocalciferol represent 400 units of vitamin D, how many 1.25-mg. ergocalciferol capsules will provide a dose of 200,000 units of vitamin D?

26. A physician prescribes 2.5 million units of potassium penicillin G daily for one week. If 1 unit of potassium penicillin G equals 0.6 mcg., how many tablets, each containing 250 mg., will provide the potassium penicillin G for the prescribed dosage regimen?

27. ℞ Potassium Penicillin G   5,000 units per ml.
      Isotonic Sodium Chloride Solution   ad   15 ml.
      Sig. Nose drops.

Using soluble penicillin tablets, each containing 200,000 units of crystalline potassium penicillin· G, explain how you would obtain the potassium penicillin G needed in compounding the prescription.

28. ℞ Potassium Penicillin G   5,000,000 units
      Water for Injection   q.s.
      M. et. ft. sol. 250,000 units per ½ ml.
      Sig. One-half ml. (250,000 units) by aerosol inhala-
          tion every three hours.

The package information enclosed with a vial containing 5,000,000 units of potassium penicillin G specifies that when 23 ml. of a sterile diluent are added to the powder the resulting concentration is 200,000 units per ml. On the basis of this information, how many milliliters of water for injection should be used in compounding the prescription?

29. ℞ Polymyxin B Sulfate   10,000 units per ml.
      Sterile Distilled Water   ad   15 ml.
      Sig. Use topically.

Using the contents of a vial (500,000 units) of polymyxin B sulfate and sterile distilled water as the diluent, explain how you would obtain the polymyxin B sulfate needed in compounding the prescription.

30. ℞ Streptomycin Sulfate   0.025 g. per tsp.
      Kaolin Mixture with Pectin   ad   120 ml.
      Sig. Tsp. t.i.d. for one week.

Using the contents of a 1-g. vial of streptomycin sulfate and distilled water as the diluent, explain how you would obtain the streptomycin sulfate needed in compounding the prescription. One g. of streptomycin sulfate accounts for 0.8 ml. of the reconstituted solution.

31. ℞ Bacitracin   1,000 units per g.
      Distilled Water   q.s.
      Hydrophilic Ointment   ad   30 g.
      Sig. Apply as directed. Store in the refrigerator.

The only source of bacitracin is a vial containing 50,000 units of the dry powder. Using distilled water as the diluent, explain how you would obtain the bacitracin needed in compounding the prescription.

32. An intravenous infusion for a child weighing 60 lb. is to contain 20 mg. of vancomycin hydrochloride per kg. of body weight in 200 ml. of sodium chloride injection. Using a 10-ml. vial containing 500 mg. of vancomycin hydrochloride (dry powder), explain how you would obtain the amount needed in preparing the infusion.

33. A medication order for an intravenous infusion for a patient weighing 110 lb. calls for 0.3 mEq of ammonium chloride per kg. of body weight to be added to 500 ml. of 5% dextrose injection. How many milliliters of a sterile solution containing 100 mEq of ammonium chloride per 20 ml. should be used in preparing the infusion?

34. An intravenous infusion for a patient weighing 132 lb. calls for 7.5 mg. of kanamycin sulfate per kg. of body weight to be added to 250 ml. of 5% dextrose injection. How many milliliters of a kanamycin sulfate injection containing 500 mg. per 2 ml. should be used in preparing the infusion?

35 Five hundred (500) ml. of a 2% sterile solution of ammonium chloride are to be administered by intravenous infusion over a period of four hours. If the dropper in the venoclysis set calibrates 20 drops per ml., at what rate, in drops per minute, should the flow be adjusted in order to administer the infusion over the desired time interval?

36. A reconstituted solution containing 500,000 units of polymyxin B sulfate in 10 ml. of water for injection is added to 250 ml. of 5% dextrose injection. The infusion is to be administered over a period of two hours. If the dropper in the venoclysis set calibrates 15 drops per ml., at what rate, in drops per minute, should the flow be adjusted in order to administer the infusion over the designated time interval?

37. Five hundred (500) ml. of an intravenous solution contain 0.2% of succinylcholine chloride in sodium chloride injection. At what flow rate should the infusion be administered to provide 2.5 mg. of succinylcholine chloride per minute?

38. A liter of a 0.3% intravenous infusion of potassium chloride is to be administered over a period of four hours. (a) How many milliequivalents of potassium are represented in the infusion? (b) If the dropper in the venoclysis set calibrates 20 drops per ml., calculate the rate of flow, in drops per minute, needed to administer the infusion over the desired time interval.

39. In preparing an intravenous infusion containing sodium bicarbonate, 50 ml. of a 7.5% sodium bicarbonate injection were added to 500 ml. of 5% dextrose injection. How many milliequivalents of sodium were represented in the total volume of the infusion?

Some Commercial Problems

DISCOUNTS

ONE of the more important discounts that the retail pharmacist encounters in everyday practice is the so-called *trade discount* which is a deduction from list prices of merchandise. Pharmaceutical manufacturers and wholesalers issue catalogues to community and hospital practitioners and allow certain discounts from the list prices that are quoted on the items appearing in their catalogues.

To compute the net cost of merchandise, given the list price and the discount:

Example:

> The list price of an elixir is $12.75 per gallon, less 40%. What is the net cost of the elixir per gallon?

List price		Discount		Net cost
100%	—	40%	=	60%
$12.75	×	0.60	=	$7.65, *answer.*

Frequently, several discounts are allowed. For example, the list price on some merchandise may be subject to deductions of *40%, 10%, and 5%.* This chain of deductions is usually referred to as a *series discount.* In such cases, the discounts in the series cannot be figured by adding them; rather, the first discount is deducted from the list price and each successive discount is taken upon the balance remaining after the preceding discount has been deducted. The order in which the discounts in a series discount are taken is immaterial.

To compute the net cost of merchandise, given the list price and the series discount:

Example:

>   A certain ointment lists at $5.00 per lb., less discounts of 40%, 10%, and 5%. What is the net cost of the ointment per lb.?

$$100\% - 40\% = 60\% \qquad 100\% - 10\% = 90\% \qquad 100\% - 5\% = 95\%$$

> $5.00 × 0.60 = $3.00, cost after 40% is deducted

> $3.00 × 0.90 = $2.70, cost after 10% is deducted

> $2.70 × 0.95 = $2.57, net cost, *answer.*

To compute a single discount equivalent to a series discount:

This is done by subtracting each discount in the series from 100% and multiplying together the net percentages. The product thus obtained is subtracted from 100% to give the single discount equivalent to the series discount.

Example:

>   Calculate the single discount equivalent to a series discount of 40%, 10%, and 5%.

$$100\% - 40\% = 60\% \qquad 100\% - 10\% = 90\% \qquad 100\% - 5\% = 95\%$$

>   0.60 × 0.90 × 0.95 = 0.513 or 51.3% = % to be paid

>   Discount = 100% − 51.3% = 48.7%, *answer.*

MARKUP

The term *markup*, sometimes used interchangeably with the term *margin of profit (gross profit)*, refers to the difference between the cost of merchandise and its selling price. For example, if a pharmacist buys an article for $1.50 and sells it for $2.50, the markup (or gross profit) as a dollars-and-cents item is $1.00.

Markup percentage (percentage of gross profit) refers to the markup (gross profit) divided by the selling price. The expression of the percent of markup may be somewhat ambiguous since it may be based on either the cost or the selling price of merchandise. In modern retail practice, this percentage is invariably based on selling price, and when reference is made to markup percentage (or % of gross profit), it means the % that the markup is of the selling price. However, if a pharmacist chooses, for the sake of convenience, to base percentage markup on the cost of merchandise, he may do so providing he does not overlook the fact that the markup on cost must yield the desired percentage of gross profit on the selling price.

To calculate the selling price of merchandise to yield a given % of gross profit on the cost:

Example:

> *The cost of 100 tablets is $1.50. What should be the selling price per hundred tablets to yield a 66⅔% gross profit on the cost?*

> Cost × % of gross profit = Gross profit

> $1.50 × 66⅔% = $1.00

> Cost + Gross profit = Selling price

> $1.50 + $1.00 = $2.50, *answer.*

To calculate the selling price of merchandise to yield a given % of gross profit on the selling price:

Example:

> *The cost of 100 tablets is $1.50. What should be the selling price per hundred tablets to yield a 40% gross profit on the selling price?*

> Selling price = 100%

> Selling price — Gross profit = Cost

> 100%   —   40%   = 60%

$$\frac{60\ (\%)}{100\ (\%)} = \frac{(\$)1.50}{(\$)x}$$

> x = $2.50, *answer.*

To calculate the percentage markup on the cost that will yield a desired % of gross profit on the selling price:

Example:

> *What should the percentage markup on the cost of an item be to yield a 40% gross profit on the selling price?*

> Selling price = 100%

> Selling price — Gross profit = Cost

> 100%   —   40%   = 60%

$$\frac{\text{Cost as}}{\text{Selling price as } \%} = \frac{\text{Gross profit as}}{\text{x } (\%)}$$

x = % gross profit on the cost

$$\frac{60 \ (\%)}{100 \ (\%)} = \frac{40 \ (\%)}{\text{x } (\%)}$$

x = $66\frac{2}{3}\%$, *answer.*

Practice Problems

1. Calculate the single discount equivalent to each of the series discounts listed below.

(a) 40%, 5%, and 5%   (d) 40%, 5%, and 2%
(b) 20%, 10%, 5%, and 5%   (e) 25%, 10%, 10%, and 2%
(c) 20%, 10%, and 5%   (f) 10%, 10%, and 2%

2. If an ointment is listed at $4.50 per pound, less 40%, what is the net cost of 10 pounds?

3. If a certain preparation is listed at $24.00 per dozen, less $33\frac{1}{3}\%$, what is the net cost per item?

4. A fluidextract is listed at $10.25 per gallon, less 40%. What is the net cost of f℥xii?

5. A pharmacist received a bill of goods amounting to $150, less discounts of 10% and 5%. What is the net amount of the bill?

6. If a gross of bottles of cough syrup costs $200, less 40% and 2%, what is the net cost per bottle?

7. A certain preparation is listed at $25.75 per dozen, less 40% and 15%. What is the net cost per unit?

8. A certain ointment is listed at $8.00 per dozen tubes, less 40%, 10%, and 5%. What is the net cost of a single tube?

9. A certain proprietary lists at $12.00 per dozen, less 40% and 15%. What is the net cost per unit?

10. The list price on a certain tablet is $25.00 per 5 M, less 40%. What is the net cost of 100 tablets?

11. Calculate the difference in the net cost of a bill of goods amounting to $500 if the bill is discounted at 40% and if it is discounted at 30% and 10%.

12. ℞ Glycerin   120.0
      Boric Acid Solution
      Witch Hazel   aa ad   500.0
      Sig. Apply to affected areas.

Witch hazel is listed at $4.50 per gallon, less 40%. What is the net cost of the amount needed in compounding the prescription?

13. ℞ Codeine Phosphate   0.3
      Hydriodic Acid Syrup
      Cosanyl   aa   120.0
      Sig. 5 ml. for cough.

Cosanyl is listed at $34.30 per gallon, less 40%. What is the net cost of the amount needed in compounding the prescription?

14. ℞ Hydriodic Acid Syrup
      Cheracol   aa ad Oi
      Sig. 5 ml. every 2 or 3 hours.

Cheracol is listed at $42.30 per gallon, less 40%. What is the net cost of the amount needed in compounding the prescription?

15. ℞ Belladonna Tincture   30.0
      Phenobarbital Elixir   ad   240.0
      Sig. 5 ml. in water a.c.

Belladonna tincture is listed at $5.00 per pint, less 40%, and phenobarbital elixir is listed at $11.50 per gallon, less 40%. Calculate the net cost of the ingredients in the prescription.

16.   Aluminum Acetate Solution   100 g.
      Lanolin   200 g.
      Zinc Oxide Paste   300 g.
      Label: Paste 123.

Zinc oxide paste is listed at $12.00 per 5 lb., less 40%. What is the net cost of the amount needed in the formula?

17. An article costs $0.75. At what price must a pharmacist sell it to realize a gross profit of $66\frac{2}{3}\%$ on the cost?

18. A certain article is listed at $4.00 per dozen, less 40%. At what price must the article be sold to yield a gross profit of $66\frac{2}{3}\%$ on the cost?

19. A bottle of tablets is listed at $3.00 with discounts of 40% and 5%. At what price must it be sold to yield a gross profit of 40% on the selling price?

20. A bottle of mouth wash costs 75 cents. At what price must it be sold to yield a gross profit of 40% on the selling price?

21. A jar of cleansing cream is sold for $3.00, thereby yielding a gross profit of 60% on the cost. What did it cost?

22. A certain proprietary is sold for 85 cents, thereby yielding a gross profit of 35% on the selling price. What did it cost?

23. A certain preparation is listed at $5.00 per dozen, less 40%. At what price must it be sold to yield a gross profit of 50% on the selling price?

24. If chloroform (specific gravity 1.475) costs $1.45 per pound, at what price per pint must it be sold to yield a gross profit of 50% on the selling price?

25. A certain fluidextract is listed at $7.50 per gallon, less 40%. At what price should f℥iv be sold in order that a gross profit of 50% on the selling price might be realized?

26. A pharmacist buys glycerin (specific gravity 1.25) for $1.00 per pound. At what price must he sell f℥viii in order to realize a gross profit of 50% on the selling price?

27. A pharmacist buys 20,000 tablets for $100.00 with discounts of 40% and 10%. At what price per hundred must he sell the tablets in order to realize a gross profit of 40% on the selling price?

28. A pharmacist buys a bottle of multiple vitamin capsules for $5.00 less discounts of 40% and 10%. At what price must the capsules be sold to yield a profit of 50% on the selling price?

29. Calculate the difference between a single discount of 40% and a series discount of 25% and 15%.

30. A pharmacist purchases an oil for 90 cents per liter. If he sold 1 pt. of it for $1.00, what percentage of gross profit on the selling price did he realize?

31. A pharmacist sells a bottle of tablets for $3.75, thereby realizing a gross profit of 60% on the cost. Calculate the cost of the tablets.

32. A pharmacist finds that he can realize a gross profit of 40% on the selling price if he sells a medicine for $1.50 per bottle. What percentage of gross profit does this represent if based on the cost of the medicine?

33. A pharmacist sells a jar of a cosmetic cream for $2.50, thereby realizing a profit of 60% on the selling price. Calculate the cost of the cosmetic cream.

34. A certain cough syrup lists at $20.00 per gallon with discounts of 40% and 15%. What is the net cost of f℥ vi of the cough syrup?

35. A pharmacist finds that he can realize a gross profit of 60% on the selling price if he sells an item for $5.00. What percentage of gross profit does this represent if based on the cost of the item?

36. A pharmacist bought 5 gallons of an elixir for $100.00, which was 20% off the list price. He sold 4 gallons of the elixir at 10% off the list and the balance at 10% above list. What was the percentage of gross profit, the basis of the calculation to be the selling price?

37. A pharmacist buys one dozen bottles of an ophthalmic solution listed at $24.00 per dozen. He receives a discount of 40% off the list price plus a 2% discount for paying the bill before the 10th of the month. At what price per unit must he sell the solution in order to realize a gross profit of 50% on the selling price?

38. At what price must a pharmacist mark an item that costs $1.30 so that he can reduce the selling price 25% for a special sale and still make 35% on the cost price?

39. A pharmacist bought a bill of goods at a discount of 30%, 10%, and 10%. The total discount amounted to $129.90. Calculate the original amount of the bill.

Dilution Table

Each column indicates the total number of parts by volume of weak solution of the ratio strength specified at the top that can be made by diluting ONE part by volume of any of the stronger solutions of the percentage strengths given in the left-hand column.

For example, a 1:4000 solution can be made by diluting 1 ml. of 1% solution to 40 ml., or by diluting 1 ml. of 2% solution to 80 ml., or 1 ml. or 3% solution to 120 ml.; and so on.

Again, when 1 ml. of 5% solution is diluted to 10 ml., you get a 1:200 solution; when 1 ml. of 5% solution is diluted to 50 ml., you get a 1:1000 solution; and so on.

%	$\frac{1}{100}$	$\frac{1}{200}$	$\frac{1}{300}$	$\frac{1}{400}$	$\frac{1}{500}$	$\frac{1}{600}$	$\frac{1}{700}$	$\frac{1}{800}$	$\frac{1}{900}$	$\frac{1}{1000}$	$\frac{1}{2000}$	$\frac{1}{3000}$
0.1	...	...	...	...	...	...	...	...	...	(1)	2	3
0.2	...	...	...	...	(1)	1.2	1.4	1.6	1.8	2	4	6
0.3	...	...	...	1.2	1.5	1.8	2.1	2.4	2.7	3	6	9
0.4	...	...	1.2	1.6	2.0	2.4	2.8	3.2	3.6	4	8	12
0.5	...	(1)	1.5	2.0	2.5	3.0	3.5	4.0	4.5	5	10	15
0.6	...	1.2	1.8	2.4	3.0	3.6	4.2	4.8	5.4	6	12	18
0.7	...	1.4	2.1	2.8	3.5	4.2	4.9	5.6	6.3	7	14	21
0.8	...	1.6	2.4	3.2	4.0	4.8	5.6	6.4	7.2	8	16	24
0.9	...	1.8	2.7	3.6	4.5	5.4	6.3	7.2	8.1	9	18	27
1	(1)	2	3	4	5	6	7	8	9	10	20	30
2	2	4	6	8	10	12	14	16	18	20	40	60
3	3	6	9	12	15	18	21	24	27	30	60	90
4	4	8	12	16	20	24	28	32	36	40	80	120
5	5	10	15	20	25	30	35	40	45	50	100	150
6	6	12	18	24	30	36	42	48	54	60	120	180
7	7	14	21	28	35	42	49	56	63	70	140	210
8	8	16	24	32	40	48	56	64	72	80	160	240
9	9	18	27	36	45	54	63	72	81	90	180	270
10	10	20	30	40	50	60	70	80	90	100	200	300
11	11	22	33	44	55	66	77	88	99	110	220	330
12	12	24	36	48	60	72	84	96	108	120	240	360
13	13	26	39	52	65	78	91	104	117	130	260	390
14	14	28	42	56	70	84	98	112	126	140	280	420
15	15	30	45	60	75	90	105	120	135	150	300	450
16	16	32	48	64	80	96	112	128	144	160	320	480
17	17	34	51	68	85	102	119	136	153	170	340	510
18	18	36	54	72	90	108	126	144	162	180	360	540
19	19	38	57	76	95	114	133	152	171	190	380	570
20	20	40	60	80	100	120	140	160	180	200	400	600
21	21	42	63	84	105	126	147	168	189	210	420	630
22	22	44	66	88	110	132	154	176	198	220	440	660
23	23	46	69	92	115	138	161	184	207	230	460	690
24	24	48	72	96	120	144	168	192	216	240	480	720
25	25	50	75	100	125	150	175	200	225	250	500	750
30	30	60	90	120	150	180	210	240	270	300	600	900
35	35	70	105	140	175	210	245	280	315	350	700	1050
40	40	80	120	160	200	240	280	320	360	400	800	1200
45	45	90	135	180	225	270	315	360	405	450	900	1350
50	50	100	150	200	250	300	350	400	450	500	1000	1500

To make up a desired quantity of dilute solution, select a quantity of the strong that when multiplied by the total number of parts will give the desired quantity or any insignificant excess. One liter of 1 : 10000 solution may be made by diluting 5 ml. of 2% solution to 200 × 5 ml. or 1000 ml.

To make very dilute solutions, proceed by steps. Dilute 1 ml. of 30% solution to 300 ml., making a 1 : 1000 or 0.1% solution; then dilute 1 ml. of this to 1000 ml. to get a 1 : 1000000 solution.

This table is valid for all solutions except if expansion or contraction occurs when active ingredient is mixed with diluent.

%	$\frac{1}{4000}$	$\frac{1}{5000}$	$\frac{1}{10000}$	$\frac{1}{25000}$	$\frac{1}{50000}$	$\frac{1}{100000}$	$\frac{1}{200000}$	$\frac{1}{500000}$	$\frac{1}{1000000}$
0.1	4	5	10	25	50	100	200	500	1000
0.2	8	10	20	50	100	200	400	1000	2000
0.3	12	15	30	75	150	300	600	1500	3000
0.4	16	20	40	100	200	400	800	2000	4000
0.5	20	25	50	125	250	500	1000	2500	5000
0.6	24	30	60	150	300	600	1200	3000	6000
0.7	28	35	70	175	350	700	1400	3500	7000
0.8	32	40	80	200	400	800	1600	4000	8000
0.9	36	45	90	225	450	900	1800	4500	9000
1	40	50	100	250	500	1000	2000	5000	10000
2	80	100	200	500	1000	2000	4000	10000	20000
3	120	150	300	750	1500	3000	6000	15000	30000
4	160	200	400	1000	2000	4000	8000	20000	40000
5	200	250	500	1250	2500	5000	10000	25000	50000
6	240	300	600	1500	3000	6000	12000	30000	60000
7	280	350	700	1750	3500	7000	14000	35000	70000
8	320	400	800	2000	4000	8000	16000	40000	80000
9	360	450	900	2250	4500	9000	18000	45000	90000
10	400	500	1000	2500	5000	10000	20000	50000	100000
11	440	550	1100	2750	5500	11000	22000	55000	110000
12	480	600	1200	3000	6000	12000	24000	60000	120000
13	520	650	1300	3250	6500	13000	26000	65000	130000
14	560	700	1400	3500	7000	14000	28000	70000	140000
15	600	750	1500	3750	7500	15000	30000	75000	150000
16	640	800	1600	4000	8000	16000	32000	80000	160000
17	680	850	1700	4250	8500	17000	34000	85000	170000
18	720	900	1800	4500	9000	18000	36000	90000	180000
19	760	950	1900	4750	9500	19000	38000	95000	190000
20	800	1000	2000	5000	10000	20000	40000	100000	200000
21	840	1050	2100	5250	10500	21000	42000	105000	210000
22	880	1100	2200	5500	11000	22000	44000	110000	220000
23	920	1150	2300	5750	11500	23000	46000	115000	230000
24	960	1200	2400	6000	12000	24000	48000	120000	240000
25	1000	1250	2500	6250	12500	25000	50000	125000	250000
30	1200	1500	3000	7500	15000	30000	60000	150000	300000
35	1400	1750	3500	8750	17500	35000	70000	175000	350000
40	1600	2000	4000	10000	20000	40000	80000	200000	400000
45	1800	2250	4500	11250	22500	45000	90000	225000	450000
50	2000	2500	5000	12500	25000	50000	100000	250000	500000

Abbreviations Commonly used in Prescriptions

Abbreviation	Meaning	Abbreviation	Meaning
aa. or $\overline{aa}$	of each	N.F.	National Formulary
a.c.	before meals	noct.	night
ad	up to	non rep.	do not repeat
a.d.	right ear	O.	pint
ad lib	at pleasure	o.d.	right eye
aq.	water	o.l.	left eye
a.s.	left ear	o.s.	left eye
a.m.	morning	o.u.	each eye
a.u.	each ear	p.c.	after meals
b.i.d.	twice a day	p.m.	afternoon; evening
c. or $\overline{c}$	with	p.o.	by mouth
cap.	capsule	p.r.n.	when required
cc.	cubic centimeter	pulv.	powder
comp.	compound	q.d.	every day
dil.	dilute	q.h.	every hour
div.	divide	q.i.d.	four times a day
d.t.d.	give of such doses	q.s.	a sufficient quantity
elix.	elixir	s. or $\overline{s}$	without
et	and	Sig.	write on label
ex aq.	in water	sol.	solution
ft.	make	s.o.s.	if there is need
g. or Gm.	gram	ss. or $\overline{ss}$	one half
gr.	grain	stat.	immediately
gtt.	drop	sup.	suppository
h. or hr.	hour	syr.	syrup
h.s.	at bedtime	tab.	tablet
i.m.	intramuscular	tbsp.	tablespoonful
inj.	injection	t.i.d.	three times a day
i.v.	intravenous	tr.	tincture
M.	mix	tsp.	teaspoonful
mcg.	microgram	u.d.	as directed
mg.	milligram	ung.	ointment
ml.	milliliter	U.S.P.	United States
N.D.	New Drugs		Pharmacopeia

Review Problems

1. A liquid contains 500 mcg. of a medicament per ml. Estimate the number of milligrams of the medicament that 1 gallon of the liquid will contain.

2. Estimate the number of $\frac{1}{120}$-gr. tablets that can be made from 62.5 mg. of atropine sulfate.

3. A pharmacist weighed 0.015 g. of a substance on a prescription balance having a sensitivity requirement of 0.004 g. Estimate the percentage of error that he may have incurred.

4. A pharmacist weighed 1 grain of atropine sulfate on a torsion prescription balance having a sensitivity requirement of 6.5 mg. Estimate the percentage of error that he may have incurred.

5. A pharmacist weighed 24 mg. of amphetamine sulfate on a prescription balance having a sensitivity requirement of 4 mg. Estimate the percentage of error that he may have incurred.

6. A sample of alcohol measured 10.3 ml. and weighed 8.05 g. Estimate the specific gravity of the sample.

7. A glass stopper loses 20.560 g. when suspended in water and 30.232 g. when suspended in a certain liquid. Estimate, to one decimal place, the specific gravity of the liquid.

8. A glass stopper loses 10.560 g. when suspended in water and 14.362 g. when suspended in a certain liquid. Estimate, to one decimal place, the specific gravity of the liquid.

9. Sulfuric acid has a specific gravity of 1.84. Estimate its specific volume.

10. A chemical costs $4.00 per lb. Estimate the approximate cost of ℥vi.

11. A prescription for 240 ml. of a liquid contains 15 mg. of atropine sulfate and has a dose of 10 ml. (a) Calculate the fraction of a grain of atropine sulfate that is contained in each dose. (b) Using a torsion prescription balance having a sensitivity requirement of 6.5 mg., explain how you would obtain the 15 mg. of atropine sulfate with an error not greater than 5%. Use distilled water as the diluent.

(341)

12. A pharmacist weighed 20 mg. of cocaine alkaloid on a prescription balance having a sensitivity requirement of 4 mg. Calculate the maximum potential error in terms of percentage.

13. Assuming that a prescription balance has a sensitivity requirement of 0.0065 g., what is the smallest amount, expressed in milligrams, that can be weighed with an error not greater than 5%?

14. A certain vehicle contains 0.15 ml. of amaranth solution per 100 ml. of finished product. Using a 10-ml. graduate, calibrated from 2 to 10 ml., in units of 1 ml., explain how you would measure the amaranth solution required for 500 ml. of the vehicle. Use water as the diluent.

15.   Ephedrine Sulfate   10.0 g.
       Chlorobutanol   5.0 g.
       Dextrose   40.0 g.
       Amaranth   0.02 g.
       Rose Water, to make   1000.0 ml.
       Label: Ephedrine nasal spray.

In preparing the spray, a pharmacist weighed the amaranth on a torsion balance having a sensitivity requirement of 2 mg. Calculate the percentage of error that he may have incurred.

16. In preparing a cough syrup containing 0.030 g. of hydromorphone hydrochloride, a pharmacist weighed the hydromorphone hydrochloride on a torsion balance having a sensitivity requirement of 4 mg. Calculate the percentage of error that he may have incurred.

17. Using a torsion prescription balance having a sensitivity requirement of 4 mg., explain how you would weigh the atropine sulfate needed to prepare 250 ml. of a solution which is to contain 120 mcg. of atropine sulfate in each 5-ml. dose.

18. In compounding a prescription for ℥ii of a 5% benzocaine cream, a pharmacist used 45 gr. of benzocaine instead of the 48 gr. that he should have used. Calculate the percentage of error that he incurred.

19. If an average No. 1 gelatin capsule weighs 90 mg., and no capsule in the lot varies in weight by more than plus or minus 10% of this average, what is the maximum percentage of error that could be incurred by using a capsule of the lot as a tare in filling other capsules of the same lot with 300 mg. of a medicinal substance?

20. In preparing one fluidounce of a saturated solution of potassium iodide, a pharmacist used ℥ vii of potassium iodide instead of the 455 gr. called for. Calculate the percentage of error on the basis of what he should have used.

21. ℞ Atropine Sulfate   gr. $\frac{1}{100}$
    Bismuth Subgallate   gr. v
    Carbowax Base   q.s.
    Make 10 such suppositories
    Sig. One at night.

   Using a torsion prescription balance having a sensitivity requirement of $\frac{1}{16}$ gr., explain how you would obtain the correct amount of atropine sulfate with an error not greater than 5%. Use bismuth subgallate as the diluent.

22. A prescription balance has a sensitivity requirement of 6.5 mg. Explain how you would weigh 60 mg. of a medicinal substance with an error not greater than 5%. Use lactose as the diluent.

23. In checking the inventory of narcotics in a hospital pharmacy, the checker found it to be kept in the metric system. The inventory showed 124.4 g. (4 one-ounce original bottles) of codeine sulfate on hand at the beginning of the inventory period. The prescriptions on file showed that 96 g. of codeine sulfate had been dispensed. On weighing the contents of the one-ounce bottle that remained, the checker found that only 17.4 g. were left, instead of 28.4 g. that apparently should have remained. What percentage of error, if any, had been made in the inventory?

24. A certain injectable solution contains 30 micrograms of vitamin B_{12} per ml. How many milligrams of vitamin B_{12} are there in a 10-ml. vial of the solution?

25. How many tablets, each containing 10 micrograms, can be made from 0.250 g. of vitamin B_{12}?

26. A vitamin liquid contains, in each 0.5 ml., the following:
    Thiamine Hydrochloride   1 mg.
    Riboflavin   400 mcg.
    Ascorbic Acid   50 mg.
    Nicotinamide   2 mg.
   Calculate the quantity, expressed in grams, of each ingredient in 30 ml. of the liquid.

27. How many milligrams of thiamine hydrochloride are required to prepare 5 liters of an elixir, each 5 ml. to contain 100 mcg. of thiamine hydrochloride?

28. The prophylactic dose of riboflavin is 2 mg. How many micrograms of riboflavin are there in a capsule containing 3 times the prophylactic dose?

29. How many grains of codeine phosphate are left in an original $\frac{1}{8}$-oz. bottle after the amount required to prepare 100 capsules each containing $\frac{1}{4}$ gr. of codeine phosphate as one of the ingredients is used?

30. How many grains of atropine sulfate are left in a $\frac{1}{2}$-oz. bottle after enough of it is used to make 10,000 tablets, each containing $\frac{1}{200}$ gr.?

31. A pharmacist bought 4 oz. of phenobarbital. How many capsules, each containing $1\frac{1}{2}$ grains, could he prepare from this amount?

32. A pharmacist bought 1 oz. of a chemical from a wholesaler. He dispensed at different times, ℥ii, 20 gr., ℈iss, and ℥ss. How many grains of the chemical were left?

33. A pharmacist purchased 5 gallons of alcohol. He used at different times Oii, 2 gallons, 8f℥, and $\frac{1}{2}$ gallon. What volume, in fluidounces, remained?

34. How many 300-mg. tablets can be made from $\frac{1}{4}$ lb. of chloral hydrate?

35. A prescription calls for 1.25 g. of phenacaine hydrochloride. If the phenacaine hydrochloride costs $8.00 per oz., what is the cost of the amount needed for the prescription?

36. A liquid preparation is to contain 0.5 mcg. of a medicament per ml. How many grams are needed to make 5 gallons of the preparation?

37. If homatropine hydrobromide costs $13.00 per oz., what is the cost of 300 mg.?

38. A pharmacist purchased 5 g. of codeine phosphate. He used it in preparing 50 capsules each containing $\frac{1}{2}$ gr. of codeine phosphate and in formulating 1 pt. of a cough syrup containing 1 gr. of codeine phosphate per fluidounce. For purposes of inventory, how many grams of codeine phosphate remained?

39. How many micrograms of nitroglycerin are contained in a $\frac{1}{200}$ gr. tablet?

40. If iodine costs $6.36 a pound, and iodine tincture contains 20 g. of iodine in a liter, what will be the cost of the iodine in one pint of the tincture?

41. A two (2)-ml. ampul solution contains 0.5 g. of aminophylline. How many minims of the solution should be used to give 25 mg. of aminophylline?

42. ℞ Podophyllum Resin   25%
    Compound Benzoin Tincture   ad   30 ml.
    Sig. Apply locally for venereal warts.

At $5.50 per oz., what is the cost of the podophyllum resin needed in compounding the prescription?

43. The dose of a certain antibiotic is 5 mg. per kg. of body weight. How many milligrams should be used for a person weighing 145 lb.?

44. How many 0.000065-g. doses can be prepared from 15 gr. of atropine sulfate?

45. If chloral hydrate costs $4.05 per lb., what is the cost of the amount needed to prepare a liter of a solution containing 300 mg. per teaspoonful?

46. ℞ Codeine Phosphate   gr. iv
    Ammonium Chloride   ℥i
    Ephedrine Sulfate Syrup   ℥iss
    Tolu Balsam Syrup   ad   ℥iv
    Sig. Teaspoonful for cough.

Convert the quantities in this prescription to the metric system.

47. An elixir is to contain 250 mcg. of an alkaloid in each teaspoonful dose. How many grams of the alkaloid will be required to prepare 5 liters of the elixir?

48. How many grains of atropine sulfate are required to make f℥ss of a solution containing $\frac{1}{1000}$ gr. of atropine sulfate in each five minims of the solution?

49. The dose of a drug is 0.5 mg. How many micrograms should be given to a child 10 years old?

50. A f℥ vi mixture contains, in each teaspoonful, $\frac{1}{6}$ gr. of codeine phosphate. How many grains of codeine phosphate are contained in the entire mixture?

51. The average adult dose of a solution is 0.2 ml. What is the dose, expressed in minims, for a child 8 years old?

52. If the adult dose of a drug is 0.03 mg., what is the dose for a child 10 years old?

53. The initial dose of a drug is 0.25 mg. per kg. of body weight. How many milligrams should be prescribed for a person weighing 154 lb.?

54. The adult dose of belladonna extract is 15 mg. Calculate the dose, in grains, for a child 8 years old.

55. The average adult dose of a certain solution is 0.3 ml. (a) What is the dose for a child 6 years old? (b) If the solution is to be dispensed in a dropper bottle, the dropper of which calibrates 30 drops per ml., how many drops should be given to obtain the correct dose for the child?

56. ℞ Atropine Sulfate   gr. $\frac{1}{10}$
     Distilled Water   ad   ℥i
     Sig. Five minims in each feeding.

Calculate the amount of atropine sulfate in each prescribed dose.

57. ℞ Lugol's Solution   30 ml.
     Sig. Ten drops in water once a day.

Lugol's solution contains 5% of iodine. If the dispensing dropper calibrates 25 drops per ml., calculate the amount, in milligrams, of iodine in each dose of the solution.

58. ℞ Cyanocobalamin   10 mcg. per ml.
     Disp. 10-ml. sterile vial.
     Sig. 1.5 ml. every other week.

(a) How many micrograms of cyanocobalamin will be administered in a period of twelve weeks?

(b) How many milligrams of cyanocobalamin are there in 10 ml. of this preparation?

59. ℞ Sol. Atropine Sulfate   10 ml.
       1:1000
     Sig. Five drops t.i.d. as directed.

Assuming that a standard N.F. dropper (20 drops per ml.) is used to measure the prescribed dose, calculate the amount, in grains, of atropine sulfate in each dose.

60. The adult dose of aureomycin is 250 mg. What would be the dose for a child 2 years old?

61. The rectal dose of sodium thiopental is 45 mg. per kg. of body weight. How many milliliters of a 10% solution should be used for a person weighing 150 lb.?

62. ℞ Digitoxin Solution (Oral) ℥ii
  Make sol.—0.01 mg. per ℳii
  Sig. ℳiv in a.m. with meals.

If the dispensing dropper calibrates 600 drops per f℥i, how many milligrams of digitoxin should be used in compounding the prescription?

63. ℞ Procaine Penicillin G   300,000 units
  Buffered Crystalline Penicillin G 100,000 units
  Crystalline Dihydrostreptomycin 1 g.
  Water for Injection ad   3 ml.
  Make a multiple-dose vial containing 5 doses.
  Sig. For intramuscular use only. Sterile.

To permit withdrawal of the five doses prescribed, an excess volume of 0.80 ml. must be present in the 15 ml. vial. How much of each of the three antibiotics should be used in compounding the prescription?

64. ℞ Sol. Atropine Sulfate   30 ml.
  (Each 5 drops = $\frac{1}{1000}$ gr.)
  Sig. Five (5) drops in each feeding.

If the dispensing dropper calibrates 20 drops per ml., how many milligrams of atropine sulfate should be used in compounding the prescription?

65. ℞ Sodium Fluoride   q.s.
  Vitamin Drops ad   50 ml.
  (10 drops = 2.2 mg. NaF)
  Sig. Ten (10) drops in orange juice.

Assuming that the dispensing dropper calibrates 25 drops per ml., how many milligrams of sodium fluoride should be used in compounding the prescription?

66. ℞ Hydromorphone Hydrochloride $\frac{1}{4}$ gr.
  Hydriodic Acid Syrup
  Tolu Balsam Syrup aa   60 ml.
  Sig. Teaspoonful every four hours.

Calculate the amount, in grains, of hydromorphone hydrochloride in each prescribed dose.

67. A physician asks you to prepare a prescription for capsules of aureomycin for a child 3 years old, each capsule to contain the calculated dose of aureomycin and 100 mg. of lactose as the diluent. He directs that one capsule be taken three times a day for 10 days. The adult dose of aureomycin is 250 mg. How many of the commercially available 250 mg. capsules should be used in preparing the prescription?

68. How many chloramphenicol capsules, each containing 250 mg., are needed to provide 25 mg. per kg. per day for 1 week for a person weighing 175 lb.?

69. The dose of piperazine citrate is 50 mg. per kg. of body weight once daily for seven consecutive days. How many milliliters of piperazine citrate syrup containing 500 mg. per teaspoonful should be prescribed for a child weighing 66 lb.?

70.   Thymol Iodide   8 g.
        Castor Oil   15 ml.
        Zinc Oxide Ointment, to make   100 g.

How much of each ingredient is required to prepare 5 lb. of the ointment?

71. A formula for capsules calls for 15 mg. of belladonna extract, 20 mg. of phenobarbital, and enough lactose to make 0.2 g. How much of each ingredient should be used in preparing 50 capsules?

72. ℞ Coal Tar   5 parts
        Zinc Oxide Paste   50 parts
        Disp. 240 g.
        Sig. Apply.

How many grams of coal tar should be used in compounding the prescription?

73.   Coal Tar   50 g.
        Bentonite   80 g.
        Water   300 ml.
        Hydrophilic Ointment   80 g.
        Zinc Oxide Paste, to make   1000 g.

How much of each ingredient should be used in preparing 1 lb. of the ointment?

74.   Aminophylline   250 mg.
           Phenobarbital Sodium   50 mg.
           Benzocaine   20 mg.
           Carbowax Base   2 g.

Calculate the quantity of each ingredient to be used in preparing 250 suppositories.

75.   Witch Hazel   120 ml.
           Glycerin   50 ml.
           Boric Acid Solution, to make   1000 ml.

How much of each ingredient should be used in preparing 5 gallons of the lotion?

76.   Starch
           Zinc Oxide   aa   10%
           Sulfur   5%
           White Petrolatum   250 g.

How many grams of each ingredient should be used in preparing 5 lb. of the ointment?

77. Set up a formula for 5 lb. of a glycerogelatin containing 10 parts, by weight, of zinc oxide, 15 parts, by weight, of gelatin, 40 parts by, weight, of glycerin, and 35 parts, by weight, of water.

78.   Salicylic Acid   0.5 g.
           Precipitated Sulfur   4.5 g.
           Hydrophilic Ointment   35.0 g.

Calculate the quantity of each ingredient to be used in making 5 lb. of the ointment.

79.   Burow's Solution   1 part
           Lanolin   2 parts
           Zinc Oxide Paste   3 parts

Calculate the quantity of each ingredient required to prepare 1 lb. of the paste.

80.   Coal Tar   10 g.
        Polysorbate 80   5 g.
        Zinc Oxide Paste   985 g.

Calculate the quantity of each ingredient required to prepare 10 lb. of the ointment.

81.   Hydrocortisone   0.1 g.
        Chlorobutanol   0.5 g.
        Normal Saline Solution   ad   100.0 ml.

How much of each ingredient should be used to prepare f℥i of the suspension?

82.   Menthol   0.2 g.
        Hexachlorophene   0.1 g.
        Glycerin   10. ml.
        Isopropyl Alcohol   35. ml.
        Purified Water   ad   100. ml.

Calculate the quantity of each ingredient required to prepare 1 gallon of the lotion.

83.   Isopropyl Alcohol   50   ml.
        Propylene Glycol   2   ml.
        Glacial Acetic Acid   0.1 ml.
        Purified Water   ad   100   ml.

Calculate the quantity of each ingredient required to prepare 1 gallon of the lotion.

84.   Benzoic Acid   6 parts
        Salicylic Acid   3 parts
        Polyethylene Glycol Ointment   91 parts

Calculate the quantity of each ingredient required to prepare 1 lb. of the ointment.

85.   Coal Tar   5 parts
        Zinc Oxide
        Starch   aa   10 parts
        Hydrophilic Ointment   50 parts

Calculate the quantity of each ingredient required to prepare 1000 g. of the ointment.

86. If 232 g. of a liquid measure 263 ml., what is its specific gravity?

87. If 4 f℥ of a liquid weigh 1932 gr., what is its specific gravity?

88. If the specific gravity of a liquid is 1.32, what is its specific volume?

89. If 5000 ml. of a syrup weigh 6565 g., calculate (a) its specific gravity and (b) its specific volume.

90. A pycnometer weighs 23.57 g. Filled with distilled water, it weighs 47.35 g. Filled with another liquid, it weighs 44.75 g. Calculate the specific gravity of the liquid.

91. The weight of a plummet in air is 10.97 g. Submerged in distilled water, it weighs 8.62 g. Submerged in another liquid, it weighs 8.12 g. Calculate the specific gravity of the liquid.

92. The specific gravity of a liquid is 1.478. Calculate its specific volume.

93. A glass plummet weighs 39.63 g. in air, 24.63 g. in water, and 28.83 g. in ether. Calculate (a) the specific gravity and (b) the volume, in ml., of 5 lb. of ether.

94. A piece of glass weighs 250 grains in air, 135 gr. when submerged in water, and 145 gr. when submerged in a certain acid. Calculate (a) the specific gravity of the acid, (b) the specific gravity of the glass, and (c) the specific volume of the acid.

95. A bottle holds 50.3 g. of water. When 8.6 g. of an insoluble powder are introduced and the bottle is filled with water, the contents weigh 55.4 g. What is the specific gravity of the powder?

96. A piece of wax weighs 12.5 g. in air, and a sinker weighs 24.6 g. when submerged in water. When submerged together in water, the wax and sinker weigh 22.4 g. What is the specific gravity of the wax?

97. A crystal of a chemical weighs 8.34 g. in air and 5.86 g. when submerged in an oil with a specific gravity of 0.825. What is the specific gravity of the crystal?

98. If a substance weighs 10.6 g. and displaces 12.5 g. of water, what is its specific gravity?

99. If the specific volume of a liquid is 1.264, what is its specific gravity?

100. A saturated solution contains, in each 100 ml., 100 g. of a substance. If the solubility of the substance is 1 g. in 0.7 ml. of water, what is the specific gravity of the saturated solution?

101. The specific gravity of strong ammonia solution is 0.897 at 25° C. Calculate the weight, in grams, of 10 pt. of the solution.

102. In making a certain syrup, 6800 g. of sucrose were dissolved in enough water to make 8 liters. Assuming the specific gravity of the syrup to be 1.313, how many milliliters of water were used?

103. Calculate the volume, in milliliters, of 0.48 g. of hydrochloric acid having a specific gravity of 1.18.

104. A formula for 200 g. of an ointment contains 10 g. of glycerin. How many milliliters of glycerin having a specific gravity of 1.25 should be used in preparing 1 lb. of the ointment?

105. What is the volume, in milliliters, of 2 kg. of a liquid with a specific volume of 1.125?

106. What is the weight, in kilograms, of 5000 ml. of a liquid with a specific gravity of 1.09?

107.   White Wax   12.5 g.
        Mineral Oil   60.0 g.
        Lanolin   2.5 g.
        Sodium Borate   1.0 g.
        Rose Water   24.0 g.
        Label: Cold cream.

How many milliliters of mineral oil having a specific gravity of 0.900 should be used in preparing 10 lb. of the cream?

108. How many milliliters of a commercially available 50% (v/v) solution of glycerin should be used to provide 2 g. of glycerin per kilogram of body weight for a person weighing 110 lb.? The specific gravity of glycerin is 1.25.

109. Given a solution of potassium permanganate prepared by dissolving sixteen 0.325-g. tablets in enough distilled water to make 2600 ml.,

   (a) What is the percentage strength of the solution?
   (b) What is the ratio strength of the solution?
   (c) How many milliliters should be used in preparing 2 liters of a
       1:8000 solution?

110. Given a salt solution of 1:1500 concentration, what is:

(a) the percentage strength?
(b) the weight, in grains, of the salt per pint?
(c) the weight, in micrograms, of the salt per ml.?
(d) the number of milliliters required to prepare 2 liters of a 1:2500 solution?

111. How many tablets, each containing 0.125 g. of mercury bichloride, should be used in preparing a liter of a 0.1% solution?

112. ℞ Potassium Iodide
     (50 mg. per tsp.)
    Ephedrine Sulfate Syrup   ad   240 ml.
    Sig. Teaspoonful as directed.

Potassium Iodide Solution, N.F., contains 100% (w/v) of potassium iodide. How many milliliters of the solution should be used to obtain the potassium iodide required in compounding the prescription?

113. ℞ Potassium Permanganate   6.0
    Distilled Water ad   250.0
    Sig. Dilute two tablespoonfuls to one quart.

What is the percentage strength of the dilution?

114. In compounding a prescription for f℥i of a $\frac{1}{2}$% solution of atropine sulfate, a pharmacist filtered the solution, losing f℥i. If he adjusted the volume to f℥i after the filtration, (a) what was the concentration of atropine sulfate in the resulting product, and (b) what percentage of error did he incur?

115. Eight hundred and seventy grams of sucrose are dissolved in 470 ml. of water, and the resulting volume is 1010 ml. Calculate (a) the percentage strength (w/v) of the solution, (b) the percentage strength (w/w) of the solution and (c) the specific gravity of the solution.

116. A formula for a cosmetic cream calls for 0.04% of a mixture of 65 parts of methylparaben and 35 parts of propylparaben. How many grams of each should be used in formulating 10 lb. of the cream?

117. On June first a pharmacist purchased 1 oz. of cocaine hydrochloride. During the month he dispensed the following:

        ℥i of an ointment containing 3% of cocaine hydrochloride
        f℥ii of a solution containing 1% of cocaine hydrochloride
        f℥iv of a solution containing 4% of cocaine hydrochloride

How many grains of cocaine hydrochloride were left in stock for the July first narcotic inventory?

118. On June first a pharmacist had in stock ½ oz. of cocaine hydrochloride. During the month he dispensed the following:

    (a) ℞ Cocaine Hydrochloride   1.25%
             Hydrophilic Ointment ad   ℥ii
             Sig. Apply.

    (b) ℞ Cocaine Hydrochloride   4%
             Distilled Water ad   ℥iv
             Sig. Use as directed.

    (c) ℞ Cocaine Hydrochloride   gr. $\frac{1}{10}$
             Cerium Oxalate   gr. iii
             Make 100 cap.
             Sig. One capsule for nausea.

How many grains of cocaine hydrochloride were left in stock for the July first narcotic inventory?

119. A prescription calls for f℥iv of a 15% solution of Neo-Silvol. (a) How many grains of Neo-Silvol should be used in compounding the prescription? (b) If Neo-Silvol costs $1.80 per oz., what is the cost of the amount needed in the prescription?

120. How many grams of mercury bichloride should be used in preparing 5 gallons of an 0.025% (w/v) solution?

121. How would you prepare f℥iv of a 4% (w/v) solution of cocaine hydrochloride?

122. If 60 gr. of silver nucleinate are dissolved in enough water to make f℥ii, what is the percentage strength (w/v) of the solution?

123. How many grams of zinc sulfate must be dissolved in 450 g. of water to make a 15% (w/w) solution?

124. How many grains of gentian violet should be used in preparing f℥vi of a 0.25% solution?

125. How much 4% (w/v) solution can be made from ⅛ oz. of cocaine hydrochloride?

126. The specific gravity of a 64.7% (w/w) solution of sucrose in water is approximately 1.313. How many grams of sucrose and how many milliliters of water will be required to make 8000 ml. of a 64.7% (w/w) aqueous solution? What will be the percentage strength (w/v) of the solution?

127. If silver nucleinate costs $4.20 per oz., what is the cost of the amount needed in preparing f℥ii of a 20% solution?

128. Camphor liniment contains 20% (w/w) of camphor in cottonseed oil. How many grams of camphor and how many milliliters of cottonseed oil having a specific gravity of 0.915 are required to make 5 kilograms of camphor liniment?

129. An ophthalmic ointment contains 1:3000 of mercury bichloride and 5:3000 of sodium chloride. Express these concentrations in terms of percentage.

130. ℞ Precipitated Sulfur   12.5%
     Zinc Oxide Ointment   ad   ℥ii
     Sig. Apply.

How many grains of precipitated sulfur should be used in compounding the prescription?

131. In preparing 750 ml. of a syrup, 550 g. of sucrose were used. If the specific gravity of the syrup was 1.25, how many milliliters of water were used in preparing it?

132. Terpin Hydrate Elixir contains 40% (v/v) of glycerin. If glycerin (specific gravity 1.25) is bought at $9.60 for 10 lb., what is the cost of the amount needed to prepare 5 gallons of the elixir?

133. ℞ Zinc Sulfate Solution ⅕%
     Holocaine Solution   1%   aa   15.0 ml.
     Sig. For the eye.

If the zinc sulfate was weighed on a balance having a sensitivity requirement of 4 mg., what percentage of error might have been incurred?

134. ℞ Belladonna Tincture   60.0
     Sodium Phenobarbital   1.0
     Peppermint Water   ad   240.0
     Sig. 5 ml. once a day.

Belladonna tincture contains 0.03% (w/v) of alkaloids. Express the amount, in micrograms, of alkaloids represented in each dose of the prescription.

135. Phenobarbital Elixir contains 0.4% of phenobarbital. Calculate the amount, in milligrams, of phenobarbital in a dessertspoonful dose of the elixir.

136. ℞   Menthol   0.25%
          Magnesia Magma
          Calamine Lotion
          Rose Water   aa   ad   120 ml.
          Sig. Apply.

How many milligrams of menthol should be used in compounding the prescription?

137. ℞   Vioform   0.1 g.
          Precipitated Sulfur   0.2 g.
          Zinc Oxide   1.0 g.
          Hydrocortisone Lotion $\frac{1}{2}$% ad   15   ml.
          Sig. For external use.

Calculate the percentage of Vioform in the finished product.

138. ℞   Precipitated Sulfur   1%
          Isopropyl Alcohol 70%
          Calamine Lotion   aa   ad   120 ml.
          Sig. Apply.

How many grams of precipitated sulfur and how many milliliters of 99% isopropyl alcohol should be used in compounding the prescription?

139. How many fluidounces of a commercially available 17% solution of benzalkonium chloride should be used to prepare 1 gallon of a 1:750 solution?

140. You are directed to prepare 10 liters of a 1:5000 solution of potassium permanganate. If the potassium permanganate is available only in the form of tablets each containing 0.2 g., how many tablets should be used in preparing the solution?

141. How many milliliters of 28% (w/w) ammonia solution having a specific gravity of 0.90 are required to prepare 1 gallon of 5% (w/v) ammonia solution?

142. How many milliliters of 85% (w/w) phosphoric acid having a specific gravity of 1.71 should be used in preparing 10 liters of a 1:2000 solution of phosphoric acid for bladder irrigation?

143. How many grams of coal tar should be added to 1 lb. of Coal Tar Ointment, U.S.P., to increase the strength to 2%? Coal Tar Ointment, U.S.P., contains 1% of coal tar.

144. ℞   Calomel   0.6
        Alcohol 70%   ad   30.0
        Sig. Use in right ear.

(a) How many milliliters of 95% (v/v) alcohol should be used in preparing 30 ml. of 70% (v/v) alcohol? (b) What is the percentage (w/v) of calomel in the prescription?

145. ℞   Precipitated Sulfur   4.0
        Calamine   8.0
        Isopropyl Alcohol 40%   200.0
        Witch Hazel   ad   240.0
        Sig. Apply.

How many milliliters of 99% isopropyl alcohol should be used in compounding the prescription?

146. How many grams of a greaseless ointment base should be added to 4500 g. of an ointment containing 675 g. of precipitated sulfur to prepare an ointment containing 5% of precipitated sulfur?

147. A preparation is to be made from opium tincture and must contain 0.06% of morphine. If opium tincture contains 10% of opium and if the opium contains 10% of morphine, how many milliliters of the tincture should be used to prepare a liter of the product?

148. A manufacturing pharmacist has on hand four lots of belladonna tincture, containing 25 mg., 27 mg., 33 mg., and 35 mg. of alkaloids per 100 ml. How many gallons of each lot should he use to prepare 16 gallons of belladonna tincture containing 30 mg. of alkaloids per 100 ml.?

149. A pharmacist wishes to prepare one pint of a potent tincture (10%) and containing 64% alcohol from the corresponding fluidextract (100%) and containing 60% of alcohol. How much 95% alcohol and how much water should he use?

150. How many milliliters of a 1:200 solution of atropine sulfate should be used in preparing 250 ml. of a solution to contain 300 mcg. of atropine sulfate per teaspoonful?

151. How many grams of silver nitrate should be used in preparing 500 ml. of a solution such that 10 ml. diluted to a liter will yield a 1:5000 solution?

152. How many milliliters of 95% (v/v) alcohol and of 30% (v/v) alcohol should be mixed to make 4000 ml. of 50% (v/v) alcohol?

153. What is the percentage (v/v) of alcohol in a mixture of 600 ml. of 78% (v/v) alcohol, 1500 ml. of 42% (v/v) alcohol, and 800 ml. of 35% (v/v) alcohol?

154. How much mercury bichloride and how much 95% (v/v) alcohol should be used in preparing 1 gallon of a 1:1000 solution of mercury bichloride in 70% (v/v) alcohol?

155. How many milliliters of 5% (w/v) solution of aluminum acetate are required to prepare 500 ml. of a $\frac{1}{20}$% (w/v) solution?

156. ℞   Resorcinol Monoacetate   10.0 ml.
          Castor Oil   5.0 ml.
          Ethyl Alcohol 85%   ad   200.0 ml.
          Sig. Apply to scalp.

How many milliliters of 95% (v/v) ethyl alcohol and how much water should be used in compounding the prescription?

157. A certain cream contains 1 part of water and 2 parts of hydrophilic petrolatum. How many milliliters of water should be added to 1000 g. of the cream to increase the water content to 50%?

158. How many grams of talc should be added to 1 lb. of a powder containing 20 g. of zinc undecylenate per 100 g. to reduce the concentration of zinc undecylenate to 3%?

159. A formula for a phenolated calamine lotion calls for 2% of bentonite. How many milliliters of a 5% bentonite magma should be used to obtain the bentonite needed in preparing 1 gallon of the lotion?

160. How many milliliters of water should be added to 10 lb. of phenol crystals (98% of phenol) to prepare liquefied phenol (88% of phenol)?

161. A hospital pharmacist has on hand 14 liters of iodine tincture (2%). How many milliliters of strong iodine tincture (7%) should he mix with it in order to get a product that will contain 3.5% of iodine?

162. ℞ Potassium Iodide Solution 10%
    Ephedrine Sulfate Solution 3% aa ad   60 ml.
    Sig. Use as directed.

How many milliliters of a saturated solution of potassium iodide (100% w/v) should be used to obtain the potassium iodide needed in compounding the prescription?

163. In preparing 15 ml. of a 1:10,000 solution of histamine phosphate, a pharmacist used 5 ml. of a solution containing 0.275 mg. of histamine phosphate per ml. Calculate the percentage of error that he may have incurred.

164. How many milliliters of 36% (w/w) hydrochloric acid having a specific gravity of 1.18 are required to prepare 5 gallons of 10% (w/v) hydrochloric acid?

165. How many grams of ephedrine sulfate and of chlorobutanol should be used to make 500 ml. of a solution such that 30 ml. diluted to 100 ml. will represent 1:500 of ephedrine sulfate and 1:3000 of chlorobutanol?

166. A formula for an ophthalmic solution calls for 500 ml. of a 0.02% solution of benzalkonium chloride. How many milliliters of a 1:750 solution should be used to obtain the amount of benzalkonium chloride needed in preparing the ophthalmic solution?

167. ℞ Phenol   600 mg.
    Boric Acid Solution
    Calamine Lotion   aa   ad   240 ml.
    Sig. Apply to affected areas.

What is the percentage of phenol in the finished product?

168. A belladonna mixture contains 60 ml. of belladonna tincture (65% of alcohol), 280 ml. of high alcoholic elixir (78% of alcohol) and enough peppermint water to make 500 ml. Calculate the percentage of alcohol in the mixture.

169. ℞ Potassium Permanganate   q.s.
    Distilled Water   ad   500 ml.
    Sig. 5 ml. diluted to a liter equals a 1:8000 solution.

How many 0.3-g. tablets of potassium permanganate should be used in compounding the prescription?

170. What is the weight, in kilograms, of 5 gallons of a mixture of equal parts of simple syrup having a specific gravity of 1.313 and distilled water?

171. How many milliliters of a syrup having a specific gravity of 1.350 should be added to 5 liters of a syrup having a specific gravity of 1.250 to make a product having a specific gravity of 1.313?

172. How many milliliters of each of two liquids with specific gravities of 0.950 and 0.875 should be used to prepare 12 liters of a liquid having a specific gravity of 0.925?

173. How many milliliters of purified water must be added to 1 lb. of wool fat to convert it to hydrous wool fat containing 25% of water?

174. If 500 g. of Aquaphor will absorb 1500 g. of water, how many milliliters of water will be absorbed by 1000 g. of Eucerin which contains 50% of Aquaphor and 50% of water?

175. How many grams of ichthammol should be added to 5 lb. of 10% ichthammol ointment to make an ointment containing 25% of ichthammol?

176. ℞ Epinephrine Bitartrate   2.0 g.
        Sodium Bisulfite   0.1 g.
        Sodium Chloride   0.7 g.
        Distilled Water   ad   100.0 ml.
        Sig. Use in the eyes.

How many milliliters of a 0.9% sodium chloride solution should be used to obtain the sodium chloride for the prescription?

177. ℞ Penicillin   60,000 units
        Streptomycin   600 mg.
        Alcohol 70%   30 ml.
        Glycerin   ad   60 ml.
        Sig. For the ear.

How many milliliters of 95% alcohol and how much water should be used in compounding the prescription?

178.   Sorbitan Sesquioleate   6.0 g.
         White Petrolatum   54.0 g.
         Methylparaben   0.1 g.
         Distilled Water   ad   100.0 g.
         Label: Hydrated petrolatum.

A mixture (1 and 9) of the first two ingredients absorbs 18 times its weight of water. How much additional water can be added to 2000 g. of the above product to obtain one containing the maximum amount of water that can be absorbed?

179. ℞   Atropine Sulfate Solution 2%   30 ml.
          Sig. For the eye.

In preparing the solution a pharmacist filtered it, losing 5 ml. If he adjusted the volume to 30 ml. after filtration, (a) what was the concentration of atropine sulfate in the resulting product and (b) what percentage of error did he incur?

180. ℞   Sodium Fluoride   q.s.
          Distilled Water   ad   60.0
          Sig. Five drops added to a liter of drinking water.

The prescriber informs you that the drinking water contains 0.4 p.p.m. of fluoride ion. How many mg. of sodium fluoride should be used in preparing the solution so that five drops of it diluted to one liter with the drinking water will yield a solution containing 1 p.p.m. of fluoride ion? The dispensing dropper calibrates 20 drops per ml.

181. ℞   Scopolamine Hydrobromide   0.25%
          Phenacaine Hydrochloride   0.5%
          Sodium Chloride   q.s.
          Sterile Distilled Water   ad   50.0
          Make isotonic sol.
          Sig. For the eyes.

How many milliliters of an 0.9% sodium chloride solution should be used in compounding the prescription?

182.   Procaine Hydrochloride   2%
          Ephedrine Hydrochloride   0.1%
          Sodium Chloride   q.s.
          Water for Injection   ad   1000 ml.
          Make isotonic sol.
          Label: Procaine and Ephedrine Injection.

How many grams of sodium chloride should be used in preparing the injection?

183. ℞ Ephedrine Sulfate   0.5%
        Phenacaine Hydrochloride   0.5%
        Dextrose   q.s.
        Distilled Water   ad   30.0
        Make isotonic sol.
        Sig. Nasal spray.

How many grams of dextrose should be used in compounding the prescription?

184. ℞ Tubocurarine Chloride   0.6
        Chlorobutanol   0.5%
        Sodium Chloride   q.s.
        Sterile Distilled Water ad   20.0
        Make isotonic sol.
        Sig. To be administered by the nurse.

Tubocurarine chloride (ml. wt.—786) is a 3-ion electrolyte, dissociating 85%. How many grams of sodium chloride should be used in compounding the prescription?

185. ℞ Phenobarbital Sodium   15 mg. per ml.
        Sodium Chloride   q.s.
        Sterile Distilled Water   ad   20 ml.
        Make isotonic sol. and sterilize.
        Sig. For office use.

How many grams of sodium chloride should be used in compounding the prescription?

186. ℞ Ephedrine Hydrochloride   2%
        Chlorobutanol   0.2%
        Dextrose   q.s.
        Distilled Water   ad   120.0
        Make isotonic sol.
        Sig. Nasal spray.

How many grams of anhydrous dextrose should be used in compounding the prescription?

187.   Papaverine Hydrochloride   50 mg. per ml.
        Sodium Chloride   q.s.
        Sterile Distilled Water   ad   30.0 ml.
        Label: Papaverine Injection: 1 ml. = 50 mg.

Papaverine hydrochloride has a molecular weight of 376. Its dissociation factor is 1.8. How many grams of sodium chloride should be used to make this solution isotonic?

188. ℞ Atropine Sulfate 2%
     Boric Acid q.s.
     Distilled Water ad 100 ml.
     Make isotonic sol.
     Sig. For the eyes.

(a) How many grams of boric acid should be used? (b) How many milliliters of a 5% boric acid solution should be used to obtain the amount of boric acid needed in the prescription? (c) You are directed to sterilize this prescription at a temperature not exceeding 105° C. Calculate the corresponding F. temperature.

189. ℞ Epinephrine 1.0%
     Sodium Bisulfite 0.2%
     Chlorobutanol 0.5%
     Sodium Chloride q.s.
     Sterile Distilled Water ad 15.0 ml.
     Make isotonic sol.
     Sig. For the eye.

(a) How many grams of epinephrine bitartrate (mol. wt.—333) should be used to obtain the amount of epinephrine (mol. wt.—183) needed in compounding the prescription?

(b) Starting with epinephrine bitartrate, how many milligrams of sodium chloride should be used in compounding the prescription?

190. ℞ Pontocaine 0.025 g.
     Zinc Sulfate 0.050 g.
     Epinephrine Solution 1:1000 5. ml.
     Boric Acid q.s.
     Sterile Distilled Water ad 15. ml.
     Make isotonic sol.
     Sig. Use in right eye.

Epinephrine solution 1:1000 is already isotonic. How many grams of boric acid should be used in compounding the prescription?

191. How many grams of 40.5% (MgO equivalent) magnesium carbonate are required to prepare 24 bottles of magnesium citrate solution so that each bottle will contain the equivalent of 6.0 g. of MgO?

192. The formula for Albright's Solution "G" calls for 4.37 g. of anhydrous sodium carbonate (Na_2CO_3—mol. wt. 106) in 1000 ml. of finished product. In preparing 5 gallons of the solution, how many grams of monohydrated sodium carbonate ($Na_2CO_3.H_2O$—mol. wt. 124) should be used?

193.   Stearic Acid   20%
         Potassium Hydroxide   q.s.
         Glycerin   10%
         Water, to make   1000 g.
         Label: Vanishing cream.

How many grams of 85% potassium hydroxide should be used to saponify 25% of the stearic acid in the formula? The saponification value of stearic acid is 208.

194. A cold cream formula calls for 350 g. of white wax. The white wax to be used has an acid value of 22. How many grams of sodium borate which has an equivalent weight of 191 should be used in formulating the cream?

195. Assuming that no potassium citrate is available, how many grams of potassium bicarbonate and how many grams of citric acid are required to prepare 5 liters of a solution to contain 0.3 g. of potassium citrate in each teaspoonful?

$$3KHCO_3 + H_3C_6H_5O_7 = K_3C_6H_5O_7 + 3H_2O + 3CO_2$$

196. How many grams of 85% potassium hydroxide are required to saponify completely 1350 ml. of a fixed oil having a specific gravity of 0.925 and a saponification value of 190?

197. A commercially available tablet contains 0.2 g. of $FeSO_4.2H_2O$. How many milligrams of elemental iron are represented in each tablet?

198. In the monograph on Ferrous Sulfate Tablets, the U.S.P. states that an "equivalent amount of exsiccated ferrous sulfate may be used in place of $FeSO_4.7H_2O$ in preparing Ferrous Sulfate Tablets." How many grams of exsiccated ferrous sulfate (mol. wt.—179) could be used to replace the $FeSO_4.7H_2O$ (mol. wt.—278) in preparing 10,000 tablets, each containing 0.3 g. of the hydrated salt?

199. The formula for Benedict's Solution calls for 100 g. of anhydrous sodium carbonate (Na_2CO_3—106) per liter of finished product. You are directed to prepare 5 liters of the solution. In checking the stock of the ingredients you find that only 250 g. of anhydrous sodium carbonate are available. How many grams of monohydrated sodium carbonate ($Na_2CO_3.H_2O$—124) should be used in addition to the anhydrous salt that is available?

200. A hospital requests you to prepare 5000 ml. of a solution of sodium p-aminosalicylate ($NH_2C_6H_3OHCOONa$—175), each 5 ml. to contain 1 g. of p-aminosalicylic acid. How many grams of p-aminosalicylic acid ($NH_2C_6H_3OHCOOH$—153) and how many grams of sodium bicarbonate ($NaHCO_3$—84) should be used in preparing the solution?

201. The formula for Sodium Phosphate Solution calls for 755 g. of sodium phosphate per liter of finished product. You are directed to prepare 4 liters of the solution. In checking the stock of the ingredients, you find that only 5 lb. of sodium phosphate are available. How many grams of exsiccated sodium phosphate (mol. wt.—142) should be used in addition to the sodium phosphate (mol. wt.—268) that is available?

202.

Stearic Acid	20%
Liquid Petrolatum	5%
Triethanolamine	5%
Coconut Oil Soap	40%
Distilled Water	25%
Glycerin	5%

How many grams of 85% potassium hydroxide should be used in preparing the coconut oil soap required for making 10 lb. of this cream? Coconut oil soap contains 40% (w/w) of coconut oil, and the saponification value of coconut oil is 260.

203. A formula for a cosmetic cream calls for 5 lb. of stearic acid. How many grams of 88% potassium hydroxide are required to saponify 25% of the stearic acid? The saponification value of stearic acid is 208.

204. The formula for Green Soap calls for 380 g. of a vegetable oil and 91.7 g. of potassium hydroxide (85%). On the basis of these figures, what must be the saponification value of a vegetable oil in order that it may be used in the manufacture of the soap?

205. Assuming that no potassium acetate is available, how many grams of potassium bicarbonate and how many milliliters of 36% (w/w) acetic acid, specific gravity 1.05, should be used in preparing 1 gallon of a 10% solution of potassium acetate?

$$KHCO_3 + HC_2H_3O_2 = KC_2H_3O_2 + CO_2 + H_2O$$

206.

Stearic Acid	50 g.
White Petrolatum	150 g.
Mineral Oil	250 g.
Triethanolamine	q.s.
Rose Water, to make	1000 g.

How many grams of triethanolamine (mol. wt.—149) are required for a complete reaction with the stearic acid (mol. wt.—284) in preparing the product?

207. One liter of ethylene at a pressure of 760 mm. of mercury and at 0° C. weighs 1.260 g. Calculate its volume at a pressure of 780 mm. and at 27° C.

208. How many grams of potassium chloride should be used in making a liter of a solution containing 5 mEq of potassium per ml.?

209. What is the percent (w/v) concentration of a solution containing 100 mEq of ammonium chloride per liter?

210. Convert 20 mg. % of calcium to mEq of calcium.

211. How many mEq of potassium are contained in each 10-ml. dose of a 5% (w/v) solution of potassium chloride (KCl)?

212. ℞   Potassium Chloride   125 g.
        Peppermint Water   ad   500 ml.
        Sig. 5 ml. as directed.

    How many mEq of potassium are represented in the prescribed dose?

213. A patient has been using one 1-g. tablet of potassium chloride twice a day. His physician now wishes to change the medication to a liquid dosage form containing 134 mEq of potassium per 100 ml. What dose of the liquid preparation should he prescribe to provide the same amount of potassium as that represented by the tablets?

214. How many grams of sodium bicarbonate should be used in preparing a liter of a solution which is to contain 8 mEq of sodium bicarbonate in each 10 ml.?

215. How many mEq of potassium are represented in 5 million units of Potassium Penicillin G ($C_{16}H_{17}KN_2O_4S$—mol. wt. 372)? One mg. of Potassium Penicillin G represents 1595 Penicillin Units.

216. The normal blood plasma calcium level is 10 mg. %. Express this concentration in terms of mEq per liter.

217. ℞ Elixir Potassium Chloride   500 ml.
          (5 mEq per tsp.)
       Sig. Teaspoonful t.i.d.

(a) How many grams of potassium chloride should be used in preparing the elixir?

(b) How many mEq of potassium are represented in the daily prescribed dose of the elixir?

218. An iron complex with vitamin D tablet contains 540 mg. of calcium gluconate ($C_{12}H_{22}CaO_{14}.H_2O$—mol. wt. 448) and 500 mg. of calcium carbonate ($CaCO_3$—mol. wt. 100). How many mEq of calcium are supplied in the daily prophylactic dose of three tablets?

219. How many grams of calcium chloride ($CaCl_2.2H_2O$) are required to prepare half a liter of a solution containing 5 mEq of calcium chloride per ml.?

220. How many milliosmols of sodium chloride are represented in 1 liter of a 3% hypertonic sodium chloride solution? Assume complete dissociation.

221. Calculate the pH of a solution in which the hydrogen-ion concentration is 5.9×10^{-6}.

222. A certain elixir has a pH value of 4.1. Calculate the hydrogen-ion concentration of the elixir.

223. The pH value of a certain buffer solution is 9.2. Calculate the hydrogen-ion concentration of the solution.

224. Calculate the pH of a solution in which the hydrogen-ion concentration is 0.000000092 gram-ion per liter.

225. The dissociation constant of benzoic acid is 6.30×10^{-5} at 25° C. Calculate the pK_a value of benzoic acid.

226. Calculate the pH of a buffer solution containing 0.8 mole of sodium acetate and 0.5 mole of acetic acid per liter. The pK_a value of acetic acid is 4.76 at 25° C.

227. What molar ratio of sodium acetate to acetic acid is required to prepare an acetate buffer solution having a pH of 5.0? The K_a value of acetic acid is 1.75×10^{-5} at 25° C.

228. Calculate the molar ratio of disodium phosphate and sodium acid phosphate required to prepare a buffer system having a pH of 7.9. The pK_a value of sodium acid phosphate is 7.21 at 25° C.

229. What molar ratio of sodium borate to boric acid should be used in preparing a borate buffer having a pH of 8.8? The K_a value of boric acid is 6.4×10^{-10} at 25° C.

230. Calculate the half-life (years) of ^{60}Co which has a disintegration constant of 0.01096 month^{-1}.

231. A Sodium Iodide ^{131}I Solution has a labeled activity of 1 millicurie per ml. as of 12:00 noon on November 17. How many milliliters of the solution should be administered at 12:00 noon on December 1 to provide an activity of 250 microcuries? The half-life of ^{131}I is 8.08 days.

232. The blood hemoglobin levels in grams per 100 ml. for a group of 25 individuals were recorded as follows:

14.0	14.6	15.8	14.5	16.0
16.2	15.0	15.7	15.4	13.5
13.3	13.4	16.1	14.8	14.8
14.7	14.5	15.6	13.9	15.1
15.9	13.3	13.2	15.7	14.5

Prepare an array of the data, calculate the mean, and find the median and the mode from the array.

233. In determining the refractive index of a volatile oil, 15 observations were made at 20° C. and the following values were recorded:

1.4590	1.4650	1.4602
1.4645	1.4595	1.4599
1.4623	1.4637	1.4605
1.4642	1.4597	1.4593
1.4639	1.4645	1.4643

Calculate the mean, the range, and the average deviation for the recorded values.

234. In determining the weight variation of 20 tablets taken at random from a manufacturer's lot, the following weights, in milligrams, were recorded:

325 mg.	320 mg.	317 mg.	315 mg.
315 mg.	335 mg.	340 mg.	325 mg.
324 mg.	340 mg.	325 mg.	330 mg.
330 mg.	325 mg.	318 mg.	323 mg
328 mg	322 mg.	322 mg.	325 mg.

Calculate the mean, the average deviation, and the standard deviation for the recorded weights.

235. The diameter of oil globules in a certain emulsion was measured in microns (μ) and recorded as follows:

5.0 μ	6.75 μ	3.75 μ	3.5 μ
4.5 μ	3.0 μ	3.25 μ	3.75 μ
2.5 μ	6.0 μ	4.5 μ	5.5 μ
6.5 μ	4.5 μ	5.0 μ	6.25 μ
4.0 μ	7.0 μ	5.25 μ	5.75 μ

Calculate the mean, and find the median and the mode for the recorded measurements.

236. In checking the melting point of a new chemical compound, analyst A made 64 determinations with an average deviation of 1.5° C. Analyst B made 36 determinations with an average deviation of 0.5° C. Compare the reliability of their results and indicate which analyst probably found a truer average.

237. A volume of gas was collected at a barometric pressure of 762 mm. and a temperature of 25° C. Calculate (a) the corresponding temperature on the F. scale and (b) the equivalent pressure in inches.

238. A manufacturer recommends that his product be stored at a temperature not exceeding 40° F. Express this temperature on the centigrade scale.

239. A patient shows a temperature of 103.5° F. on a clinical thermometer. What would this temperature be on the centigrade scale?

240. A table of specifications states that a certain substance must congeal at −30±5° C. A sample of the substance was found to congeal at −37° F. Did the sample conform to specifications?

241. A manufacturer states that his product is stable at temperatures not over 45° C. Would the product be stable at 100° F.?

242. A hospital pharmacist has in stock 24 pints of 90 proof brandy and 10 fifths of 88 proof whisky. How many proof gallons are represented by this inventory?

243. A manufacturing pharmacist bought 50 proof gallons of spirits. How many wine gallons does this represent if the purchase was 70% (v/v) alcohol?

244. A hospital pharmacist had 54 gallons of 95% alcohol on hand on the first of the month. During the month he prepared 50 gallons of 50% (v/v) alcohol and 50 gallons of 25% (v/v) alcohol. How many proof gallons were left at the end of the month?

245. How many proof gallons are represented by 27 wine gallons of 190 proof alcohol?

246. If alcohol is taxed at $10.50 per proof gallon, what is the tax on 30 wine gallons of 70% (v/v) alcohol?

247. A blood sample is taken from a 150-lb. person. Chemical examination shows the sample to contain 0.2% of ethyl alcohol. Assuming that the alcohol is carried in the body fluids and that 70% of the body weight consists of fluids, how many fluidounces of 100 proof whisky would have to be absorbed to produce this blood level?

248. Using the alcoholometric table find the specific gravity of a sample of alcohol whose percentage strength is 25.75% (v/v) at 15.56° C.

249. A sample of alcohol has a specific gravity of 0.8038 at 15.56° C. By reference to the alcoholometric table find its percentage strength (v/v).

250. The solubility of magnesium sulfate is 1 g. in 1 ml. of water at 25° C., and the volume of the resulting solution is 1.5 ml. How many grams of magnesium sulfate and how many milliliters of water should be used in preparing 1 gallon of a saturated solution of magnesium sulfate?

251. What is the solubility of a chemical if 500 g. of an aqueous saturated solution yield a residue of 70 g. upon evaporation?

252. The solubility of salicylic acid in water is 1 g. in 460 ml. Calculate the percentage strength (w/w) of a saturated solution of salicylic acid.

253. In a solubility determination, 100 g. of a chemical were dissolved in 300 ml. of distilled water at 25° C., and the volume of the resulting solution was 340 ml. Calculate the percentage strength (w/v) of the solution.

254. What is the solubility of a chemical if 1200 g. of a saturated alcoholic solution yield a residue of 75 g. upon evaporation? The specific gravity of alcohol is 0.8.

255. You are directed to prepare 5 liters of a 50% emulsion of mineral oil. How many grams of acacia and how many milliliters of water should be used in preparing the primary of the emulsion?

256. The formula for a castor oil emulsion calls for 25% of castor oil. In formulating 1 gallon of the emulsion, how many grams of acacia and how many milliliters of water should be used in preparing the nucleus or primary emulsion?

257. What is the HLB of an emulsifier blend consisting of 25% of Span 20, 20% of Arlacel 83, and 50% of Tween 20?

258. In what proportion should Span 20, Span 40, and Tween 20 be blended to give a "required HLB" of 13.7?

259.

Mineral Oil	30%
Cetyl Alcohol	2%
Lanolin, Anhydrous	3%
Emulsifier	5%
Propylene Glycol	10%
Preserved Water ad	100%

(a) Calculate the "required HLB" of the oil phase.

(b) How many grams of Span 60 and how many grams of Tween 20 should be used in formulating 5 lb. of the product?

260.

Stearic Acid	10.0%
Lanolin	2.0%
Mineral Oil	3.0%
Emulsifier	5.0%
Propylene Glycol	10.0%
Purified Water ad	100.0%

The emulsifier blend is to consist of Span 80 and Tween 20. How many grams of each should be used in formulating 5 lb. of the product?

261. A hospital pharmacist purchased 1 gallon of belladonna fluidextract containing 60% of alcohol from which he desires to prepare belladonna tincture (10%) containing 70% of alcohol.

(a) If 1 gram of the drug yields 1 ml. of the fluidextract, how many milliliters of the tincture can be prepared from the quantity of fluidextract which he purchased?

(b) How many milliliters of 95% alcohol and how much water should be used in preparing this volume of the tincture?

262. ℞ Belladonna Extract   10 mg.
        Phenobarbital   30 mg.
        Demerol   100 mg.
        Make 20 such capsules
        Sig. One for pain.

Only belladonna tincture (10%) is available. If 1 g. of belladonna extract represents 4 g. of the drug, how many milliliters of belladonna tincture should be used in compounding the prescription?

263. ℞ Ephedrine Sulfate   0.150 g.
        Hyoscyamus Extract   0.015 g
        Carbowax Base   q.s.
        Make 10 such suppositories
        Sig. Insert one at night.

Hyoscyamus tincture (10%) is the only preparation of hyoscyamus available. If 1 g. of the extract represents 4 g. of the drug, how many milliliters of the tincture should be used in compounding the prescription?

264. ℞ Atropine Sulfate   gr. $\frac{1}{200}$
        Codeine Phosphate   gr. $\frac{1}{4}$
        Aspirin   gr. v
        Make 24 such capsules
        Sig. One capsule p.r.n.

The atropine sulfate is available only in the form of $\frac{1}{150}$ gr. tablets. Explain how you would obtain the correct amount of atropine sulfate.

265. ℞ Sodium Phenobarbital   gr. $\frac{1}{8}$ per tsp.
        Atropine Sulfate   gr. $\frac{1}{500}$ per tsp.
        Syrup   ad   ℥iv
        Sig. Teaspoonful in each feeding.

The atropine sulfate is available only in the form of $\frac{1}{150}$ gr. tablets Explain how you would obtain the correct amount of atropine sulfate.

266. ℞ Atropine Sulfate   300 mcg.
        Phenobarbital   30 mg.
        Dexedrine   3 mg.
        Make 20 such capsules
        Sig. One capsule as directed.

If the atropine sulfate is available only in the form of tablets, each containing $\frac{1}{150}$ gr., how many tablets should be used in compounding the prescription?

267. ℞ Hycodan   2 mg.
     Colchicine   gr. $\frac{1}{100}$
     Aspirin   300 mg.
     Make 24 such capsules
     Sig. One capsule t.i.d.

Only colchicine granules, each containing $\frac{1}{120}$ grain, are available. Explain how you would obtain the colchicine needed in compounding the prescription.

268. ℞ Hydrocortisone   1.5%
     Neomycin Ointment
     Emulsion Base aa ad   30 g.
     Sig. Apply.

If the hydrocortisone is available only in the form of 20 mg. tablets, how many tablets should be used to obtain the hydrocortisone needed in compounding the prescription?

269. ℞ Penicillin G   10,000 units per ml.
     Isotonic Sodium Chloride Solution ad   15 ml.
     Sig. For the nose. Store in the refrigerator.

Only soluble penicillin tablets, each containing 400,000 units of penicillin G, are available. Explain how you would obtain the penicillin G needed in compounding the prescription.

270. If 1 mg. of potassium phenoxymethyl penicillin represents 1530 penicillin units, what weight, in micrograms, represents one unit?

271. How many milliliters and how many minims of U-80 isophane insulin suspension will provide 54 units of insulin?

272. One penicillin unit is the antibiotic activity of 0.6 mcg. of F.D.A. Sodium Penicillin G Master Standard. How many penicillin units are represented by 1 mg. of the standard?

273. ℞ Bacitracin   1,000 units per g.
     Hydrophilic Petrolatum ad   30 g.
     Sig. Apply as directed.

The only source of bacitracin is a vial containing 50,000 units of the dry powder. Using hydrophilic petrolatum as the diluent (levigating agent, in this case), explain how you would obtain the bacitracin needed in compounding the prescription.

274. ℞ Penicillin G   10,000 units per ml.
     Streptomycin Sulfate   250 mg.
     Isotonic Sodium Chloride Solution   ad   15 ml.
     Sig. For topical application.

The penicillin G is available in tablets, each containing 200,000 units. The streptomycin sulfate is available in 1-g. vials as the dry powder, and, when dissolved in a suitable diluent, it accounts for 0.8 ml. of the final volume of the solution. Using isotonic sodium chloride solution as the diluent, explain how you would obtain the penicillin G and the streptomycin sulfate needed in compounding the prescription.

275. A certain hyperalimentation solution contains 600 ml. of a 5% protein hydrolysate, 400 ml. of 50% dextrose injection, 35 ml. of a 20% sterile potassium chloride solution, 100 ml. of sodium chloride injection, and 10 ml. of a 10% calcium gluconate injection. The solution is to be administered over a period of six hours. If the dropper in the venoclysis set calibrates 20 drops per ml., at what rate, in drops per minute, should the flow be adjusted in order to administer the solution during the designated time interval?

276. A phosphate solution for intravenous infusion contains 40 millimoles of sodium phosphate (Na_2HPO_4) and 10 millimoles of potassium acid phosphate (KH_2PO_4) per liter. Calculate (a) the amount, expressed as mEq, of sodium ion, (b) the amount, expressed as mEq, of potassium ion, and (c) the amount, in grams, of phosphorus represented in the infusion.

277. A solution prepared by dissolving 500,000 units of polymyxin B sulfate in 10 ml. of water for injection is added to 250 ml. of 5% dextrose injection. The infusion is to be administered over a period of two hours. If the dropper in the venoclysis set calibrates 25 drops per ml., at what rate, in drops per minute, should the flow be adjusted in order to administer the total volume over the designated time interval?

278. If a lubricating jelly is listed at $9.60 per dozen tubes, with discounts of 40% and 10%, what is the net cost per tube?

279. Calculate the net amount of a bill of good for $1240, with discounts of 40%, 5% and 5%.

280. A certain nasal preparation is listed at $10.00 per dozen, less 40% and 10%. At what price per unit must the preparation be sold to yield a gross profit of $66\frac{2}{3}\%$ on the cost?

281. A pharmacist buys a bottle of vitamin capsules at $7.50 less a discount of 40%. At what price must the capsules be sold to yield a gross profit of 40% on the selling price?

282. If some toothbrushes are bought at $6.50 a dozen, less 40% and 2%, what is the net cost of one toothbrush, and at what price must it be sold so that a gross profit of 50% on the selling price will be realized?

283. A pharmacist buys 5000 capsules for $45.00 with a discount of 40%. At what price per hundred must he sell the capsules in order to realize a gross profit of 50% on the selling price?

284. The state collects a 3% sales tax on sales at retail. If the tax and selling price are recorded as one transaction on the cash register, calculate the taxable sales on receipts of $14,500.00.

285. A prescription specialty lists at $14.50 per pint, less a discount of 40%. At what price must 60 ml. of the specialty be sold to yield a gross profit of 50% on the selling price?

Answers to Practice Problems

NOTE: *Answers are given to all problems in Chapter 1 (Some Fundamentals of Measurement and Calculation) and Chapter 14 (Exponential and Logarithmic Notation); elsewhere, only the answers to odd-numbered problems are given.*

Chapter 1

BUILDING ON A BASE

(Page 6)

1. (a) Three
   (b) Six
   (c) Nine
   (d) Twelve
   (e) Five
   (f) Ten
   (g) Twenty-five
   (h) Thirty
   (i) Twelve
   (j) Twenty-four
   (k) One hundred forty-four
   (l) One hundred fifty-six
2. (a) 11
   (b) 21
   (c) 101
   (d) 120
   (e) 12
   (f) 22
   (g) 103
   (h) 200
   (i) 13
   (j) 26
   (k) 148
   (l) 1000

THE BINARY-DIMIDIAL SYSTEM

(Page 10)

1. See text, p. 7.
2. See text, p. 8.
3. (a) 1000
   (b) 111
   (c) 1010
   (d) 10000
   (e) 1101
   (f) 10110
4. (a) 100
   (b) 10
   (c) 100
   (d) 101
   (e) 1
   (f) 111
5. (a) 110
   (b) 1100
   (c) 11001
   (d) 10010
   (e) 1001
   (f) 10101
6. (a) 11
   (b) 101
   (c) 100
   (d) 11
   (e) 10
   (f) 100

ROMAN NUMERALS

(*Page 13*)

1. (a) xviii
   (b) lxiv
   (c) lxxii
   (d) cxxvi
   (e) xcix
   (f) xxxvii
   (g) lxxxiv
   (h) xlviii
   (i) MCMLXXXIV
2. (a) Part 4
   (b) Chapter 19
   (c) 1959
   (d) 1814
3. (a) 45
   (b) 1000
   (c) 48
   (d) 64
   (e) 16
   (f) 84
4. (a) 5, 15, 80, 4
   (b) $1\frac{1}{2}$, 40, 6, $\frac{1}{2}$

SIGNIFICANT FIGURES

(*Page 20*)

1. (a) Six
   (b) Four
   (c) Three
   (d) Three
   (e) Seven
   (f) One
2. (a) Two
   (b) Three
   (c) Two
   (d) Four
   (e) Five
   (f) Two
   (g) Four

SIGNIFICANT FIGURES (*continued*)

   (h) Three
   (i) Two
   (j) Two
3. (a) 32.8
   (b) 200
   (c) 0.0363
   (d) 21.6
   (e) 0.00944
   (f) 1.08
   (g) 27.1
   (h) 0.862
   (i) 3.14
   (j) 1.01
4. (a) 0.001
   (b) 34.795
   (c) 0.005
   (d) 6.130
   (e) 14.900
   (f) 1.006
5. 330.8 gr.
6. 420.5 g.
7. 38 gr.
8. 40 gr.
9. (a) 6.38
   (b) 1.0
   (c) 90.2
   (d) 240 gr.
   (e) 6.0 g.
   (f) 210.55 g.
   (g) 0.068 gr.
   (h) 0.054 g.
   (i) 630
   (j) 230
   (k) 2.6
   (l) 0.0267
   (m) 140
   (n) 23.808
10. 473 milliliters means $\pm$ 0.5 ml.
    473.0 milliliters means $\pm$ 0.05 ml.
11. 0.65 gram means $\pm$ 0.005 g.
    0.6500 grams means $\pm$ 0.00005 g.

SIGNIFICANT FIGURES (*continued*)

12. (a) 4.0 gr.
    (b) 0.43 gr.
    (c) 14.819 g.
    (d) 12 minims
    (e) 350 gr.

ESTIMATION

(*Page 27*)

NOTE: *Estimated answers will vary with methods used. Some calculated answers are here given in parentheses for comparison.*

1. Six zeros
2. Four zeros
3. Three zeros
4. Two zeros
5. 20,500
   (*19,881*)
6. 22,000
   (*21,405*)
7. 14,500
   (*14,320*)
8. 36,000
   (*35,314*)
9. $240.00
   (*$253.19*)
10. $160.00
    (*$169.99*)
11. 20 × 20 = 400
    (*374*)
12. 30 × 30 = 900
    (*868*)
13. 8 × 50 = 400
    (*384*)
14. 20 × 38 = 760
    (*722*)
15. 30 × 60 = 1800
    (*1736*)
16. 40 × 77 = 3080
    (*3003*)

ESTIMATION (*continued*)

17. 40 × 40 = 1600
    (*1638*)
18. 120 × 90 = 10,800 or 11,000
    (*11,500*)
19. 360 × 100 = 36,000
    (*35,770*)
20. 473 × 100 = 47,300
    (*48,246*)
21. 600 × 200 = 120,000
    (*121,584*)
22. 600 × 120 = 72,000
    (*73,688*)
23. 650 × 20 = 13,000
    (*12,825*)
24. 1000 × 13 = 13,000
    (*12,974*)
25. 7000 × 800 = 5,600,000
    (*5,435,670*)
26. 1000 × 1000 = 1,000,000
    (*1,042,956*)
27. 8000 × 10,000 = 80,000,000
    (*82,286,560*)
28. 7000 × 20 = 140,000
    (*136,477*)
29. 5000 × 1000 = 5,000,000
    (*4,917,078*)
30. 2300 × 6000 = 13,800,000
    (*13,875,543*)
31. $2\frac{1}{2}$ × 14 = 35
    (*$36\frac{1}{4}$*)
32. 800 ÷ 3 = 266
    (*$266\frac{2}{3}$*)
33. 21 × 7 = 147
    (*$142\frac{2}{9}$*)
34. $\frac{3}{4}$ × 800 = 600
    (*612*)
35. 840 ÷ 3 = 280
    (*283.76*)
36. 6 × 7000 = 42,000
    (*41,557*)
37. 2 × 700 = 1400
    (*1438.812*)

ESTIMATION (*continued*)

38. $0.02 \times 500 = 10$
    (*9.4304*)
39. $(7 \times 7000) \div 100 = 490$
    (*504.6426*)
40. $100 \times 0.0031 = 0.31$
    (*0.3038*)
41. $6 \times 70 = 420$
    (*411.079*)
42. $7500 \div 10 = 750$
    (*728.8947*)
43. $170 \div 20 = 8.5$
    (*9.0*)
44. $(\frac{2}{3} \times 165)$ or $110 \div 10 = 11$
    (*11*)
45. $180 \div 100 \div 20 = 0.09$
    (*0.08*)
46. $300 \div 15 = 20$
    (*21.39*)
47. $16 \div 320 = \frac{1}{20}$ or 0.05
    (*0.05*)
48. $3600 \div 4 = 900$
    (*900*)
49. $8400 \div 7 = 1200$
    (*1200.7*)
50. $1100 \div 100 = 11$
    (*11*)
51. $9800 \div 5 = 1960$
    (*2000*)
52. $1700 \div 6 = 283$
    (*298.5*)
53. $0.01 \div 5 = 0.002$
    (*0.002149*)
54. $200 \div 4 = 50$
    (*48.6*)
55. $19 \div 0.25 = 19 \times 4 = 76$
    (*73.9*)
56. $19 \div 50 = 38 \div 100 = 0.38$
    (*0.409*)
57. $460 \div 8 = 57.5$
    (*57.3*)
58. $4500 \div 0.50 = 4500 \times 2 = 9000$
    (*9340*)
59. 90,000

ESTIMATION (*continued*)

60. 300
61. 3
62. 0.01 or $\frac{1}{100}$
63. 3.5
64. 100
65. 100
66. 20
67. 160
68. $1,250
69. $400
70. $225
71. $400
72. 0.9 g.
73. 750 doses
74. $15
75. $10

PERCENTAGE OF ERROR

(*Page 31*)

1. 5%
2. 8%
3. 5%
4. 2.4%
5. 6.3%
6. 1.4%
7. 0.1%
8. 5.2%
9. 6.7%
10. 0.24 g.
11. $3\frac{1}{8}$ gr.
12. 0.2 g.
13. 8.33%
14. 2.4 gr.
15. 10%
16. (a) No; (b) Yes; (c) Yes
    (d) No; (e) No; (f) Yes
17. 4.6%
18. $3\frac{1}{3}$%
19. 1.1%
20. 0.1%
21. 0.02 g.
22. 0.1 mg.

Aliquot Method of Measuring

(Page 37)

1. (a) 100 ml.
   (b) 3 mg.
2. Weigh .... 120 mg.
   Dilute to .... 1500 mg.
   Weigh .... 150 mg.
3. Weigh .... 80 mg.
   Dilute to .... 1600 mg.
   Weigh .... 100 mg.
4. Weigh .... 2 gr.
   Dilute to .... 40 gr.
   Weigh .... 2 gr.
5. Weigh .... 400 mg.
   Dilute to .... 8000 mg.
   Weigh .... 400 mg.
6. Weigh .... 4 gr.
   Dilute to .... 20 gr.
   Weigh .... 5 gr.
7. Weigh .... 160 mg.
   Dilute to .... 4000 mg.
   Weigh .... 200 mg.
8. Weigh .... 3 gr.
   Dilute to .... 16 gr.
   Weigh .... 4 gr.
9. Measure .... 3 ml.
   Dilute to .... 10 ml.
   Measure .... 2 ml.
10. Measure .... 3 ml.
    Dilute to .... 8 ml.
    Measure .... 2 ml.
11. Measure .... 2 ml.
    Dilute to .... 10 ml.
    Measure .... 4 ml.
12. Measure .... 5 ml.
    Dilute to .... 8 ml.
    Measure .... 2 ml.
13. Measure .... 15 ℳ
    Dilute to .... 50 ℳ
    Measure .... 20 ℳ

Aliquot Method of Measuring
(continued)

14. Weigh .... $1\frac{1}{2}$ gr.
    Dissolve in enough
    alcohol to make .... 10 ml.
    Measure .... 2 ml.
15. Weigh .... 0.100 g.
    Dissolve in enough
    water to make ..... 10 ml.
    Measure .... 2 ml.

Common and Decimal Fractions
(Page 46)

1. (a) $\frac{37}{32}$ gr. or $1\frac{5}{32}$ gr.
   (b) $\frac{13}{600}$ gr.
   (c) $\frac{77}{480}$ gr.
2. (a) $\frac{209}{64}$ or $3\frac{17}{64}$ gr.
   (b) $\frac{1}{120}$ gr.
   (c) $\frac{5}{6}$ gr.
3. (a) $\frac{225}{48}$ or $4\frac{11}{16}$
   (b) $\frac{105}{4}$ or $26\frac{1}{4}$
   (c) $\frac{9}{2500}$
4. (a) $\frac{10}{1}$ or 10
   (b) $\frac{3}{10}$
   (c) $\frac{1}{12}$
   (d) $\frac{2}{3}$
   (e) $\frac{8}{15}$
   (f) $\frac{64}{1}$ or 64
5. (a) $\frac{48}{3}$ or 16
   (b) $\frac{1}{60000}$
   (c) $\frac{25}{2}$ or $12\frac{1}{2}$
6. (a) $62\frac{1}{2}$
   (b) 15
   (c) 64
   (d) 12,500
7. (a) $\frac{1}{32}$
   (b) $\frac{4}{5}$
   (c) $\frac{64}{1}$
8. $\frac{189}{200}$ gr.
9. 75 doses

COMMON AND DECIMAL FRACTIONS
(*continued*)

10. $\frac{59}{160}$ gr.
11. $\frac{223}{60}$ or $3\frac{43}{60}$ gr.
12. $\frac{1}{90}$ gr.
13. $\frac{1}{300}$ gr.
14. 80 doses
15. (a) 0.125
    (b) 0.0002
    (c) 0.0625
16. 2.048
17. 1.565
18. 2000 doses
19. $\frac{1}{240}$ gr.
20. $\frac{1}{96}$ gr.
21. $\frac{8}{75}$ gr.
22. 2 gr.
23. 0.0785 g.
24. 4.481 g.
25. $\frac{1}{120}$ gr.
26. $\frac{1}{24}$

RATIO, PROPORTION, VARIATION

(*Page 55*)

1. (a) $\dfrac{3 \text{ (gallons)}}{\frac{1}{2} \text{ (gallon)}}$ or $\dfrac{12 \text{ (quarts)}}{2 \text{ (quarts)}}$

   (b) $\dfrac{1 \text{ (yard)}}{\frac{2}{3} \text{ (yard)}}$ or $\dfrac{3 \text{ (feet)}}{2 \text{ (feet)}}$

   (c) $\dfrac{\frac{1}{2} \text{ (mile)}}{\frac{1}{3} \text{ (mile)}}$ or $\dfrac{2640 \text{ (feet)}}{1760 \text{ (feet)}}$

   (d) $\dfrac{4 \text{ (hours)}}{2 \text{ (hours)}}$ or $\dfrac{240 \text{ (minutes)}}{120 \text{ (minutes)}}$

   (e) $\dfrac{2 \text{ (feet)}}{\frac{1}{2} \text{ (foot)}}$ or $\dfrac{24 \text{ (inches)}}{6 \text{ (inches)}}$

RATIO, PROPORTION, VARIATION
(*continued*)

2. (a) $32.40
   (b) $316.67
   (c) 0.91 g.
   (d) $\frac{9}{50}$ gr.
   (e) $7.59
   (f) 2500 tablets
   (g) 40 pounds
   (h) $1.93
   (i) 25.6 g.
   (j) 41.25 g.
   (k) 80 gr.
   (l) 115.4 liters
   (m) 14 gr.
   (n) $\frac{25}{96}$ gr.
   (o) $72\frac{1}{2}$ pounds
   (p) 0.547 g.
   (q) 2%
   (r) $2\frac{1}{2}$ hours
   (s) 1333 ml.
   (t) 0.02% or $\frac{1}{50}$%
   (u) 40 tablets
   (v) 10 minims
   (w) 3000 ml.
   (x) 0.15 ml.
   (y) 125,000 units

Chapter 2

THE METRIC SYSTEM

(*Page 65*)

1. 502.550 g., or 503 g.
3. 0.000025 g.
5. 0.0005 g.
7. 400 doses
9. 0.1125 mg.
11. 1006.650 g., or 1007 g.
13. 250 ml.

The Metric System (*continued*)

15. 0.0985 g., or 98.5 mg.
17. 83.33 ml.
    5.4 mg.
19. 1,256,000 mcg.
    1256 mg.
    0.001256 kg.
21. 2.69375 or 2.694 g.
23. 114 g.
25. 30 mg.
27. 3999.5 mg.—which rounds off to what you started with: 4000 mg., or 4 g.
29. 152.625 or 152.6 g.
31. 4.60 g.
33. 23.88 mg.
35. 20,410 g. per 25.4 mm.
37. 0.125 mg.
39. 134.759 g.
41. 0.625 mg.
43. 35.09 g.
45. 9 g.
    13 g.
    0.26 g.
47. 363.025 or 363.0 mg.
49. 368.25 or 368 mg.
51. 20 tablets
53. 0.0125 g.
    12.5 g.
    0.125 g.
55. 13 mcg.
57. 1.538 g.

Chapter 3

The Common Systems

(Page 74)

1. (a) 150 gr.
   (b) 1050 gr.
   (c) 530 gr.
   (d) 90 gr.

The Common Systems (*continued*)

3. (a) ℥ $\frac{1}{2}$ʒ 8 gr., or
       ℥ 1℈ 18 gr.
   (b) ℥ 2℈ $\frac{1}{2}$℈ 5 gr., or
       ℥ $\frac{1}{2}$ʒ 1℈ 5 gr.
   (c) ℥ 1ʒ 1℈ $\frac{1}{2}$℈, or
       ℥ 1$\frac{1}{2}$℈
   (d) 1ʒ $\frac{1}{2}$℈ 5 gr.
   (e) 1ʒ $\frac{1}{2}$ʒ 6 gr., or
       1ʒ 1℈ 16 gr.
5. 84 fʒ
7. 16 doses
9. 320 bottles
11. 350 capsules
13. 218.75 or 218 tablets
15. 8 f℥
17. $\frac{1}{2}$ gr.
    1$\frac{1}{2}$ gr.
    6 gr.
19. 72 cents
21. 6562 doses
23. 1750 tablets
25. 84.4 gr.
27. 370 gr.

Chapter 4

Conversion

(Page 82)

1. $3\frac{3}{20}$ in.
   $4\frac{7}{10}$ in.
3. $31\frac{1}{2}$ in.
5. 4.93 ml.
7. 8.161 liters
9. 0.0000394 in., or $\frac{1}{25400}$ in.
11. 3.94 or 4 in.
13. 12,123.7 or 12,120 ml.
15. 30.9 or 31 gr.
    2.76 or $2\frac{3}{4}$ in.
17. 308 tablets

Conversion (*continued*)

19. (a) $\frac{1}{926}$ g., or
    1.08 or 1.1 mg.
    (b) 7.39 or 7.4 ml.
    (c) 24.375 or 24 mg.
    (d) 1.84 or 1.8 ml.
    (e) 0.325 mg.
21. 44.9 lb. per 1.0 in.
23. 0.00077 or $\frac{1}{1300}$ gr.
25. 12 cents
27. 2392 or 2400 tablets
29. 65 mcg.
31. 0.65 mg.
33. 50 doses
35. 1.04 g.
37. $\frac{1}{2540}$ in.

Chapter 5

CALCULATION OF DOSES

(*Page 95*)

NOTE: *In calculating the number of doses contained in a specified quantity of medicine, disregard any fractional remainder.*

1. 800 doses
3. 30 doses
5. 48 doses
7. 2 teaspoonfuls
9. 2 teaspoonfuls
11. 16 f℥
13. $\frac{1}{130}$ gr.
15. $\frac{1}{240}$ gr.
17. $\frac{1}{4}$ gr.
19. $\frac{1}{13}$ gr.
21. $\frac{1}{130}$ gr.
23. 25 mg.
    0.5 ml.
25. $\frac{2}{13}$ gr.
27. 5 ℳ
    $\frac{1}{6}$ gr.

CALCULATION OF DOSES (*continued*)

29. $\frac{4}{5}$ gr.
31. 180 gr. or ℥iii
    360 ℳ or f℥vi
33. 40 mg.
35. 6 ml.
37. 7.2 g.
39. 2 teaspoonfuls
41. $\frac{19}{65}$ gr.
43. 187.5 to 375 mg.
45. 0.025 g.
47. 2 gr.
49. 0.2 mg.
51. $\frac{1}{13}$ gr.
53. $\frac{1}{550}$ gr.
55. 0.02 mg.
57. (a) 0.125 ml.
    (b) 3 drops
59. 42 capsules
61. 180 mcg.

Chapter 6

REDUCING AND ENLARGING FORMULAS

(*Page 107*)

1.   45.   ml.
        0.9 g.
        3.6 g.
    ad 180.   ml.
3.   0.57 g.
        0.34 g.
        22.7 g.
        272. g.
        568. g.
        568. g.
    ad 2270. g., or 5 lb.
5.   1725. g.
        90.8 g.
        416. g.
        227. ml.
    ad 4540. g., or 10 lb.

REDUCING AND ENLARGING
FORMULAS (*continued*)

7.   4.73 g.
                2.36 g.
                2.36 g.
     9.46 or   9.5   ml.
                2.36 g.
             14.2   g.
     0.47 or   0.5   ml.
        ad 473.   ml., or 1 pt.

9.   113.5 g.
               113.5 g.
               227.   g.
    Total: 454.   g., or 1 lb.

11.   200 ml.
                50 ml.
              750 ml.
    Total: 1000 ml., or 1 liter

13.   430 ml.
              860 ml.
            1075 ml.
    Total: 2365 ml., or 5 pt.

15. 118.3 or   118 ml.
     59.13 or   59 ml.
    177.4 or   177 g.
         ad   2365 ml., or 5 pt.

17. 353.1 or   353 g.
                25 g.
    100.9 or   101.g.
    201.8 or   202 g.
              1589 g.
    Total: 2270 g., or 5 lb.

19.   192 gr., or ʒiii gr. xii
              96 gr., or ʒiss gr. vi
         1632 gr., or
                 ʒiii ʒiii gr. xii
    Total: 1920 gr., or ʒiv

21.   0.180 g.
        2.340 g.
        0.036 g.
        0.288 g.
    ad 3.60   g.

REDUCING AND ENLARGING
FORMULAS (*continued*)

23. 2649.5   or 2650 ml.
     8516.25 or 8516 g.
        ad 18925 ml., or 5 gal.

25. 2499   or 2500 g.
     454.4   or   454 g.
     170.4   or   170 g.
               852 g.
        ad 11.36 kg., or 25 lb.

27.   0.062 g.
        0.034 g.
    ad 240.   ml.

29.   1.60 g.
   0.667 or   0.68 g.
             1.20 g.
           13.3   g.

31.   0.744 g.
        0.444 g.
    ad 60.   ml.

33.   37.85 g.
        56.78 g.
       113.6   g.
       2650.   ml.
    ad 3785.   ml., or 1 gal.

35.   9.46 g.
       166.   ml.
        47.   ml.
    ad 473.   ml , or 1 pt.

37.   22.7 g.
       431.3 g.
       385.9 g.
    3700.1 g.

Chapter 7

DENSITY, SPECIFIC GRAVITY, AND SPECIFIC VOLUME

(*Page 121*)

1. 0.812 g. per ml.
3. 1.83   g. per ml.
5. 0.9375
7. 1.313

Density, Specific Gravity, and Specific Volume
(continued)

9. 1.18
11. 1.235 or 1.24
13. 1.169 or 1.17
15. 0.8633
17. 1.831
19. 3.237
21. 2.498 or 2.50
23. 0.237
25. 2.00
27. 1.110
29. 1.096, or 1.10
31. 0.5476
33. 1.212 or 1.21

Chapter 8

Weights and Volumes of Liquids

(Page 128)

1. 116 g.
3. 190.4 or 190 g.
5. 9.2 kg.
7. 8.12 kg.
9. 7.37 or 7.4 lb.
11. 205.8 or 206 g.
13. 4.97 kg.
15. 13.17 or $13\frac{1}{5}$ lb.
17. 58.47 or 58.5 ml.
19. 546.4 or 546 ml.
21. 367.9 or 368 ml.
23. 4348 or 4350 ml.
25. 1101 or 1100 ml.
27. 4.73 or $4\frac{7}{10}$ pt.
29. 29.2 or $29\frac{1}{5}$ pt.
31. $23.23
33. $100.02
35. $0.65
37. 1938 ml.
39. 181.05 or 181.1 ml.
41. 15.5 ml.
    120.77 or 120.8 ml.

Chapter 9

Percentage Preparations

(Page 147)

1. 12.5 g.
3. 0.48 g.
5. 0.3 g.
7. 7.5 g.
9. 15 mg.
11. 1.82 gr.
13. 45.5 gr.
15. 9.1 gr.
17. 4.55 gr.
19. 25 g.
21. 0.35%
23. 0.2%
    1.5%
25. 0.44%
    4.4%
27. 6.15 liters
29. 50,444 or 50,400 ml.
31. 20 f℥
33. 378.5 or 379 ml.
35. 2838 or 2840 ml.
37. 709.5 or 710 ml.
39. 250 mg.
    7.5 ml.
41. 96 ℳ
43. 2.2%
45. 5%
47. 20.8%
49. 30 mg.
51. 18.75%
53. 1600 ml.
55. 1.875 or 1.88 g.
57. 882.1 or 882 g.
59. 100 g.
61. 20 g.
63. 25%
65. 16.5%
67. 25 g.
69. 2.4 gr.
71. 30.6%

PERCENTAGE PREPARATIONS
(*continued*)

73. 600 mg.
75. 7.2 gr.
    232.8 or 233 gr.
77. 5.9%
79. 9.5%
81. 5%
83. (a) 1:800
    (b) 1:40
    (c) 1:125
    (d) 1:166$\frac{2}{3}$ or 6:1000
    (e) 1:300
    (f) 1:2000
85. 1:2000
87. 1:588
89. 1:1182 or 1:1200
91. 1:1,000,000
93. 0.25 g.
95. 625 mg.
97. 1:8000
99. 100 mg.
    2.5 mg.
101. 60 mg.
    37.5 mg.

Chapter 10

DILUTION AND CONCENTRATION

(*Page 183*)

1. 1:3200
3. 4%
5. 15%
7. 32%
9. 20,000 ml.
11. 425 ml.
13. 544 g.
15. 84.6 or 84$\frac{3}{5}$ lb.
17. 6944 or 6940 ml.
19. 1600 ml.
21. 12 f℥

DILUTION AND CONCENTRATION
(*continued*)

23. 40 ml.
25. 4.7 ml.
27. 248 ml.
29. 1.8 ml.
31. 461𝕞 or 7 f℥ 40𝕞
33. 3 ml.
35. 5.45 or 5.5 ml.
37. 48 ml.
    32 ml.
39. 7.5 ml.
41. 28.8 or 29𝕞
43. (a) 10 g.
    (b) 400 ml.
45. 92.1 or 92 gr.
47. 28.2 ml.
49. 12.5 g.
51. 500 ml.
53. 1667 ml.
55. Enough to make 4150 ml.
57. 101 ml.
    Enough to make 240 ml.
59. 115.7 or 116 ml.
61. 245.6 or 246 ml.
63. 770.4 or 770 ml.
65. 14.5%
67. 4.95% (w/w)
    4.125 or 4.13% (w/v)
69. 5.36 g.
71. 1 g.
    9 g.
73. 1000 g.
75. 4.76%
77. 59.04 or 59 g.
79. 0.050 g.
81. 5 mg.
83. 3 gr.
85. 1.25%
87. 2.575 or 2.58%
89. 25.36 or 25.4%
91. 39.4%

DILUTION AND CONCENTRATION
(*continued*)

93. 56.88 or 56.9%
95. 12:70, or 6:35
97. 3:5
99. 1.5:27, or 3:54, or 1:18
101. 12:5:5
103. 300 ml.
105. 300 g.
      2200 g.
107. 800 g.
      1200 g.
      2400 g.
       400 g.
109. 66.66 or 66.7 g.
111. 300 ml.
113. 100 g.
115. 166.7 g.
117. 22,500 ml.
119. (a) 8%
     (b) 164.7 or 165 g.
121. 0.855
123. 44.2 or 44 ml.
     55.8 or 56 ml.
125. 4500 ml.

Chapter 11

ISOTONIC SOLUTIONS

(*Page 205*)

1. 1.73%
3. —0.52° C.
5. —0.036° C.
7. 3.3 gr.
9. 0.500 g.
11. 2.35 or 2.4 gr.
13. 0.1095 or 0.110 g.
15. 0.467 g.
17. 0.690 g.
19. 17.8 or 18 ml.

ISOTONIC SOLUTIONS (*continued*)

21. 0.7 gr.
23. 0.290 g.
25. 4.5 g.
27. 13 ml.

Chapter 12

CHEMICAL PROBLEMS

(*Page 224*)

1. 74.096, or 74.10
3. 46.068, or 46.07
5. 60.052, or 60.05
7. C: 64.81%
   H: 13.60%
   O: 21.59%
9. Na: 16.66%
   H: 2.92%
   P: 22.45%
   O: 57.97%
11. 1024 g.
13. 25.45%
15. 73.88%
17. 181 mg.
19. 55.2 or 55 mg.
21. 0.165 g.
23. 530.5 or 531 mg.
25. 555.5 or 556 g.
    388.8 or 389 g.
27. 6786 g.
    2323 g.
29. 585 g.
31. 2.1 g.
33. 66.88 or 66.9 g.
35. 80 mg.
37. 571 g.
39. 18.2 g.
41. 225 g.
43. 11.8 or 12 g.
45. 200

CHEMICAL PROBLEMS
(continued)

47. (a) 8.59 or 8.6 g.
    (b) 19.3 g.
49. 11.36 or 11.4 g.
51. 7.5 g.
53. 1.452 or 1.45 g.
55. 19.9 liters
57. 140 liters
59. 218.7 or 219 g.
61. 365.7 or 366 g.
63. 112 liters
    113.5 liters
65. 7 liters
    7.69 or 7.7 liters
67. 110 ml.

Chapter 13

ELECTROLYTE SOLUTIONS

(Page 237)

1. 372.8 mg.
3. 4 mEq
5. 0.298%
7. 200 mEq
9. 9.009 g.
11. 20 ml.
13. 2.5 mEq per ml.
15. 10 mEq per liter
17. 14 mOsm
19. (a) 17.880 g.
    (b) 5 mEq
21. 4.36 mEq per liter
23. 25 mEq
25. 74.5 g.
27. 4.5 mEq
    2.25 mOsm
29. 154 mOsm
31. 139 mOsm

Chapter 14

EXPONENTIAL NOTATION

(Page 243)

1. (a) 1.265×10^4
   (b) 5.5×10^{-9}
   (c) 4.51×10^2
   (d) 6.5×10^{-2}
   (e) 6.25×10^{-8}
2. (a) 4,100,000
   (b) 0.0365
   (c) 0.00000513
   (d) 250,000
   (e) 8695.6
3. (a) $17.5 \times 10^7 = 1.75 \times 10^8$
   (b) $16.4 \times 10^{-4} = 1.64 \times 10^{-3}$
   (c) 6.0×10^0
   (d) $12 \times 10^7 = 1.2 \times 10^8$
   (e) $36 \times 10^2 = 3.6 \times 10^3$
4. (a) 3.0×10^3
   (b) 3.0×10^{-10}
   (c) 3.0×10^9
5. (a) 8.52×10^4, or 8.5×10^4
   (b) 3.58×10^{-5}, or 3.6×10^{-5}
   (c) 2.99×10^3, or 3.0×10^3
6. (a) 6.441×10^6, or 6.4×10^6
   (b) 6.6×10^{-3}
   (c) 6.94×10^3, or 6.9×10^3

LOGARITHMIC NOTATION

(Page 249)

1. (a) 3.3512
   (b) 0.7214
   (c) 3.8451
   (d) 2.2739
   (e) $\overline{3}.4675$
   (f) $\overline{1}.8600$
   (g) 5.3324
   (h) $\overline{4}.1373$

Logarithmic Notation
(continued)

    (i) 1.8375
    (j) 6.7924
2. (a) $2.827 \times 10^4 = 28{,}270$
    (b) $1.42 \times 10^1 = 14.2$
    (c) $2.139 \times 10^0 = 2.139$
    (d) $1.29 \times 10^{-1} = 0.129$
    (e) $6.154 \times 10^2 = 615.4$
    (f) $1.468 \times 10^2 = 146.8$
    (g) $1.062 \times 10^0 = 1.062$
    (h) $7.766 \times 10^{-3} = 0.007766$
    (i) $8.383 \times 10^1 = 83.33$
    (j) $1.329 \times 10^{-2} = 0.01329$
3. (a) 22,790
    (b) 7315
    (c) 14.76
    (d) 822.6
    (e) 17,090
4. (a) 7517
    (b) 197.6
    (c) 0.00517
    (d) 35.37
    (e) 13.75 or 13.8
5. (a) 79.36 or 79.4
    (b) 108.5 or 109
    (c) 292.8 or 293

Chapter 15

Some Calculations Involving Hydrogen-ion Concentration and pH

(Page 254)

1. 10.6
3. 6.22 or 6.2
5. 7.36 or 7.4
7. 6.31×10^{-3}, or 6.3×10^{-3}
9. 7.94×10^{-6}, or 7.9×10^{-6}
11. 3.98×10^{-7}, or 4.0×10^{-7}

Chapter 16

Some Calculations Involving Buffer Solutions

(Page 261)

1. 3.86
3. 4.56
5. 5.5
7. 6.91
9. 2.82:1
11. 0.03 unit
13. 8.2 g.
    6.0 g.

Chapter 17

Some Calculations Involving Radioisotopes

(Page 269)

1. 152 days
3. 0.0541 hour^{-1}
5. $\lambda = 0.04794$ day^{-1}
    $T\frac{1}{2} = 14.5$ days
7. $\lambda = 0.01084$ day^{-1}
    $T\frac{1}{2} = 64$ days
9. 77.3 microcuries
11. 0.17 ml.

Chapter 18

Basic Statistical Concepts

(Page 283)

1. Mean: 127.8
   Median: 126
   Mode: 125
3. Mean: 100.7
   A.D.:   2.62
   S.D.:   3.22
5. Mean: 5.02
   Median: 5.02
   Mode: 5.05

BASIC STATISTICAL CONCEPTS
(*continued*)

7. Yes. Since every button has an equal chance of being drawn, every subject has an equal chance of being selected for the experiment.
9. 1:3 in favor of the later check.

APPENDIX A

THERMOMETRY

(*Page 292*)

1. 50° F.
3. 39.2° F.
5. 25° C.
7. 37° C.
9. 23° F. to 572° F.
11. 159.8° F.
13. −40° C.
15. 86° F. to 95° F.
17. 68° F.
19. 35.6° F. to 41° F.
21. 176° F.
    179.6° F.
23. 198° C.
    −111.1° C.

APPENDIX B

PROOF STRENGTH

(*Page 296*)

1. 102.6 proof gallons
3. 490 proof gallons
5. 83⅓ wine gallons
7. 125 wine gallons
9. $99.65
11. $324.90
13. $27.80
15. 36.1 proof gallons

APPENDIX C

ALCOHOLOMETRIC TABLES

(*Page 301*)

1. 53.10% (v/v)
3. 26.50% (v/v)
5. 87.226 or 87.23% (v/v)
7. 0.82575 or 0.8258
9. 0.96998 or 0.9700

APPENDIX D

SOLUBILITY RATIOS

(*Page 304*)

1. 1:5.25, or 1 g. in 5.25 ml. of water
3. 1:2.67, or 1 g. in 2.67 ml. of water
5. 5.714 or 5.70% (w/w)
7. 59.5 g.
   178.57 or 178.6 ml.
9. 1 g. in 0.7 ml.

APPENDIX E

EMULSION NUCLEUS

(*Page 307*)

1. (a) 125 g.
   (b) 250 ml.
3. (a) 625 g.
   (b) 1250 ml.
5. (a) 2 g.
   (b) 4 ml.
7. (a) 17.5 g.
   (b) 35 ml.

APPENDIX F

HLB SYSTEM:
PROBLEMS INVOLVING HLB VALUES
(*Page 312*)

1. 14.7
3. 10.7

PROBLEMS INVOLVING HLB VALUES
(*continued*)

5. 12.2
7. 73% of Tween 40
   27% of Span 40
9. 5 6 g. of Span 60
   19.4 g. of Tween 20

APPENDIX G

MISCELLANEOUS PROBLEMS IN
DISPENSING PHARMACY

(*Page 324*)

1. 4.8 ml.
3. 180 mg.
5. 2 ml.
7. Dissolve 1 tablet in enough distilled water to make 60 ml., and take 10 ml. of the dilution.
9. 2500 ml.
11. 15 tablets
13. 24 tablets
15. 15 tablets
17. 16 granules
19. 0.45 ml.
21. 9.6 or 10 minims
23. 400,000 units
25. 4 capsules
27. Dissolve 1 tablet in enough isotonic sodium chloride solution to make 8 ml., and take 3 ml. of the dilution.
29. Dissolve 500,000 units of polymyxin B sulfate in enough sterile distilled water to make 10 ml., and take 3 ml. of the dilution.
31. Dissolve 50,000 units of bacitracin in enough distilled water

MISCELLANEOUS PROBLEMS IN
DISPENSING PHARMACY (*continued*)

to make 5 ml., and take 3 ml. of the dilution.
33. 3 ml.
35. 41.7 or 42 drops per minute
37. 1.25 ml. per minute
39. 44.6 mEq

APPENDIX H

SOME COMMERCIAL PROBLEMS

(*Page 334*)

1. (a) 45.85 or 45.9%
   (b) 35%
   (c) 31.6%
   (d) 44.14 or 44.1%
   (e) 40.465 or 40.5%
   (f) 20.62 or 20.6%
3. $1.33
5. $128.25
7. $1.09
9. 51 cents
11. $15
13. 64 cents
15. 57 cents
17. $1.25
19. $2.85
21. $1.88
23. 50 cents
25. 28 cents
27. 45 cents
29. 3.75%
31. $2.34
33. $1.00
35. 150%
37. $2.35
39. $300

Index

Reference in *italics* indicates that a term is defined, illustrated, or otherwise explained.

(393)